week 1
Intro 2-4
Econ 6-47
Global Impact 88-103

106-123
126-134

HIV/AIDS Pandemic

52-65 78-85
136-149
152-163
173-180
190-201

206-213
218-220

360-434

222-236
238-252

256-279
288-331
336-339

HIV/AIDS Pandemic

Origins, Science, and Global Impact

Revised Third Edition

Edited by Cindy Gustafson-Brown
University of California – San Diego

cognella
SAN DIEGO

Bassim Hamadeh, CEO and Publisher
Seidy Cruz, Specialist Acquisitions Editor
Carrie Montoya, Manager, Revisions and Author Care
Kaela Martin, Project Editor
Casey Hands, Production Editor
Jess Estrella, Senior Graphic Designer
Alexa Lucido, Licensing Manager
Natalie Piccotti, Director of Marketing
Kassie Graves, Vice President of Editorial
Jamie Giganti, Director of Academic Publishing

Printed in the United States of America.

cognella® ACADEMIC PUBLISHING
3970 Sorrento Valley Blvd., Ste. 500, San Diego, CA 92121

Contents

Section I

Introduction

1.1

Introduction to HIV and AIDS

HIV IS THE **HUMAN IMMUNODEFICIENCY VIRUS.** This virus primarily infects two types of white blood cells, known as **macrophages** and **$CD4^+$ T cells** (or "T helper cells"). The virus disables or kills these cells, resulting in progressive deterioration of the immune system. The immune system fights back with some success initially, often resulting in several years of a stalemate between the virus and the body. In the absence of treatment, an infected person may live 8–12 years without significant symptoms of illness.

The gradual decline in $CD4^+$ T cells will eventually disable the immune system so severely that the patient will begin to succumb to "**opportunistic**" infections. These are infections which rarely cause problems for those with healthy immune systems, but when one is **immunosuppressed**, opportunistic viruses, bacteria, fungi, and protozoa take advantage of the weakened immunity and become deadly. (In addition, the patient is more susceptible to infectious diseases that could sicken anyone.) When an HIV-infected person reaches this point, we say they have AIDS—**acquired immunodeficiency syndrome**. It is called a syndrome because it encompasses a collection of illnesses and conditions caused by different infections, any subset of which may afflict a given patient.

The definition of AIDS, discussed later in this reader, is dependent on the presence of HIV, the types of other infections threatening the patient's health (known as AIDS-defining illnesses), and the concentration of $CD4^+$ T cells in the blood.

Having HIV is not the same as having AIDS. When a person is infected with HIV, we say they are "HIV-positive." This means they will test positive on an HIV test. However, in most cases, they do not have AIDS until several years after infection when their immune system is severely compromised and they become susceptible to life-threatening opportunistic infections. The term "HIV/AIDS" is used to refer to both conditions—HIV infection or AIDS. It is another way of saying, "HIV infection with or without AIDS."

While HIV was nearly always a death sentence when it came to the attention of the medical establishment in 1981, anti-HIV medications have changed the outlook for patients. Such drugs are known as **antiretroviral** drugs, or ARVs. The first antiretroviral drug was AZT (also known as zidovudine or

Retrovir), which came on the market in 1987. Starting in the 1990s, a plethora of additional drugs were developed, attacking the virus at several points in its life cycle. It was found that treatment was more effective and the virus less likely to develop resistance if the patient took three ARVs together in what is known as a "drug cocktail." Physicians originally referred to this as **highly active antiretroviral therapy, or HAART**, although now it is simply called **ART**. HIV cannot be cured, but improvements in ART have transformed HIV infection, in the best of circumstances, into a chronic, manageable illness. It is still too early to know for sure, but with effective treatment, many HIV-infected people may now live nearly a normal life span. Furthermore, ART has made it possible to virtually eliminate mother-to-child transmission of HIV.

In the last thirty-six years, over 77 million people globally have been infected with HIV, and 35 million people have died. Although treatment is now possible, it is not available to nearly half of the 37 million people in the world who are currently infected. In the absence of universal treatment, it is critical for people to be educated about how to prevent HIV transmission and empowered to make decisions that will preserve their health.

Transmission of HIV requires an infected bodily fluid to be transferred from the infected person to an uninfected person. This infectious fluid must be deposited on a mucous membrane or gain entry to the bloodstream through a break in the skin. The bodily fluids that are likely to harbor infectious virus are:

globally: 77 mill infect
35 mill died

- blood
- semen
- cervical fluid
- breast milk

HIV is most commonly transmitted:

- by sex with an infected person
- by sharing contaminated needles/syringes while injecting drugs
- from mother to child

Although great strides have been made by researchers toward understanding the biology of the virus and developing treatments, there is still much to be done. A challenge that still faces the scientific community is the rapid mutation rate of HIV which leads to the evolution of drug-resistant strains. While antiretroviral medications are effective, they are expensive, may have serious side effects, and require faithful adherence every day for the rest of one's life. In addition, the decades-long search for a vaccine has been littered with disappointments. It is unlikely there will be an effective HIV vaccine available for at least a decade, perhaps longer. Research into microbicides (creams or gels to prevent sexual transmission) has also been plagued with numerous failed trials; although, recently there has been a glimmer of hope on this front.

As it perplexes biologists, HIV also poses significant challenges to public health officials. It has become increasingly apparent that an effective response to the epidemic must focus on prevention as well as treatment. Although access to ARVs is expanding in many countries, for every person who begins treatment, two more are infected. Furthermore, HIV has complicated other global health issues, driving the resurgence of additional epidemics, such as tuberculosis—the leading cause of AIDS-related death in the world. Finally, the 2008 global recession strained the budgets of governments and non-profit organizations, which have struggled to recover. AIDS is expensive, and the economic downturn dealt a blow to public health efforts to fight the epidemic. No doubt, HIV will continue to be a source of grievous human suffering for some time to come.

There is, however, good news as well. The rate of growth of the global epidemic peaked in 1997 and is now declining. The number of *new* infections per year has fallen by nearly half since then (although the total number of people with HIV in the world is still increasing). Enhanced access to ARVs has reduced the rate of AIDS deaths in low-income countries. And finally, some of the hardest hit nations in Africa have significantly reduced the proportion of their citizens who are infected.

HIV/AIDS is scientifically and medically fascinating. I hope you will find the subject as engaging as I do. However, the study of HIV/AIDS may take you to some dark places where people confront illness, pain, stigma, loneliness, marginalization, poverty, injustice, and death. This *should* be distressing. But don't be paralyzed by despair. When overwhelmed by the weight of AIDS in the world, take courage by recalling the tremendous scientific advances in knowledge which HIV research has yielded and the epidemiological corner we have turned after the peak of the epidemic. And finally, be inspired by reflecting on the quiet moments of hope and grace which occur thousands of times a day throughout the world when one individual reaches out to help another with AIDS.

↑ AIDS related death

↓ # new infections / year] due to ↑ access ARVS
↓ rate of growth globally

Section II

Economics

2.1

Mechanisms for HIV/AIDS Funding

Cindy Gustafson-Brown

Funding for HIV/AIDS in low- and middle-income countries was $19.1 billion in 2016 (Kates et al., 2017, p. 2). These funds primarily come from:

- domestic spending (57%)
- donations from national governments (40%)
    - bilateral funding
    - multilateral funding
- private donations (3%)

Domestic Spending

Domestic spending is provided by affected individuals and their governments. In low- and middle-income countries, the proportion of funding provided by the budgets of national governments varies considerably, from 4% in Mozambique (UNAIDS, 2016) to 77% in South Africa (PREFAR, 2015). Since the economic crisis of 2008, domestic spending has increased, as donor spending has become less reliable. The scaling up of domestic programs and budgets has been significant and will contribute to the sustainability of the response.

Donations From National Governments

In 2016, 80% of donations from national governments were provided by five countries: the United States, the United Kingdom, France, the Netherlands, and Germany (PEPFAR, 2015). The United States government allocates its global AIDS funding through a program known as **PEPFAR**, the President's Emergency Plan for AIDS Relief, established in 2003 by President George W. Bush.

- **Bilateral funding** is assistance transferred directly from one government to another. This is the most common (74%) funding mechanism for donations from national governments. PEPFAR

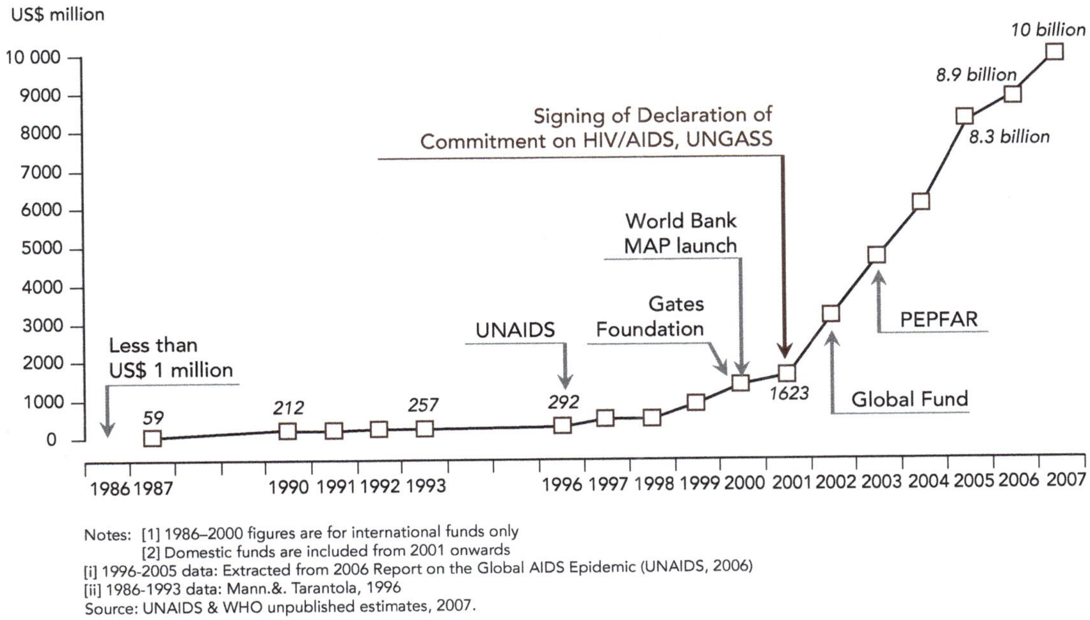

FIGURE 2.1.1 Total annual resources available for AIDS, 1986–2007

Source: UNAIDS & WHO.

bilateral funding targets "focus countries" typically characterized by large populations and high HIV prevalence.

- **Multilateral funding organizations** distribute 21% of the funding from donor nations. These international bodies receive donations from many different governments and distribute the funds independently. The largest multilateral organization providing AIDS relief is the **Global Fund to fight AIDS, TB and Malaria** followed by the **World Bank**.

Private Donations

Sources of private funding include charitable giving by corporations, foundations, philanthropists, religious groups, and non-governmental organizations (NGOs). The most significant of these is the Bill and Melinda Gates Foundation, which provides 34% of all private donations to the fight against HIV/AIDS.

References

PEPFAR. (2015). *Country operational plan.* http://www.pepfar.gov/documents/organization/250301.pdf.

Kates, J., Wexler, A., Lief, E., & UNAIDS. (2017). *Donor government funding for HIV in low- and middle-income countries in 2016.* http://www.unaids.org/en/resources/documents/2017/20170721_Kaiser_donor_funding_HIV_LMIC_2016

UNAIDS. 2016. *Prevention gap report.* http://www.unaids.org/sites/default/files/media_asset/2016-prevention-gap-report_en.pdf

2.2

The Global HIV/AIDS Epidemic

Kaiser Family Foundation

Key Facts

[...]

- Under Sustainable Development Goal 3, the global community agreed to aim to end the AIDS epidemic by 2030. However, while gains have been made, they have been uneven, and the interim "90-90-90" targets were missed. A U.N. high-level meeting reviewing progress toward the 2030 goals will take place in June 2021.
- The U.S. government (U.S.), through PEPFAR (the President's Emergency Plan for AIDS Relief), is the single largest donor to international HIV efforts in the world, including the largest donor to the Global Fund to Fight AIDS, Tuberculosis and Malaria (Global Fund).
- As COVID-19 continues to spread globally, its detrimental effects on HIV/AIDS efforts worldwide have already been seen, including disruptions of essential health services, such as testing, treatment, and prevention programs.

[...]

Global Resources

UNAIDS estimates that **$19.8 billion** was available from all sources (domestic, donor governments, multilaterals, and foundations) to address HIV in low- and middle-income countries in 2019.[1] Of this, donor governments provided $7.8 billion, representing a reduction from the $8 billion in 2018 and nearly the same as the funding levels of a decade ago (see Figure 2).[2] Other governments and organizations that contribute substantially to funding the global response include:

- hard-hit countries, which have also provided resources to address their epidemics;
- the Global Fund, which has approved over $23 billion for HIV efforts in more than 100 countries to date;[3] and
- the private sector, including foundations and corporations, which also plays a major role (the Bill & Melinda Gates Foundation, for one, has committed more than $3 billion in HIV grants to

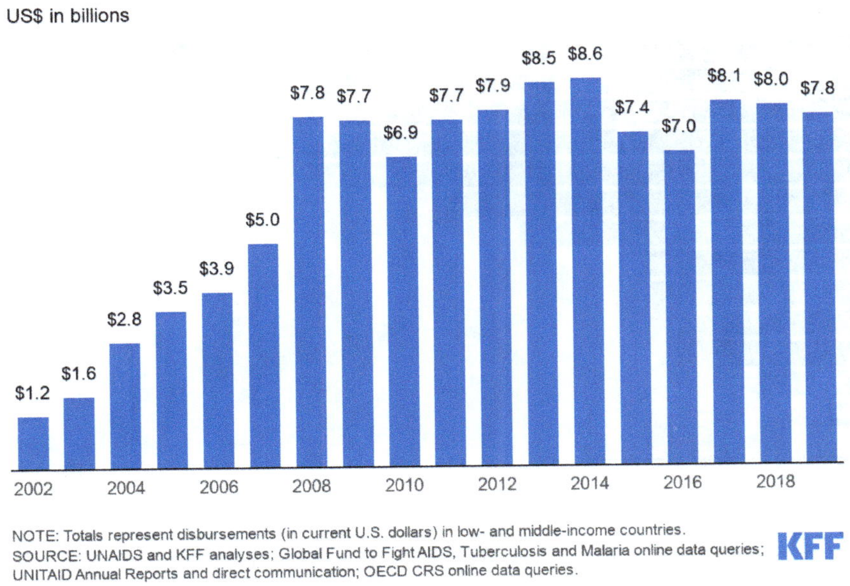

FIGURE 2.2.1 HIV Funding from Donor Governments, 2002–2019

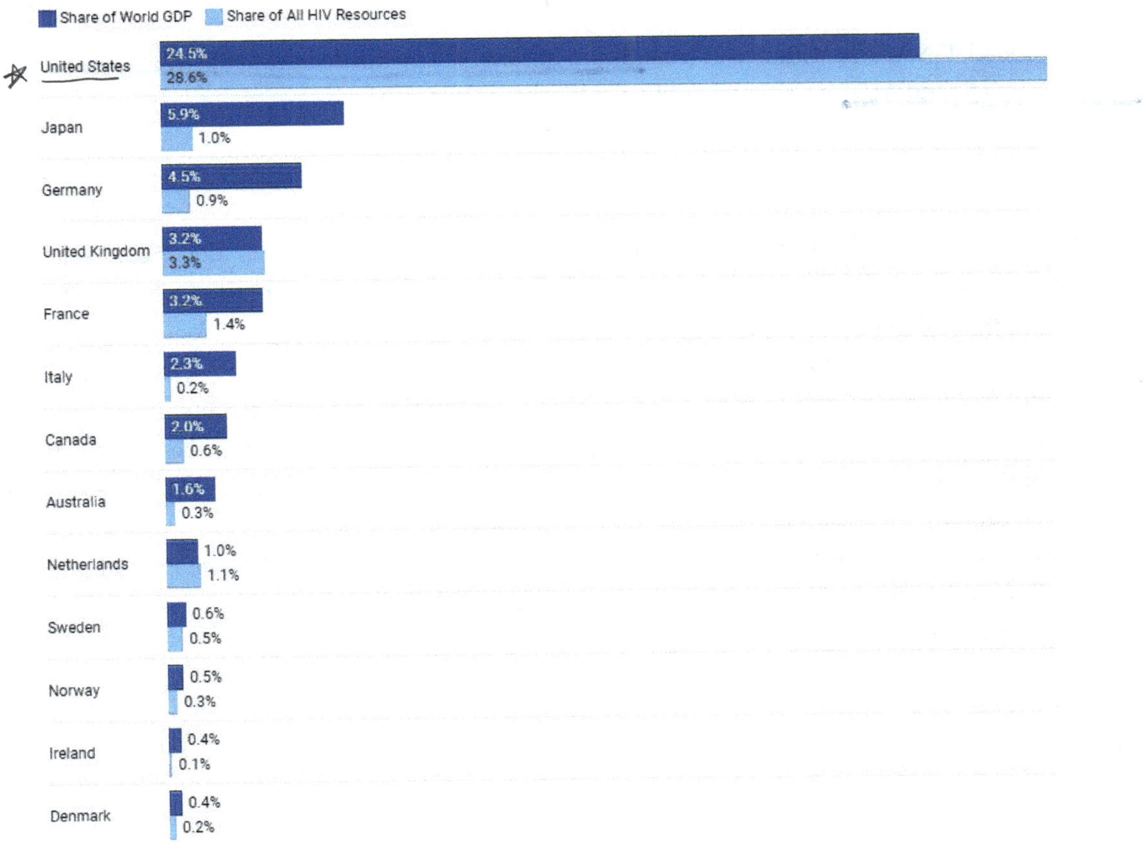

NOTES: Donor funding totals represent disbursements (in current U.S. dollars) in low- and middle-income countries. "GDP" represents gross domestic product. UNAIDS estimates that US$18.6 billion was available for HIV from all sources in 2019, expressed in 2016 USD. For purposes of this analysis, the estimate was converted to 2019 USD, or $19.8 billion. SOURCES: UNAIDS and KFF analysis, July 2020; Global Fund to Fight AIDS, Tuberculosis and Malaria online data query, January 2020; UNITAID direct communication; OECD CRS online data queries.

FIGURE 2.2.2 Donor Government Share of Resources Available for HIV Compared to Share of GDP, 2019

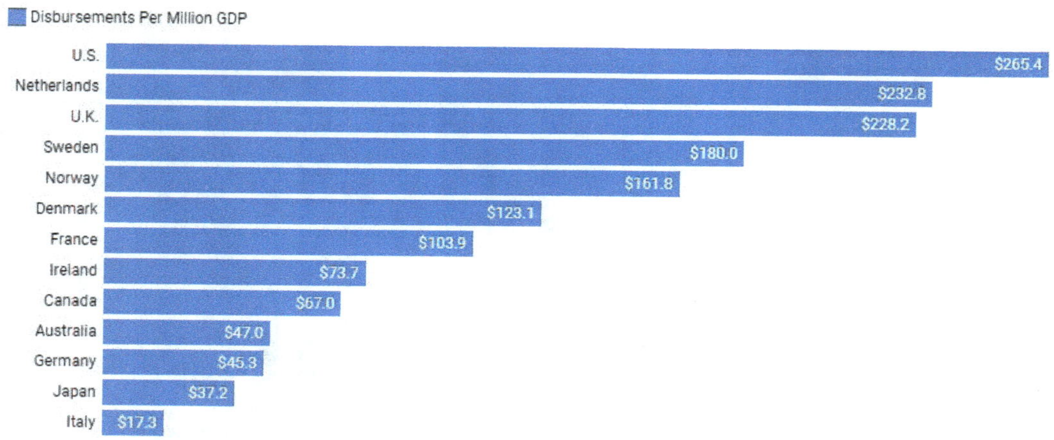

NOTES: Donor funding totals represent disbursements (in current U.S. dollars) in low- and middle-income countries. "GDP" represents gross domestic product. SOURCES: UNAIDS and KFF analysis, July 2020; Global Fund to Fight AIDS, Tuberculosis and Malaria online data query, January 2020; UNITAID direct communication; International Monetary Fund, 2019 World Economic Outlook Database, accessed June 2020.

FIGURE 2.2.3 Donor Government Ranking by Funding for HIV per US$1 Million GDP, 2019

organizations addressing the epidemic, as well as provided additional funding to the Global Fund).[4]

Looking ahead, UNAIDS estimates at least **$26.2 billion** will be needed annually by 2020 to meet global targets to end AIDS as a global public health threat by 2030.[5]

Endnotes

1. UNAIDS estimates that US$18.6 billion was available for HIV from all sources (donor governments, domestic spending, multilateral organizations, and foundations) in 2019, expressed in 2016 USD. For purposes of this fact sheet, this estimate was converted to 2019 USD, or $19.8 billion. KFF/UNAIDS. Donor Government Funding for HIV in Low- and Middle-Income Countries in 2019; July 2020.
2. KFF/UNAIDS. *Donor Government Funding for HIV in Low- and Middle-Income Countries in 2019*; July 2020.
3. Global Fund. *The Global Fund Data Explorer*; accessed December 2020, https://data.theglobalfund.org.
4. Bill & Melinda Gates Foundation. *HIV Strategy Overview*; accessed January 2021, http://www.gatesfoundation.org/What-We-Do/Global-Health/HIV#OurStrategy.
5. Total funding needed is in constant 2016 dollars. KFF/UNAIDS. *Donor Government Funding for HIV in Low- and Middle-Income Countries in 2019*, July 2020. UNAIDS. 2020 *Global AIDS Update: Seizing the Moment*; July 2020.

2.3

The U.S. President's Emergency Plan for AIDS Relief (PEPFAR)

Kaiser Family Foundation

Key Facts

- Although the U.S. has been involved in efforts to address the global AIDS crisis since the mid-1980s, the creation of the President's Emergency Plan for AIDS Relief (PEPFAR) in 2003 marked a significant increase in funding and attention to the epidemic.
- PEPFAR is the largest commitment by any nation to address a single disease in the world; to date, its funding has totaled more than $90 billion, including funding for the Global Fund to Fight AIDS, Tuberculosis and Malaria (Global Fund), to which the U.S. government is the largest donor. PEPFAR is credited with saving millions of lives and helping to change the trajectory of the global HIV epidemic.
- First authorized in 2003, the program has been reauthorized three times: in 2008, 2013, and most recently in December 2018.
- U.S. funding for PEPFAR was $6.9 billion in FY 2020, up from $2.19 billion in FY 2004; this includes contributions to the Global Fund.
- While viewed as one of the most significant and successful global health initiatives ever undertaken, PEPFAR faces several issues and challenges, including how best to: accelerate progress toward epidemic control in the context of flat or potentially reduced budgets; support and strengthen country ownership and sustainability; address the needs of young women and adolescents, as well as key populations; and leverage partnerships with the public and private sectors.

[...]

U.S. Government Efforts

Although the U.S. has been involved in efforts to address the global HIV/AIDS crisis since the mid-1980s,[1] the creation of the President's Emergency Plan for AIDS Relief (PEPFAR) in 2003 marked a significant increase in funding and attention to the epidemic.[2] PEPFAR, the U.S. government's global effort to combat

TABLE 2.3.1 PEPFAR Legislation

Full Title	Authorization Level	Public Law #	Years
United States Leadership Against HIV/AIDS, Tuberculosis, and Malaria Act of 2003 *"The Leadership Act"*	$15 billion	P.L. 108-25	FY04-FY08
Tom Lantos and Henry J. Hyde United States Global Leadership Against HIV/AIDS, Tuberculosis, and Malaria Reauthorization Act of 2008 *"The Lantos-Hyde Act"*	$48 billion	P.L. 110-293	FY09- FY13
PEPFAR Stewardship and Oversight Act of 2013 *"The PEPFAR Stewardship Act"*	Did not specify authorization for funding*	P.L. 113-56	FY14- FY18
PEPFAR Extension Act of 2018 *"The PEPFAR Extension Act"*	Did not specify authorization for funding*	P.L. 115-305	FY19-FY23

NOTES: * Congress effectively authorizes funding when it appropriates funding for a purpose. See the KFF brief on PEPFAR Reauthorization, https://www.kff.org/global-health-policy/issue-brief/pepfar-reauthorization-side-by-side-of-existing-legislation/.

HIV and the largest global health program devoted to a single disease, is credited with saving millions of lives and helping to change the trajectory of the global HIV epidemic. It was announced in January 2003 during President George W. Bush's State of the Union and authorized by Congress that same year through the Leadership Act (see Table 2.3.1). The Leadership Act governs PEPFAR's HIV response, as well as U.S. participation in the Global Fund (an independent, international multilateral financing institution that provides grants to countries to address HIV, TB, and malaria) and bilateral assistance for TB and malaria programs.[3] Congress has updated, extended, and made changes to the program through the Lantos-Hyde Act of 2008, the PEPFAR Stewardship Act of 2013, and the PEPFAR Extension Act of 2018, which goes through FY 2023. See Table 2.3.1 (see KFF brief on PEPFAR reauthorization).

[...]

Strategy

PEPFAR is currently guided by two main strategies: the overarching strategy laid out in *PEPFAR 3.0—Controlling the Epidemic: Delivering on the Promise of an AIDS-free Generation* and a complementary, more targeted strategy for accelerating implementation of PEPFAR efforts in certain high-burden countries laid out in *The PEPFAR Strategy for Accelerating HIV/AIDS Epidemic Control* (2017–2020).[4] PEPFAR 3.0 focuses on achieving epidemic control (defined by the program to be reached when the total number of new HIV infections falls below the total number of deaths from all causes among people with HIV) of the global HIV epidemic through a focus on transparency, accountability, and impact.[5] PEPFAR's 2017–2020 strategy outlines its plan to accelerate implementation in a subset of 13 PEPFAR countries that, according to PEPFAR data, show the greatest potential to achieve epidemic control by 2020: Botswana, Côte d'Ivoire, Haiti, Kenya, Lesotho, Malawi, Namibia, Rwanda, Swaziland, Tanzania, Uganda, Zambia, and Zimbabwe.[6] The strategy emphasizes accelerating testing and treatment strategies, expanding prevention, using quality data, engaging with faith-based organizations and the private sector, and strengthening policy and financial contributions by partner countries.[7] It is also intended to align with the UNAIDS 90-90-90 targets.[8]

TABLE 2.3.2 Key PEPFAR-Funded HIV Interventions

Prevention	Treatment & Care	Other Activities
• Blood supply safety • Injection safety • Prevention of mother-to-children transmission (PMTCT) of HIV • Risk reduction for youth, including sexual violence prevention • Sexual prevention programs, including condoms, contraceptive counseling, and pre-exposure prophylaxis (PrEP) • Harm reduction efforts for injecting drug users (IDUs) and non-injecting drug use • Voluntary medical male circumcision (VMMC)	• Antiretroviral (ARV) drugs for adults and children • Care and support for adults and children living with HIV • HIV testing services • TB screening and TB preventative therapy for people living with HIV	• Support for orphans and vulnerable children (OVC) • Health systems strengthening (health workforce, strategic information systems, laboratory infrastructure)

Key Activities and Results

PEPFAR activities focus on expanding access to HIV prevention, treatment, and care interventions. These include provision of antiretroviral treatment, pre-exposure prophylaxis, voluntary male circumcision, and condoms (see Table 2.3.2).[9] In addition, PEPFAR has launched specific initiatives in key strategic areas. For example, in 2015, PEPFAR launched DREAMS, a public-private partnership that aims to reduce HIV infections in adolescent girls and young women.

The latest results reported by PEPFAR indicate that it has, as of September 2019:

- supported testing services for nearly 79.6 million people in FY 2019;
- prevented more than 2.6 million babies from being born with HIV, who would have otherwise been infected;
- provided care for more than 6.3 million orphans and vulnerable children (OVC);
- supported training for more than 280,000 new health care workers; and
- supported antiretroviral treatment for more than 15.7 million people.[10]

Among the 15 countries implementing the DREAMS initiative, the latest results show a 25% or greater decline in new HIV diagnoses among adolescent girls and young women in nearly all of the regions implementing DREAMS across 10 high-burden African countries.[11]

Countries Reached

PEPFAR bilateral programs span more than 50 countries (see Figure 2.3.1).[12] More countries are reached through U.S. contributions to the Global Fund.

PEPFAR requires 25 countries[13] and the Asia, Western Hemisphere, and West Africa regional programs to develop "Country Operational Plans" (COPs) and "Regional Operational Plans" (ROPs), respectively, to document annual investments and anticipated results.[14] OGAC reviews and the Global AIDS Coordinator approves COP/ROPs.

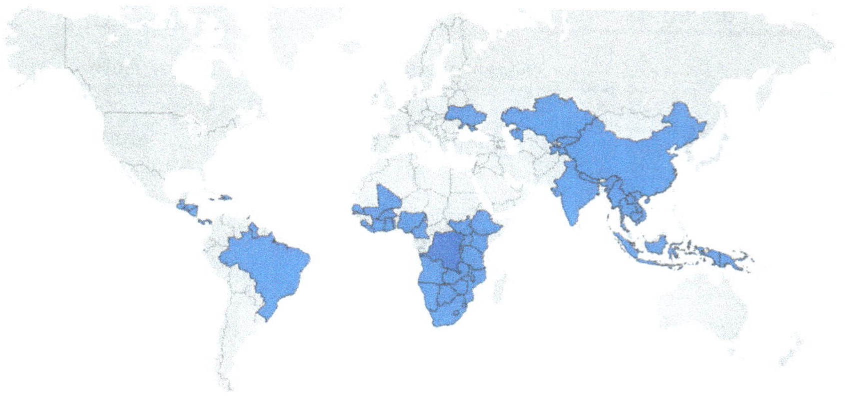

FIGURE 2.3.1 U.S. President's Emergency Plan for AIDS Relief (PEPFAR) Countries

Funding[15]

Total PEPFAR funding[16] includes all bilateral funding for HIV as well as U.S. contributions to the Global Fund and UNAIDS.[17] It represents the majority of U.S. global health funding (62% in FY 2020, or $6.9 billion[18]) and is the largest commitment by any nation to address a single disease in the world. To date, PEPFAR funding has totaled more than $90 billion (see Figure 2.3.2).

PEPFAR's creation marked a significant increase in the amount of funding provided by the U.S. for HIV. Bilateral HIV funding, which accounts for the majority of PEPFAR funding (averaging approximately 80% each year), rose rapidly from $1.1 billion in FY 2003 (the year before PEPFAR) to a peak of $5.57 billion in FY 2010. Between FY 2010 and FY 2013, it declined by more than $800 million. While it has risen since then, it is still $226 million below its peak level and has been mostly flat for the past several years. Funding for the Global Fund also increased rapidly, rising from $347 million in FY 2003 (the year before PEPFAR) to a peak level of $1.65 billion in FY 2014 before declining to $1.35 billion in FY 2015 where it remained for several years until it increased in FY 2020 to $1.56 billion.[19]

Of the approximately $6.9 billion appropriated for PEPFAR in FY 2020:

mostly bilateral

- $5.35 billion (77%) is for bilateral HIV and $1.56 billion (23%) for the Global Fund.[20]
- The majority of PEPFAR funding is channeled by Congress to the State Department ($5.93 billion, which includes $4.37 billion for bilateral HIV, most of which is then transferred to other agencies, and a $1.56 billion contribution to the Global Fund), followed by NIH ($511 million), USAID ($330 million), CDC ($128.4 million), and a small amount to DoD ($8 million).
- As in the past three years, the current Administration has proposed significantly reduced PEPFAR funding in FY 2021 ($4.42 billion) (see KFF fact sheets on the S. Global Health Budget: HIV/PEPFAR and the U.S. Global Health Budget: The Global Fund). Congress has thus far rejected proposed spending cuts.

[...]

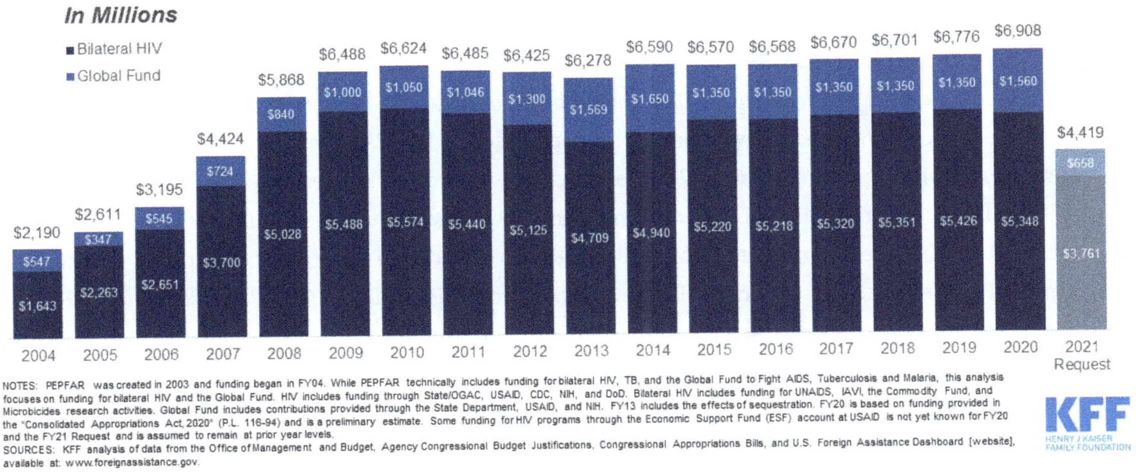

FIGURE 2.3.2 U.S. Funding for the President's Emergency Plan for AIDS Relief (PEPFAR), FY 2004—FY 2021 Request

PEPFAR & The Global Fund

The U.S. is the single largest donor to the Global Fund. Congressional appropriations to the Global Fund totaled approximately $19.5 billion from FY 2001 through FY 2020.[21] The Global Fund provides another mechanism for U.S. support by funding programs developed by recipient countries, reaching a broader range of countries, and supporting TB, malaria, and health systems strengthening (HSS) programs in addition to (and beyond their linkage with) HIV.[22] To date, over 150 countries have received Global Fund grants; 53% of Global Fund support has been committed to HIV and HIV/TB programs,[23] 29% to malaria, 16% to TB, and 2% to other health issues.[24] The original authorization of PEPFAR, and subsequent reauthorizations, included a limit on annual U.S. contributions to the Global Fund that prevented them from causing cumulative U.S. contributions to exceed 33% of the Global Fund's total contributions;[25] this requirement is in effect through FY 2023 (see the KFF fact sheet on the Global Fund).[26]

[...]

Endnotes

1. The U.S. first provided funding to address the global HIV epidemic in 1986. Then, in 1999, President Bill Clinton announced the Leadership and Investment in Fighting an Epidemic (LIFE) Initiative to address HIV in 14 African countries and in India. Later, in 2002, President George W. Bush announced the International Mother and Child HIV Prevention Initiative focused on 12 African and two Caribbean countries.
2. PEPFAR. 2009 *Annual Report to Congress*; Jan. 2009. KFF. *The U.S. Government Engagement in Global Health: A Primer*; Feb. 2019.
3. U.S. Congress. P.L. 108–25; May 27, 2003.
4. PEPFAR, *PEPFAR 3.0 Controlling the Epidemic: Delivering on the Promise of an AIDS-free Generation*, Dec. 2014. PEPFAR. *Strategy for Accelerating HIV/AIDS Epidemic Control (2017–2020)*; Sept. 2017.

5. PEPFAR, *PEPFAR 3.0 Controlling the Epidemic: Delivering on the Promise of an AIDS-free Generation*, Dec. 2014. PEPFAR. *PEPFAR 2020 Country Operational Plan Guidance for all PEPFAR Countries*, January 2020.
6. PEPFAR. *Strategy for Accelerating HIV/AIDS Epidemic Control (2017–2020)*; Sept. 2017. In 2016, PEPFAR reported that evidence had shown that, in large part due to PEPFAR support, five African countries were approaching control of their HIV epidemics; these five countries were Eswatini (formerly known as Swaziland), Lesotho, Malawi, Zambia, and Zimbabwe. These and other countries that showed the potential to achieve epidemic control by 2020 were then included in the 2017–2020 strategy for accelerating PEPFAR efforts toward control. PEPFAR. *Fact Sheet: PEPFAR Latest Global Results*, 2016. PEPFAR. "Five African Countries Approach Control of Their HIV Epidemics as U.S. Government Launches Bold Strategy to Accelerate Progress," press release; Sept. 2017.
7. PEPFAR. *PEPFAR Strategy for Accelerating HIV/AIDS Epidemic Control* (2017–2020); Sept. 2017.
8. The 90-90-90 targets were set in 2014 and aim to achieve, by 2020, "90% of people living with HIV knowing their HIV status; 90% of people who know their HIV-positive status on treatment; and 90% of people on treatment with suppressed viral loads." UNAIDS. *Fast-Track: ending the AIDS epidemic by 2030*; 2014. See also United Nations. *Transforming our world: the 2030 Agenda for Sustainable Development*; 2015, which discusses the Sustainable Development Goals (SDGs) adopted in 2015 and include a target aiming to end the AIDS epidemic by 2030 under SDG Goal 3 ("ensure healthy lives and promote well-being for all at all ages").
9. Table 2.3.2 categorization is based on PEPFAR's COP Guidance budget codes. PEFPAR. *PEFPAR 2020 Country Operational Plan Guidance for Standard Process Countries.*
10. PEPFAR. *Fact Sheet: PEPFAR Latest Global Results*; 2019.
11. The 15 African countries that are implementing DREAMS include Botswana, Cote d'Ivoire, Eswatini, Haiti, Kenya, Lesotho, Malawi, Mozambique, Namibia, Rwanda, South Africa, Tanzania, Uganda, Zambia, and Zimbabwe. PEPFAR. *Fact Sheet: PEPFAR Latest Global Results*; 2019. PEPFAR, *Dreaming of an AIDS-Free Future*, Nov. 2018. PEPFAR, "DREAMS Partnership" webpage, https://www.state.gov/pepfar-dreams-partnership/.
12. KFF analysis of data from congressional budget justification documents; PEPFAR, "Where We Work" webpage, https://www.state.gov/where-we-work-pepfar/; PEPFAR 2020 Country Operational Plan Guidance for all PEPFAR Countries; 2018 PEPFAR Progress Report on the PEPFAR Strategy for Accelerating HIV/AIDS Epidemic Control (2017–2020); and CDC's "Where We Work" webpage, https://www.cdc.gov/globalhivtb/where-we-work/index.html. PEPFAR. Press release, "Secretary Pompeo Announces Latest Lifesaving PEPFAR Results," November 27, 2018.
13. The 25 countries that are required to complete a COP are Angola, Botswana, Burundi, Cameroon, Cote d'Ivoire, Democratic Republic of the Congo, Dominican Republic, Eswatini, Ethiopia, Haiti, Kenya, Lesotho, Malawi, Mozambique, Namibia, Nigeria, Rwanda, South Africa, South Sudan, Tanzania, Uganda, Ukraine, Vietnam, Zambia, and Zimbabwe. Of these 25 countries, 14 were "focus countries" targeted in PEPFAR's first phase: Botswana, Cote d'Ivoire, Ethiopia, Haiti, Kenya, Mozambique, Namibia, Nigeria, Rwanda, South Africa, Tanzania, Uganda, Vietnam, and Zambia. Guyana, the 15th initial PEPFAR focus country, is now supported through a PEPFAR regional program. KFF analysis of data from: Congressional appropriations bills and reports; Federal Agency Budget and Congressional Justification documents; ForeignAssistance.gov; Office of Management and Budget, personal communication; PEPFAR. *2009*

Annual Report to Congress; Jan. 2009; and PEPFAR. "Where We Work" webpage, https://www.state.gov/where-we-work-pepfar/.
14. PEPFAR. *PEPFAR 2020 Country Operational Plan Guidance for all PEPFAR Countries*; Jan. 2020.
15. KFF analysis of data from: Congressional appropriations bills and reports; Federal Agency Budget and Congressional Justification documents; ForeignAssistance.gov; Office of Management and Budget, personal communication.
16. While overall PEPFAR funding technically includes bilateral funding for HIV, TB, and the Global Fund to Fight AIDS, Tuberculosis and Malaria, this analysis focuses on funding for bilateral HIV and the Global Fund.
17. UNAIDS is the Joint United Nations Programme on HIV/AIDS, the U.N. system's coordinating body that serves to help galvanize worldwide attention to AIDS.
18. Includes bilateral funding for HIV as well as U.S. contributions to the Global Fund to Fight AIDS, Tuberculosis and Malaria.
19. U.S. Congress. Public Law No: 112–25; Aug. 2, 2011. White House Office of Management and Budget (OMB). *OMB Report to the Congress on the Joint Committee Sequestration for Fiscal Year 2013*; March 1, 2013. KFF analysis of data from: Congressional appropriations bills and reports; Federal Agency Budget and Congressional Justification documents; ForeignAssistance.gov; Office of Management and Budget, personal communication.
20. KFF analysis of data from: Congressional appropriations bills and reports; Federal Agency Budget and Congressional Justification documents; ForeignAssistance.gov; Office of Management and Budget, personal communication.
21. KFF analysis of data from: Congressional appropriations bills and reports; Federal Agency Budget and Congressional Justification documents; ForeignAssistance.gov; Office of Management and Budget, personal communication.
22. Congress states that the Global Fund is the multilateral component of PEPFAR in the following: U.S. Congress. Public Law No: 110–293; July 30, 2008. U.S. Congress. Public Law No: 113–56; Dec. 2, 2013.
23. Of the 53% committed to HIV and HIV/TB programs, 46.6% was for HIV activities and 6.6% was for HIV/TB activities.
24. The Global Fund. Data Explorer; accessed May 2020: https://data.theglobalfund.org/investments/home.
25. U.S. Congress. Public Law No: 108–25; May 27, 2003. U.S. Congress. Public Law No: 110–293; July 30, 2008. U.S. Congress. Public Law No: 113–56; Dec. 2, 2013. KFF. *PEPFAR Reauthorization*, brief.
26. See the KFF. *The U.S. & The Global Fund to Fight AIDS, TB and Malaria*, fact sheet; and KFF. *PEPFAR Reauthorization*, brief.

2.4

PEPFAR—15 Years and Counting the Lives Saved

Anthony S. Fauci, M.D., and Robert W. Eisinger, Ph.D.

In the long history of successful public health initiatives, such as those leading to the eradication of smallpox, the elimination of polio throughout most of the world, and the marked reduction globally in vaccine-preventable childhood diseases, few programs have matched the impact of one that began in 2003, the President's Emergency Plan for AIDS Relief, or PEPFAR. This innovative program has had an unprecedented impact on the pandemic of HIV and AIDS.

The major scientific and clinical advances that made PEPFAR possible were the development and approval of highly effective combinations of antiretroviral medications that suppressed the replication of HIV. These drugs, generally administered in combinations of three or more, have transformed the lives of people living with HIV/AIDS, providing them with the possibility of a near-normal life expectancy and, in most cases, the ability to return to normal daily activities. Although HIV-infected people in resource-rich countries almost immediately benefited from these medications when they were licensed in the mid-1990s, a dramatic discrepancy in access to these drugs soon became apparent. More than 90% of all HIV infections were occurring in resource-limited countries, particularly in sub-Saharan Africa, where patients had little or no access to antiretroviral medications. Millions of people who could have been saved were needlessly dying.

PEPFAR was created by President George W. Bush, who felt strongly that as a resource-rich and privileged country, the United States was morally obligated to help people in low-income countries with diseases for which there were effective interventions that were unavailable to them. HIV/AIDS in the resource-limited world, particularly in southern and eastern Africa, was a stark example of such a disease. Early in his administration, Bush articulated his belief that the United States could and should design and implement a transformational and accountable program to address the HIV/AIDS pandemic in low-income countries. At that time, an estimated 30 million people were living with HIV/AIDS in Africa, where more than one third of adults in some countries were infected.[1]

After consulting scientific advisors, faith-based organizations, and others from both inside and outside his administration, Bush tasked trusted officials, including one of us (A.S.F.) and an inner circle of White House staff, with determining the feasibility of developing a program for the prevention, treatment, and care of people living with or at risk for HIV/AIDS in Africa and other low-income regions. The proposed goal would be to supply lifesaving drugs to HIV-infected people and provide the means of preventing new infections, such as the distribution of condoms to at-risk individuals.

In 2002, Bush sent members of his administration and federal officials, including one of us (A.S.F.), on a fact-finding mission to several of the hardest-hit African countries to determine whether such a program was feasible. In those countries, philanthropic and other organizations were efficiently and effectively providing antiretroviral drugs to small numbers of patients, and it was clear that patients there understood and embraced the critical need for treatment and adherence to treatment regimens. The firsthand observation of what was attainable in sub-Saharan Africa directly contradicted the notion expressed by some that HIV-infected people in southern Africa were incapable of adhering to a daily treatment regimen for a potentially lethal disease. When the delegation returned, the President, through his immediate staff, gave the go-ahead (to A.S.F. and Dr. Mark Dybul) to begin designing the program.

The challenge was to provide HIV prevention, treatment, and care for as many people as possible. Multiple versions and iterations of the proposed program were labored over by White House and other government officials, with the encouragement of the President and his senior staff. There were intense discussions concerning the size and magnitude of the program; which countries would be included; and how best to allocate effort and resources among prevention, treatment, and care; as well as several other considerations. After months of discussion and debate, Bush announced the formation of PEPFAR in his State of the Union Address on January 28, 2003. The original proposal for PEPFAR, authorized with strong bipartisan support from Congress under the United States Leadership Against HIV/AIDS, Tuberculosis, and Malaria Act of 2003, was for a program costing $15 billion over 5 years and aiming for ambitious goals, including preventing 7 million new HIV infections, treating 2 million HIV-infected persons, and providing care—including basic medical services, education, and social support—for 10 million HIV-infected people, including children who have lost one or both parents to AIDS.

Shortly after President Bush signed the legislation in May 2003, PEPFAR was officially launched in 14 countries in Africa and the Caribbean that were severely affected by HIV/AIDS: Botswana, Ethiopia, Guyana, Haiti, Ivory Coast, Kenya, Mozambique, Namibia, Nigeria, Rwanda, South Africa, Tanzania, Uganda, and Zambia. These countries collectively accounted for nearly 20 million HIV-infected men, women, and children.[1] With the addition of Vietnam in July 2004, the PEPFAR partner countries were home to more than 50% of all HIV-infected people in the world.[2] The program was an interagency effort spanning the administration and the U.S. government, coordinated by the Department of State.

PEPFAR has received continuous bipartisan support from Congress since 2003 and is the largest global health initiative for a single infectious disease that has ever been implemented. The amount of funds appropriated for PEPFAR in fiscal year 2017 totaled $6.8 billion to provide HIV/AIDS treatment, prevention, and support programs in more than 50 countries. Four PEPFAR directors—Ambassadors Randall Tobias (2003–2006), Mark Dybul (2006–2009), Eric Goosby (2009–2013), and Deborah Birx (2014–present)—reporting directly to the U.S. Secretary of State, have guided and shaped PEPFAR into a remarkable global health success. As of September 2017, PEPFAR-funded programs have provided 13.3 million HIV-infected men, women, and children with antiretroviral therapy; supported

15.2 million voluntary medical male circumcisions in eastern and southern African countries to reduce the risk of HIV transmission; averted nearly 2.2 million perinatal HIV infections; and provided care for more than 6.4 million orphans and vulnerable children.[3]

Major hurdles of lack of health systems, pervasive stigma and discrimination, and limited access to and uptake of treatment and prevention programs, as well as socioeconomic, cultural, and demographic barriers at the local, regional, and national levels, had to be overcome in order to realize these achievements. Recent PEPFAR data indicate that five African countries—Lesotho, Malawi, Swaziland, Zambia, and Zimbabwe—are on track to achieve the Joint United Nations Program on HIV/AIDS (UNAIDS) targets for treatment implementation by 2020.[4]

PEPFAR has also provided some of the critical workforce, organizational, and physical infrastructure to address other concerns—such as malaria, tuberculosis, maternal and child health, immunizations, and unanticipated infectious disease outbreaks—that affect the geographic areas where patients with HIV are treated. Specifically, the program has contributed to building sustainable health system capacity in host countries by investing in the critical infrastructure of laboratories and training more than 220,000 health care workers.[5] With regard to international public relations, PEPFAR has done as much as or more than any other program in enhancing the humanitarian image of the United States and has firmly established it as a key player in the response to a historic global public health crisis.

Over the past 15 years, PEPFAR has demonstrated the transforming results that can be realized by strong government leadership in the global health arena. It is entirely possible to bring the HIV/AIDS pandemic to an end, and PEPFAR will undoubtedly play an essential role in this endeavor. However, it is vital that support for this transformative program continue both to meet the immediate challenge of HIV/AIDS and to serve as the model for the control and elimination of other globally devastating infectious diseases.

Disclosure forms provided by the authors are available at NEJM.org.

Author Affiliations

From the National Institute of Allergy and Infectious Diseases, National Institutes of Health, Bethesda, M.D.

References

1. Office of the Press Secretary. Fact sheet: the President's Emergency Plan for AIDS Relief. Washington, DC: White House, 2003 (https://georgewbush-whitehouse.archives.gov/news/releases/2003/01/20030129-1.html).
2. Goosby E, Dybul M, Fauci AS, et al. The United States President's Emergency Plan for AIDS Relief: a story of partnerships and smart investments to turn the tide of the global AIDS pandemic. J Acquir Immune Defic SynDr. 2012; 60:Suppl 3:S51-S56.
3. President's Emergency Plan for AIDS Relief. New PEPFAR results reach historic highs in HIV prevention and treatment. November 2017 (https://www.pepfar.gov/press/releases/2017/276082.htm).

4. President's Emergency Plan for AIDS Relief. Five African countries approach control of their HIV epidemics as U.S. government launches bold strategy to accelerate progress. September 2017 (https://www.pepfar.gov/press/releases/2017/274155.htm).
5. Office of the U.S. Global AIDS Coordinator and the Health Diplomacy. PEPFAR: 2017 annual report to Congress. 2017 (https://www.pepfar.gov/documents/organization/267809.pdf).

Citing Articles

1. Gabrielle O'Malley, Gena Barnabee, Kenneth Mugwanya. (2019) Scaling-up PrEP Delivery in Sub-Saharan Africa: What Can We Learn from the Scale-up of ART?. *Current HIV/AIDS Reports* **378**.
2. Brian J. Morris, Catherine A. Hankins, Joya Banerjee, Eugenie R. Lumbers, Adrian Mindel, Jeffrey D. Klausner, John N. Krieger. (2019) Does Male Circumcision Reduce Women's Risk of Sexually Transmitted Infections, Cervical Cancer, and Associated Conditions?. *Frontiers in Public Health* 7.

2.5

The U.S. & The Global Fund to Fight AIDS, Tuberculosis and Malaria

Kaiser Family Foundation

Key Facts

- The Global Fund to Fight AIDS, Tuberculosis and Malaria (Global Fund), founded in 2002, is an independent, multilateral, financing entity designed to raise significant resources and accelerate efforts to end the AIDS, tuberculosis, and malaria epidemics.
- The U.S. government (U.S.) provided the Global Fund with its founding contribution and is its largest single donor; between FY 2001 and FY 2019 Congressional appropriations to the Global Fund totaled nearly $18 billion. The U.S. also plays a key role in the organization's governance and oversight.
- As of July 2019, the Global Fund had approved more than $49 billion in funding and disbursed more than $42 billion to over 120 countries;[1] these investments have helped to save 27 million lives.
- The Global Fund's recently completed Sixth Replenishment Conference reached its goal of raising $14 billion for the next three-year period, which included an increased funding pledge from the U.S. While both the House and Senate appropriations bills include funding for the first year of this pledge (FY 2020), Congress has not yet finalized the FY 2020 budget.

[...]

TABLE 2.5.1 Total Global Fund Pledges and Contributions as of July 2019 (US$billions)

	Total Pledges to the Global Fund	% of Total Pledges	Total Paid to the Global Fund	%
Total	**$54.7**	**100.0%**	**$49.2**	
United States	$17.5	32.1%	$15.0	
France	$6.5	11.9%	$6.0	
United Kingdom	$5.3	9.7%	$4.5	
Germany	$3.9	7.1%	$3.6	
Japan	$3.5	6.3%	$3.5	
European Commission	$2.7	4.9%	$2.6	
Canada	$2.6	4.8%	$2.4	
All Other Countries	$9.2	16.8%	$8.3	
Other Donors	$3.5	6.4%	$3.4	

Notes: Includes pledges made for the period 2001–2019 as well as those made with year of commitment yet to be confirme includes contributions made by the private sector and nongovernmental organizations, Debt2Health, and the Affordable Me malaria (AMFm). Pledge and Paid amounts, if listed by the Global Fund in the currency of origin, were converted to U.S. dollar Fund using fixed replenishment exchange rates (for the years 2014–2019) and spot exchange rates (for years earlier than 20).

Sources: The Global Fund: https://www.theglobalfund.org/en/updates/other-updates/2019-04-03-updated-pledge contributions-report/ (https://www.theglobalfund.org/en/updates/other-updates/2019-04-03-updated-pledges-an report/); accessed July 31, 2019, Kaiser Family Foundation Analysis.

[...]

Endnote

1. Does not include countries that may have received funding through regional programs.

2.6

U.S. Federal Funding for HIV/AIDS

Kaiser Foundation

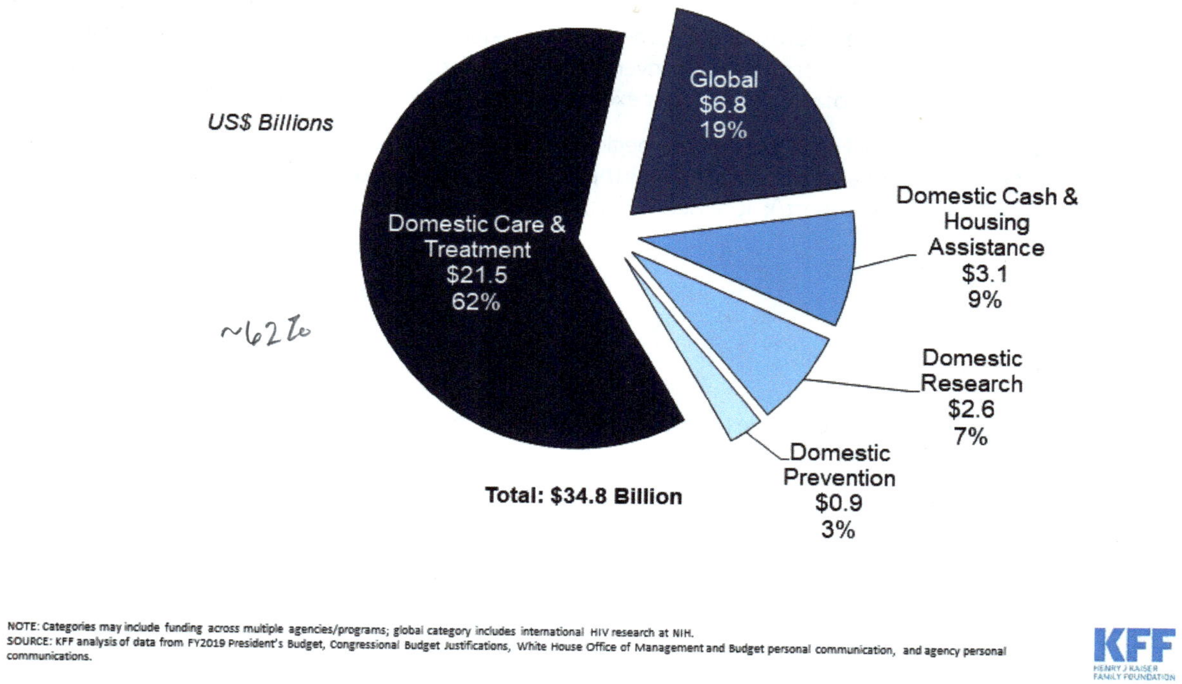

FIGURE 2.6.1 U.S. Federal Funding for HIV/AIDS, by Category, FY 2019

2.6a Medicaid and HIV

Key Facts

- Medicaid is the largest source of insurance coverage for people with HIV, estimated to cover 42% of the adult population, compared to just 13% of the adult population overall.[1,2]
- The number of Medicaid beneficiaries with HIV has grown over time as people with HIV are living longer and new infections continue to occur.[3,4] In 2013, there were 282,100 beneficiaries

with HIV compared to 212,900 in 2007, a 33% increase. The expansion of the program under the Affordable Care Act (ACA) has also increased coverage for people with HIV.

- Medicaid spending on HIV accounts for 30% of all federal spending on HIV care and it is the second largest source of public financing for HIV care in the U.S.[5] Spending has increased over time, reflecting growing numbers of beneficiaries with HIV and the rising cost of care.
- Medicaid beneficiaries with HIV are more likely to be male, Black, dually eligible for Medicare and to qualify based on disability, compared to beneficiaries overall.
- Medicaid covers a broad range of services, many of which are important for people with HIV and those at risk, including prescription drugs, inpatient and outpatient care, and preventive services.

Overview

Medicaid, the largest public health insurance program in the United States, covering health and long-term care services for 73 million low-income individuals, has played a critical role in HIV care since the epidemic began.[6,7] It is the single largest source of coverage for people with HIV in the U.S., and its role has grown over time as people with HIV are living longer, new infections continue to occur, and the program was expanded under the Affordable Care Act (ACA).[8,9] Medicaid is estimated to cover 42% of adults with HIV.[10] By comparison, just 13% of adults in the general population are covered by the program.[11]

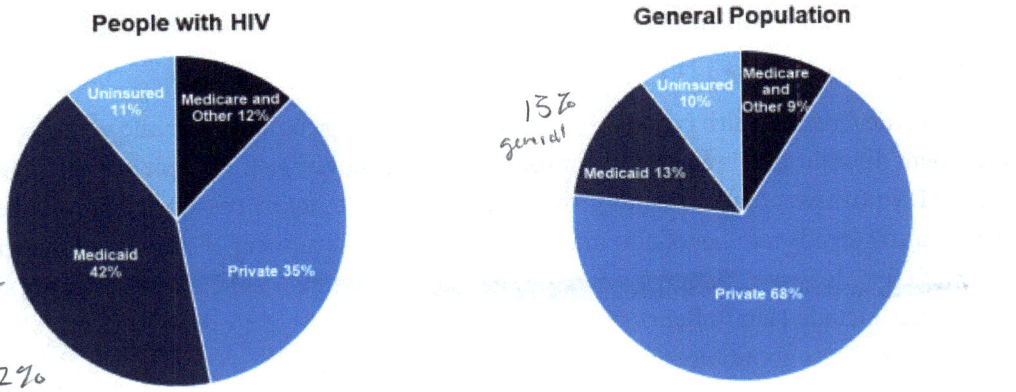

Sources: Data on people with HIV: Analysis of data from the CDC's Medical Monitoring Project (MMP), 2017 Cycle ; Data on general population: KFF analysis of the 2017 American Community Survey.
Notes: Data from both sources are limited to all adults (18+). The hierarchy used to establish insurance coverage sources in both cases was: Private coverage; Medicaid; and Medicare combined with other public coverage; and uninsured.

FIGURE 2.6.2 Insurance Coverage Among People with HIV and the General Population, 2017

[...]

Medicaid Spending on HIV

In FY 2019, federal Medicaid spending on HIV is estimated to total $6.3 billion, accounting for 30% of all federal spending on HIV care and representing the second largest source of public financing for HIV care in the U.S, after Medicare (see Figure 3).20 In addition, the states' share of Medicaid spending on HIV was estimated to be an additional $3.8 billion in FY 2019.21 Medicaid spending on HIV has increased over time, reflecting growing numbers of beneficiaries with HIV and the rising cost of care and treatment. Between 2013 and 2019, federal Medicaid spending on HIV increased by 60%, rising from $3.97 billion to $6.3 billion.22 Still, in FY 2019 federal Medicaid spending on HIV represents less than 2% of total federal Medicaid spending.

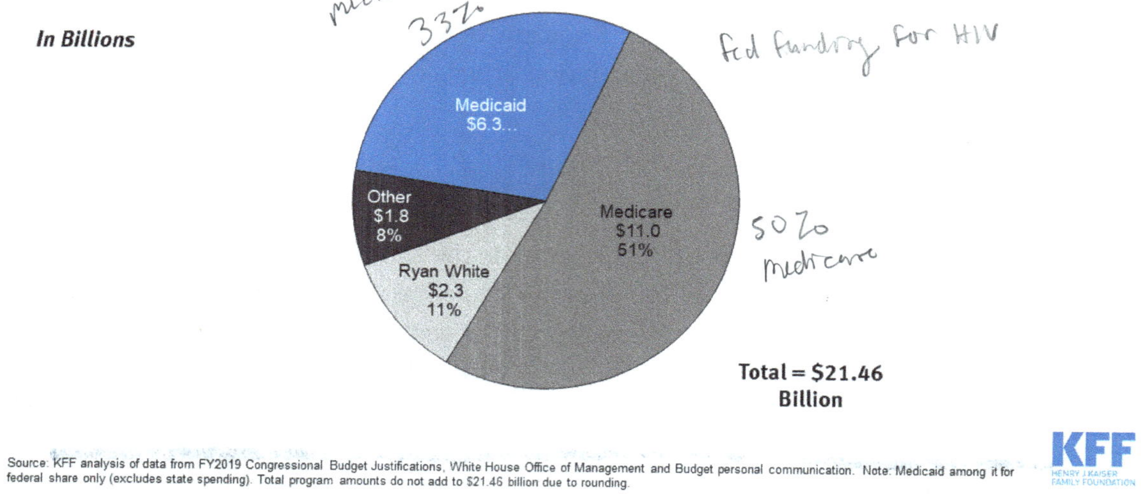

FIGURE 2.6.2 Federal Funding for HIV/AIDS Care in the U.S., by Program, FY 2019

2.6b Medicare and HIV

Medicare, the federal health insurance program for people age 65 and older and younger adults with permanent disabilities,[12] is an important source of health coverage for people with HIV.[13] As the size of U.S. HIV positive population has grown over time, due to an increased lifespan for people with HIV but also a steady number of new infections, so too has the number of Medicare beneficiaries with HIV. Both the Medicare Modernization Act of 2003 and the Affordable Care Act (ACA), signed into law in 2010, included a number of important provisions related to Medicare and its role for people with HIV. Key facts about Medicare and HIV include:

- The number of Medicare beneficiaries with HIV has tripled since the 1990s, rising from 42,520 in 1997 to 120,000 in 2014.[14]
- Approximately one quarter of people with HIV in care get their health insurance coverage through Medicare.[15]
- Medicare spending for HIV has also increased over time, and the program is now the single largest source of federal financing for HIV care and treatment.[16]
- While most people with HIV on Medicare are under age 65 and qualify because of a disability, a growing share is 65 and older, many of whom aged onto the program.

- The majority of Medicare beneficiaries with HIV are dually eligible for Medicare and Medicaid, and receive low-income subsidies under Part D.

2.6c The Ryan White HIV/AIDS Program: The Basics

Key Facts

- The Ryan White HIV/AIDS Program, first enacted in 1990, is the largest federal program designed specifically for people with HIV, serving over half of all those diagnosed.[17, 18] It is a discretionary, grant program dependent on annual appropriations from Congress"
- It is the nation's safety net for people with HIV providing outpatient HIV care and treatment to those without health insurance and filling in gaps in coverage and cost for those with insurance.
- Most Ryan White clients are low-income, male, people of color, and sexual minorities.
- The program is the third largest source of federal funding for HIV care in the U.S., following Medicare and Medicaid. In FY20 it was funded at $2.5 billion which includes new funding for the federal "Ending the HIV Epidemic" initiative and supplemental funding related to the COVID-19 response.[19] Funding is distributed to states/territories, cities, and HIV organizations in the form of grants.
- While the Affordable Care Act (ACA), has expanded coverage for many people with HIV, Ryan White continues to remain a critical component of the nation's response to HIV, providing HIV care and treatment to those who remain uninsured and bolstering access for those with insurance.

Overview

The Ryan White HIV/AIDS Program (Ryan White), the largest federal program designed specifically for people with HIV in the United States, serves over half of those in the country diagnosed with the disease.4 First enacted in 1990, the Ryan White Program has played an increasingly significant role as the number of people living with HIV has grown over time and people with HIV are living longer. It provides outpatient care and support services to individuals and families affected by the disease, functioning as the "payer of last resort" by filling the gaps for those who have no other source of coverage or face coverage limits or cost barriers.

The program has been reauthorized by Congress four times since it was first created (1996, 2000, 2006, and 2009) and each reauthorization has made adjustments to the program. The current authorization lapsed in FY 2013, but the program has continued to be funded through the annual appropriations process as there is no "sunset" provision or end date attached to the legislation. The program is administered by the HIV/AIDS Bureau (HAB) at the Health Resources and Services Administration (HRSA) of the Department for Health and Human Services (HHS), and programs and services are delivered by grantees and sub-grantees at the state and local levels.

[...]

Endnotes

1. Centers for Disease Control and Prevention. Behavioral. Medical Monitoring Project, United States, 2017 Cycle.
2. Kaiser Family Foundation analysis of American Community Survey data, 2017.
3. Kaiser Family Foundation. State Health Facts. *Medicaid Enrollment and Spending on HIV/AIDS. (FY07-FY11).* http://kff.org/hivaids/state-indicator/enrollment-spending-on-hiv/.
4. Kates, J. and Dawson, L. Kaiser Family Foundation. *Insurance Coverage Changes for People with HIV Under the ACA.* 2017. https://www.kff.org/health-reform/issue-brief/insurance-coverage-changes-for-people-with-hiv-under-the-aca/.
5. Kaiser Family Foundation. U.S. Federal Funding for HIV/AIDS: Trends Over Time. March 2019. https://www.kff.org/hivaids/fact-sheet/u-s-federal-funding-for-hivaids-trends-over-time/.
6. CMS. March 2019 Medicaid & CHIP Enrollment Data Highlights. https://www.medicaid.gov/medicaid/program-information/medicaid-and-chip-enrollment-data/report-highlights/index.html.
7. Kaiser Family Foundation. State Health Facts. Total Monthly Medicaid and CHIP Enrollment. December 2018. https://www.kff.org/health-reform/state-indicator/total-monthly-medicaid-and-chip-enrollment/?currentTimeframe=0&sortModel=%7B%22colId%22:%22Location%22,%22sort%22:%22asc%22%7D.
8. Kaiser Family Foundation. State Health Facts. *Medicaid Enrollment and Spending on HIV/AIDS. (FY07-FY11).* http://kff.org/health-reform/state-indicator-enrollment-spending-on-hiv.
9. See current status of state Medicaid expansion decisions: http://kff.org/health-reform/state-indicator/state-activity-around-expanding-medicaid-under-the-affordable-care-act/
10. Centers for Disease Control and Prevention. Behavioral. Medical Monitoring Project, United States, 2017 Cycle.
11. Kaiser Family Foundation analysis of American Community Survey data, 2017.
12. Kaiser Family Foundation. *An Overview of Medicare. 2016.* Available at: http://files.kff.org/attachment/issue-brief-an-overview-of-medicare
13. Unless otherwise noted, data on the number and characteristics of Medicare beneficiaries with HIV in this fact sheet are based on Kaiser Family Foundation analysis of 2014 data from the Medicare 5 percent sample, a claims-based dataset obtained from the Chronic Conditions Data Warehouse (CCW) of the Centers for Medicare & Medicaid Services (CMS), 2014. The 5% sample includes beneficiaries in traditional (fee-for-service) Medicare only, and therefore does not include those enrolled in Medicare Advantage plans. Beneficiaries in fee-for-service Medicare account for 69% of all Medicare beneficiaries.
14. The 1997 estimate is from Gilden DE, Kubisiak JM, Gilden DM. Managing Medicare's HIV Caseload in the Era of Suppressive Therapy, *AJPH*. Vol. 97, No. 6; June 2007. The 2014 estimate is based on Kaiser Family Foundation's analysis.
15. Kaiser Family Foundation analysis of the 5% sample (see endnote 2) and CDC. (2014) *Vital Signs: HIV Diagnosis, Care, and Treatment Among Persons Living with HIV—United States, 2011.* MMWR. 63(47); 1113–1117. Available at: http://www.cdc.gov/mmwr/preview/mmwrhtml/mm6347a5.htm?s_cid=mm6347a5_w
16. Personal communication, CMS, April 2016
17. Kaiser Family Foundation. *U.S. Federal Funding for HIV/AIDS: Trends Over Time.* November 2017. Available at: http://kff.org/global-health-policy/fact-sheet/u-s-federal-funding-for-hivaids-trends-over-time/.

18. Ryan White HIV/AIDS Program Annual Client-Level Data Report 2018. December 2019. Available at: https://hab.hrsa.gov/sites/default/files/hab/data/datareports/RWHAP-annual-client-level-data-report-2018.pdf
19. Kaiser Family Foundation analysis of FY20 HHS omnibus spending bill.
20. Ryan White HIV/AIDS Program Annual Client-Level Data Report 2018. December 2019. Available at: https://hab.hrsa.gov/sites/default/files/hab/data/datareports/RWHAP-annual-client-level-data-report-2018.pdf.

2.7

Priority-Setting in Health: Building Institutions for Smarter Public Spending

A Report of the Center for Global Development's Priority-Setting Institutions for Global Health Working Group

Amanda Glassman and Kalipso Chalkidou, Co-chairs

Executive Summary

Data, methods, and evidence on the costs, effectiveness, and equity of health interventions and technologies are increasingly available, but there is a persistent gap between this evidence and the uses of scarce public budgets for health in low- and middle-income countries. This is illustrated by low coverage of highly cost-effective health care interventions, dependency on donor finance for the most basic health care interventions, and—sometimes—public subsidies for care considered ineffective in the world's wealthiest countries. These anomalies that reduce the impact of public and donor spending on health are the result of ad hoc decision making on budgets, driven more by inertia and interest groups than science, ethics, and the public interest.

Many more lives could be saved and health equity enhanced by reallocating part of public and donor monies toward the most cost-effective and equity-enhancing health interventions and technologies. Yet too many countries lack the fair processes and institutions needed to make the connection between evidence and decisions on public spending and spell out the opportunity costs of one decision versus another, while managing the myriad interest groups and ethical conundrums that revolve around new technologies and scarce budgets.

In this report, the Center for Global Development's Priority-Setting Institutions for Health Working Group has identified core features of priority-setting processes and institutions worldwide, recommending direct substantive support for creating fair and evidence-based national and global health technology assessment systems that will be applicable in any kind of health system.

Finite Resources, Unlimited Demand, Unfair Process

Decisions on public and donor spending on health are controversial because they affect who receives what, when, and at what cost, often with life-or-death consequences. In low- and middle-income countries facing highly constrained budgets, the conflicting pressures are acute.

Allocating funding to treat HIV/AIDS is among the most visible dilemmas facing donors and policy makers. Only 53 percent of those needing antiretroviral therapy were receiving treatment in Africa in December 2009.[1] Countries and their development assistance partners decide who will receive life-saving therapy, when, and under what circumstances, yet neither have defined explicit criteria to make such decisions—leading to nontransparent processes rife with opportunities for abuse by those with influence, and partly or completely void of ethical considerations. Further, current HIV/AIDS allocation strategies do not optimize for disease reduction either.

As countries spend more on health and population demands grow, public spending begins to respond even more to interest groups and wealthy populations, and cost-effective health interventions are often the opportunity cost of that response when priorities are not explicitly set. In India, for example, only 44 percent of children 1–2 years old are fully vaccinated, yet open-heart surgery is subsidized in national public hospitals. In Colombia 58 percent of children are fully vaccinated, but in 2011 the legal system ordered the use of public monies to subsidize treating breast cancer with Avastin, a brand name medicine considered ineffective and unsafe for that purpose in the United States.[1]

The Moral Case

People who decide how to spend health budgets hold the lives and livelihoods of many other people in their hands, and they must literally make life-or-death decisions. Most such decisions take little account of the cost-effectiveness of the interventions they choose to finance, or the human costs and tradeoffs implied by choosing to fund less cost-effective interventions.

The cost-effectiveness of interventions funded by global health agencies varies greatly. For example, some of the least effective interventions for HIV/AIDS produce less than 0.1 percent of the value of the most effective (in disability-adjusted life years). And looking across multiple disease burdens, this fraction drops to less than 0.01 percent.

As a result, ignoring cost-effectiveness can easily mean losing 99 percent or more of the potential value that a health budget could have achieved. Even choosing the median intervention, as analyzed by the Disease Control Priorities in Developing Countries project, can mean losing 85 percent of the potential value.[2] In practical terms this can mean hundreds, thousands, or millions of additional deaths from the failure to set effective priorities. The moral case for considering the relative value of health interventions implies the need to divert the bulk of funds to the very best interventions.

Case Study: Uganda

Uganda, a low-income country, spends about $12.50 per capita on health care. The government uses priority-setting processes (both formal and informal) to inform health coverage decisions supported by public spending. It recently offered Ugandans access to a national health care package, but the cost is almost four times the funds available for its provision. Moreover, policy makers have voiced complaints that the complex priorities in the health care package are donor-driven and do

1 Using the WHO 2006 guidelines to initiate treatment at a CD4 cell count below 200 cells/uL (Institute of Medicine of the National Academies 2011).

not fully consider the Ugandan context.[1] The government is committed to providing essential care to its people, but it faces issues in setting priorities fairly and justifying its decisions to the public. A Ugandan physician observes:

Somebody can have malaria, and there are no drugs for malaria, and you find there are drugs for cryptococcal meningitis, and then you say to yourself, "If I come with malaria, and cannot be treated, another (patient) comes with cryptococcal meningitis and can be treated, where is the fairness?"[2]

Notes

1. Kapiriri (2012).
2. Kapiriri, Norheim, and Martin (2009).

[...]

Chapter 3. Considering Cost-Effectiveness: The Moral Perspective

The first draft of this chapter was written by Toby Ord, Balliol College, Oxford University.

Achieving good value with scarce resources is a substantial moral issue for global health. This claim may be surprising to some, since conversations on the ethics of global health often focus on moral concerns about justice, fairness, and freedom. But outcomes and consequences are also of central moral importance in setting priorities. In this chapter we explore the moral relevance of cost-effectiveness, a major tool for capturing the relationship between resources and outcomes, by illustrating what is lost in moral terms for global health when cost-effectiveness is ignored.

The Cost-Effectiveness Landscape in Global Health

The moral importance of cost-effectiveness is illustrated by its substantial variation between different interventions. A simplified example will help clarify how this becomes a moral consideration. Suppose we have a $40,000 budget that we can spend as we wish on the health condition of blindness in an African country. One option is to provide blind people with guide dogs to help them overcome their disability. This costs approximately $40,000 per person due to the training required for the dog and its recipient.[2] Another option is to pay for surgeries to reverse the effects of trachoma. This costs less than $20 per patient cured, with the cost of the surgery itself less than $10.[3] Many other options exist, but for simplicity, let us just consider these two.

We could thus use the entire budget to provide a single guide dog, helping one person overcome the challenges of blindness, or we could use it to cure more than 2,000 people of blindness. By allocating all the resources to purchase a guide dog for one person we are ignoring the legitimate claims of 2,000 other people. Some would reframe the choice by arguing that the second option is more than 2,000 times better than the first, or, even more starkly, that the first option squanders about 99.95 percent of the value that could have been produced.

---

2 Guide Dogs of America estimates $19,000 for the training of the dog. When the cost of training the recipient to use the dog is included, the cost doubles to $38,000. Other guide dog providers give similar estimates, for example, Seeing Eye estimates a total of $50,000 per person/dog partnership, while Guiding Eyes for the Blind estimates a total of $40,000.

3 Cook et al. (2006) estimate their figure to be $7.14 per surgery, with a 77 percent cure rate.

This example illustrates the basic point, but it is also unrealistic in at least two ways. First, we often have an expansive spectrum of options—with greater variation in scope and complexity than just the two previously considered. Second, and more importantly, the class of interventions under consideration is often broad enough that it is difficult to make direct "apples to apples" comparisons between the effects of two interventions.

Health economists have an answer to the second issue. They use measures that transform all health benefits into a single metric, thus allowing for direct comparisons between interventions that are aimed at different threats to health and that affect different health outcomes. The standard measure in global health is the disability-adjusted life year (DALY), which gauges the disvalue of health conditions by the number of years of life lost due to the condition plus the number of years lived with disability multiplied by a number representing the severity of the disability. For example, a condition that caused one to die 5 years prematurely and to live the past 10 years with deafness would be valued as 5 + (10 × 33.3 percent) = 8.33 DALYs.

There are a number of methodological complications and choices for calculating DALYs, which give rise to a number of different versions of DALYs and the closely related units—quality-adjusted life years. Chief among these choices is the question of the size of the weightings representing how bad it is on average to suffer from a particular disability. There are also considerations on discount rates and age weightings.

These methodological choices have ethical implications. People disagree on the appropriateness of particular disability weights, or about the method for eliciting these weights, or about discounting health benefits, or weighting benefits depending on the age of the recipients, or whether other issues such as equal moral consideration need to be factored in. Members of the Working Group and the author of this chapter have many of the same concerns and agree that DALYs should be considered only as a rough measure of the disvalue of different conditions.

In most cases, however, different reasonable choices on these parameters change the number of DALYs due to a condition by a few percent or by as much as a factor of two. By contrast, the difference in cost-effectiveness between interventions is often a factor of 100 or more. Thus, even a rough measure of DALYs saved can supply information of critical moral importance in informing key comparisons.

The two concerns raised in the hypothetical blindness case can be addressed by looking at a real-world example of funding the prevention or treatment of HIV/AIDS. Let us consider five intervention types: surgical treatment for Kaposi's sarcoma (an AIDS defining illness), antiretroviral therapy to fight the virus in infected people, prevention of transmission of HIV from mother to child during pregnancy, condom distribution to prevent transmission more generally, and education for high-risk groups such as sex workers. It is initially very unclear which of these interventions would be best to fund, and one might assume that they are roughly equal in importance. However, the most comprehensive compendium on cost-effectiveness in global health, *Disease Control Priorities in Developing Countries*, 2nd edition (2006), hereafter *DCP2*, lists their estimated cost-effectiveness as follows (Figure 2.7.1).

Note the wide discrepancies between the effectiveness obtained for the same amount of money. Treatment for Kaposi's sarcoma cannot be seen on the chart at this scale, but that says more about the other interventions being good than about this treatment being bad: treatment for Kaposi's

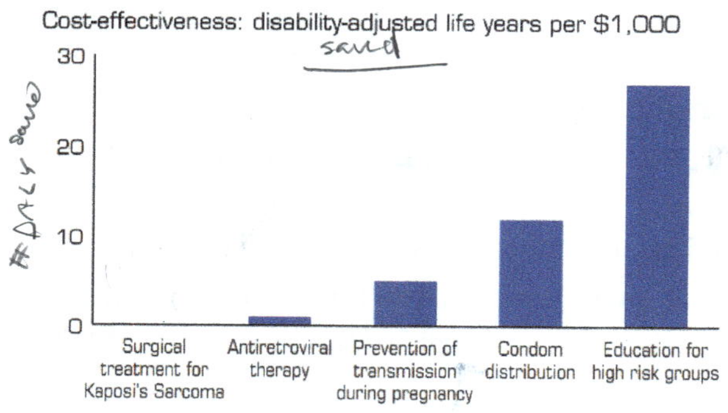

FIGURE 2.7.1 *Cost-effectiveness of HIV-related health services*

Source: Jamison et al. (2006).

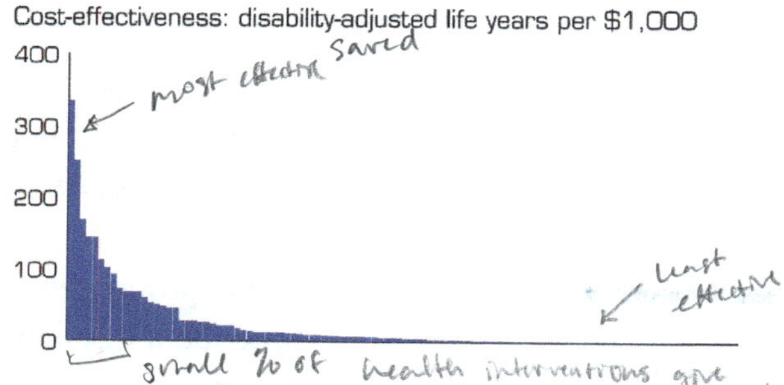

FIGURE 2.7.2 *Cost effectiveness of 108 health interventions evaluated in DCP2*

Source: Jamison et al. (2006).

sarcoma is often considered cost-effective in high-income countries. But antiretroviral therapy is estimated to be 50 times as effective as treatment for Kaposi's sarcoma, prevention of transmission during pregnancy is 5 times as effective, condom distribution is about twice as effective, and education for high-risk groups is again about twice as effective. In total the best of these interventions is estimated to be 1,400 times as cost-effective as the least good, or more than 1,400 times better than it would need to be in order to be funded in rich countries.

This discrepancy becomes even larger if we make comparisons between interventions targeted at different types of illness. *DCP2* includes cost-effectiveness estimates for 108 health interventions, arranged from least effective to most effective (Figure 2.7.2).

This larger sample of interventions is even more disparate in cost-effectiveness. The least effective intervention analyzed is still the treatment for Kaposi's sarcoma, but some other interventions are up to 10 times more cost-effective than education for high-risk groups. In total the interventions are spread over more than four orders of magnitude, ranging from 0.02 to 300 DALYs per $1,000, with a median of 5 DALYs. Thus, moving money from the least effective intervention to the most effective would theoretically produce about 15,000 times the benefit, and even moving it from the median intervention to the most effective would produce about 60 times the benefit.

It can also be seen that due to the skewed distribution, the most effective interventions produce a disproportionate amount of the benefits. According to the *DCP2* data, if we funded all of these interventions equally, 80 percent of the benefits would be produced by the top 20 percent of the interventions. It must be noted that these are merely estimates of cost-effectiveness and there may be less variance between the real, underlying cost-effectiveness values. However, even if the most effective interventions are one-tenth as effective as these figures suggest and the least effective are 10 times better than they appear, there would still be a factor of 150 between them.

Moreover, there have been health interventions that are even more effective than any of those studied in the *DCP2*. For example, consider the progress that has been made on saving lives lost to immunization-preventable illness, diarrhea, malaria, and smallpox (Figure 2.7.3).

In all cases these interventions have led to at least 2.5 million fewer deaths per year. To aid the reader in comprehending the scale of these achievements, a final bar in the graphic shows the average

1 DALY = lose 1 year of full health
↑ DALY = ↑ Disease burden
rough estimate

number of deaths per year due to war and genocide together over the 20th century (2.3 million).

Moreover, these gains have been achieved very cheaply. For instance, with smallpox, the total cost of eradication was about $400 million.[1] Since more than 100 million lives have been saved so far, this has come to less than $4 per life saved—significantly superior to all interventions in the *DCP2*. Moreover, the eradication also saved large amounts of money. About $70 million was being spent across developing countries per year in routine vaccination and treatment for smallpox, and more than $1,000 million was lost per year in reduced productivity.[2] Even just in the United States, smallpox vaccination and vigilance cost $150 million per year before eradication.[3] The eradication program thus saved an enormous number of lives per year, while saving money for both donors and recipients, paying back its entire costs every few months. It serves as an excellent proof of just how cost-effective global health can be.

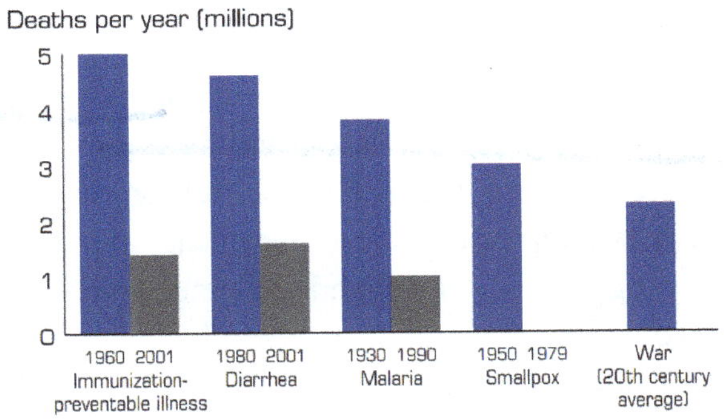

FIGURE 2.7.3 *Preventable deaths from immunization-preventable illness, diarrhea, malaria, smallpox, and war*

Note: Estimates for the death toll from all acts of war and genocide in the 20th century vary from about 160 million to 240 million, differing in which deaths they include (Leitenberg 2006).

Source: Jha et al. (2004).

The main effect of understanding the moral need of consideration of cost-effectiveness is spending our budgets to produce greater health benefits, saving many more lives and preventing or treating more disabling conditions. However, it also shows a very interesting fact about global health funding. If we can save 1,000 lives with one intervention and 10,000 with another at an equal price, then merely moving our funding from the first intervention to the second saves 9,000 lives. As such, moving funding from one intervention to a more cost-effective one can produce almost as much benefit as adding an equal amount of additional funding to the more cost-effective intervention. This is counterintuitive since it is not the case when one option is merely 10 percent or 30 percent better than another. However, when one option is 10 times or 100 times better, as is often the case in global health, redirecting funding is so important that it can be equivalent to new funding directed toward the superior intervention. In times of global austerity and shrinking budgets, it is good to know how much more can be done within current resources.

The Moral Case

In these examples we have seen how incredibly variable cost-effectiveness can be within global health. The least effective intervention in the HIV/AIDS case produces less than 0.1 percent of the value of the most effective, and if we are willing to look at different kinds of disease, this fraction drops to less than 0.01 percent. Ignoring cost-effectiveness thus does not mean losing 10 or 20 percent of the potential value that a health budget could have achieved, but it can easily mean losing 99 percent or more. Even choosing the median intervention can involve losing 85 percent of the potential value. In human and moral terms this can mean hundreds, thousands, or millions of people who will lose their lives due to the failure to take cost-effectiveness into account in allocating health resources.

since public health $ limited, dedicate $ to most effective to help most people

In non-life-saving contexts it means thousands or millions of people who will live with significant disabilities that could be prevented, mitigated, or cured.

In this chapter we make the case that considering cost-effectiveness is a necessary condition for making decisions on global health spending, but on its own, it is not enough. Other moral values similarly need to be factored into a decision-making framework; these include, but are not limited to, fairness, impact on unjust inequalities and systematic disadvantage, and other dimensions of well-being such as respect and self-determination, as well as proximity, financial protection, and the like.

Learning how to factor these other ethical considerations correctly into our decision making is an important and challenging problem. But it is important to recognize that we are failing at one terribly important moral imperative—how to achieve good value with limited resources—at the expense of untold human suffering, and not because we are intentionally forgoing securing more good in the interests of acting virtuously or avoiding violating people's rights.

Challenges Addressed

Some people do not see cost-effectiveness as advancing ethical considerations, perhaps because its empirical methodology makes it appear more like a technical or scientific matter. This is misguided. People who decide how to spend health budgets hold the lives and well-being of many other people in their hands. They are literally making life-or-death decisions. Most decisions of this sort take dramatically insufficient account of cost-effectiveness. As a result, thousands or millions of people die who otherwise would have lived. The few are saved at the expense of the many, without any justification or compelling rationale. It is typically done out of ignorance about the significance of the cost-effectiveness landscape rather than out of prejudice, but the effects are equally serious.

Another reason people might be initially suspicious of using cost-effectiveness to guide prioritization is through confusion with cost-benefit analysis. The latter is an economic method for prioritization that involves determining the benefits for each person by how many dollars they would be willing to pay, adding these up, and then dividing by the total costs in order to produce a benefit-cost ratio in units of dollars. This method is ethically suspect as it considers benefits to wealthy people (or groups) to be worth more than comparable benefits to poorer people (or groups), since the wealthy are willing to pay more for a given benefit.

However, the cost-effectiveness discussed in this chapter is very different, a type of analysis known as cost-effectiveness analysis. This method does not convert benefits into dollars but provides a raw measure of the benefits in units such as DALYs per dollar, or lives saved per dollar. Thus this method is not biased toward interventions favored by the wealthy.

Concern may be an inevitable response to cost-effectiveness since it makes a connection between dollars and health (or even life itself). Making tradeoffs between sacred values such as life and nonsacred values such as money strikes many people as morally problematic. However, no such tradeoff is made in cost-effectiveness analysis. Instead there is a budget constraint of some fixed number of dollars and the cost-effectiveness ratios help to illustrate how much benefit could be produced if this money were spent on a given intervention—for example, saving 1,000 lives or saving 10,000 lives.

Conclusions

Ignoring cost-effectiveness altogether in assessing global health risks means losing much if not most of the value that we could potentially create. For this reason alone the cost-effectiveness of interventions needs to be considered on moral grounds. This does not simply mean implementing current interventions in the most cost-effective way possible, for the improvements to be gained within a single intervention are quite small in comparison. It also does not mean just doing retrospective measures of the cost-effectiveness of the interventions you fund as part of program evaluation. It does mean expanding the domain of interventions under consideration to include all those whose cost-effectiveness has been established and that are currently underfunded. And, above all, it means allocating funds to interventions that correspond to all relevant moral considerations, including, as a core ethical priority, the moral value of producing the good of global health efficiently. Without a commitment to making value for money central to priority setting, we will continue to fail to honor obligations to improve the life prospects of those in need and to act justly.

Notes

1. Fenner et al. (1988).
2. Fenner et al. (1988).
3. Fenner et al. (1988).

2.8

Is Poverty or Wealth at the Root of HIV?

James D. Shelton, Michael M. Cassell, and Jacob Adetunji

POVERTY AND LACK OF ECONOMIC OPPORTUNITY are commonly cited as important contributors to the AIDS epidemic. Indeed an essay in *The Lancet last* year asked whether poverty reduction was the only sustainable solution to preventing AIDS.[1] Thus recent findings from the Tanzania 2003–04 HIV/AIDS indicator survey may come as a surprise.[2] The evidence is just the opposite. This nationally representative survey measured wealth in terms of physical characteristics of the household and household possessions. Household wealth is strongly positively related to HIV prevalence. Indeed the difference in prevalence for women between the lowest and highest wealth quintile is four-fold. These findings are similar to those reported for Kenya[3] last year. Notably, HIV prevalence is highest in some of the most economically advanced countries in Africa (e.g., South Africa, Botswana). A positive relation between wealth and HIV risk has been noted before,[4] but has been upstaged by the focus on poverty.[1]

The poor, especially women, are vulnerable to sexual exploitation. So why this strong relation in the opposite direction? Part of the reason must be that household wealth relates to urban residence, and HIV is higher in urban areas. Also, HIV prevalence is partly a function of survival, and wealthier people with HIV probably survive somewhat longer. On the other hand, people with HIV eventually tend to lose wealth because of loss of employment and increased expenses related to disease, thus blunting a positive relation between wealth and HIV. Perhaps wealth simply enables people and especially men to have more sexual partners. However, in Tanzania neither number of partners nor sex with a prostitute in the past 12 months were related to HIV prevalence in men. Thus none of these explanations appear adequate to explain the observed wealth–HIV relation.

Another explanation seems crucially important—the role of established concurrent sexual partnerships in generalised heterosexual epidemics.[5] According to this idea, serial monogamy and sporadic one-off sexual encounters might not contribute as much to new infections as networks of longer-term concurrent or overlapping partnerships. For example, a person may have a primary relationship, and an additional stable secondary relationship in another town. The primary partner might have no other partner, but the secondary partner might have one or more concurrent partners, and thus link to a larger network. Even though the average number of partners per person may not be especially high, HIV risk is.

Once one person in a network characterised by concurrent partnerships has HIV, everyone becomes at high risk, both because more people are more often exposed to the virus and because recently infected individuals have many-fold higher viral loads and are much more infectious.

Wealth is the key for such networks, because wealth is associated with the mobility, time, and resources to maintain concurrent partnerships. Clearly such relationships might often have a strong economic element, but poverty itself may not be a major factor. Similarly, wealth and social interaction are inextricably linked, and wealth might increase the number of opportunities for partnerships to develop.

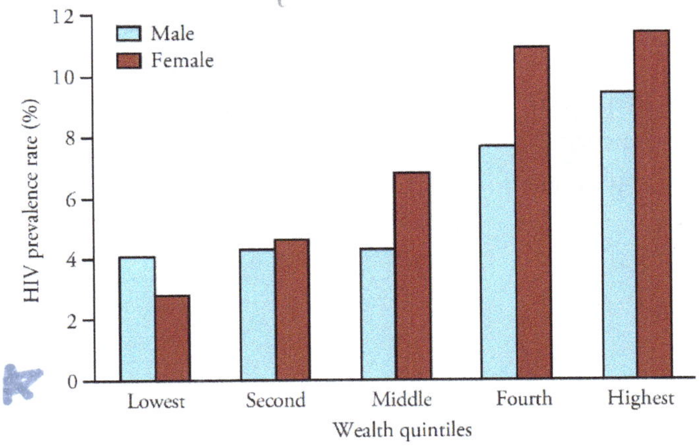

FIGURE 2.8.1 *Sex differences in HIV prevalence rates by wealth quintiles (Tanzania, 2003–04)*

It is interesting that in both Tanzania and Kenya the positive relation between HIV and wealth is if anything stronger for women. We tend to think of men using their economic means to achieve more partners, and better-off wives may be infected by their better-off husbands. But it appears women to some extent also have concurrent relationships.[5] Indeed a concurrent heterosexual network must include both men and women. Perhaps wealth allows for such behaviour in women as well, in part by increasing mobility and social interaction. Or women might improve their economic situation by having more than one concurrent partner. In any case it appears that paradoxically both wealth and economic disadvantage (or at least desire for economic advancement) play pivotal roles in HIV transmission.

What does this relationship mean for HIV programmes? First, it calls for increased attention to the economic dynamic of sexual risk in a wide variety of HIV interventions including behaviour change, condom promotion, voluntary counselling and testing, treatment, and support. But perhaps even more importantly, as described by Halperin and Epstein,[5] it reinforces the importance of promoting social norms to foster fidelity and specifically supporting a franker discussion and understanding of the dangers of having overlapping sexual partnerships.

References

1. Fenton L. Preventing HIV/AIDS through poverty reduction: the only sustainable solution? *Lancet* 2004; **364**: 1186–87.
2. Tanzania Commission for AIDS (TACAIDS), National Bureau of Statistics (NBS), and ORC Macro. Tanzania HIV/AIDS indicator Survey 2003–04. Calverton, Maryland: TACAIDS, NBS and ORC Macro, 2005: http://www.measuredhs.com/pubs/pdftoc.cfm?ID=496 (accessed April 22, 2005).

3. Central Bureau of Statistics (CBS) [Kenya], Ministry of Health (MOH) [Kenya], ORC Macro. 2004. Kenya demographic and health survey 2003. Calverton, Maryland: CBS, MOH, and ORC Macro, 2003: http://www.measuredhs.com/pubs/pdftoc.cfm?ID=462 (accessed April 22, 2005).
4. Halperin D.T., Allen A. Is poverty the root cause of African AIDS? *AIDS Anal Afr* 2000; **11**: 1–15.
5. Halperin D.T., Epstein H. Concurrent sexual partnerships help explain Africa's high HIV prevalence: implications for prevention. *Lancet* 2004; **364**: 4–6.

2.9

Squaring the Circle

AIDS, Poverty, and Human Development

Peter Piot, Robert Greener, and Sarah Russell

IT IS OFTEN ASSERTED THAT AIDS is at the core of a "vicious circle", whereby the impacts of AIDS increase poverty and social deprivation, while poverty and social deprivation increase vulnerability to HIV infection. In examining this view, it is important to distinguish between what might be called the "downstream" effects of AIDS on poverty, and the "upstream" effects of poverty upon the risk of acquiring HIV.

The "Upstream Effects": Poverty and Vulnerability to HIV

Generally speaking, there is a strong association between poverty and ill health—wealthier countries and wealthier individuals enjoy better health as measured by a variety of indicators such as life expectancy or incidence of waterborne diseases. Many researchers have had the same expectation about AIDS, which has often been described as a "disease of poverty" [1].

There is one fundamental difference, however, between AIDS and other health problems generally linked with poverty. Unlike diseases such as tuberculosis and malaria, HIV is mostly transmitted through sex. This brings into play the economic perspective around reward and dependency, which influences the extent to which individuals are able to make and exercise choices about sexual behaviour. Recent evidence clearly indicates that AIDS is a disease of inequality, often associated with economic transition, rather than a disease of poverty in itself.

Undeniably, more people live with HIV in poor countries than in rich ones. More than 60% of people living with HIV inhabit the world's poorest region: sub-Saharan Africa. Nevertheless, studies during the early stage of the epidemic suggested that HIV incidence initially occurred not amongst the poorest, but among better-off members of society in this region. A decade later, infections still appear more concentrated among the urban employed and more mobile members of society, and consequently the more wealthy groups, as can be seen in Table 2.9.1 [2].

It is important to note that HIV prevalence is very high in all of the wealth quintiles—including quintile 1, the poorest (the wealthiest is quintile 5). While there is abundant research that documents the mechanisms that lead from extreme poverty to HIV vulnerability [3], the data now indicate that the less well-studied risk factors among the better-off in fact dominate the aggregate picture. The fact that most people living with HIV in the region today are poor simply reflects the fact that the epidemic has now spread throughout the generalized population in a region that has a high proportion of poor people.

Whether the patterns observed in this part of Africa will also emerge elsewhere remains to be seen. In Asia, for example, epidemics have so far been mostly concentrated in sex workers (and their clients) and drug users, who are often very poor. Infection patterns are now influenced by rapid economic development, which has increased the movement of both men and women in search of opportunities within and across borders. And here, as in Africa, mobility correlates to higher rates of HIV infection.

Many researchers now point not to poverty itself but to economic and gender inequalities and weakened "social cohesion" [4] as factors influencing sexual behaviour and hence the potential for HIV transmission. Some, notably Amartya Sen [5], have looked at poverty as an outcome of poor governance. It has been suggested that, by extension, regimes that do not focus on the well-being of populations impoverish their citizens, deny their enjoyment of basic human rights, and erode public health—exacerbating both the upstream and downstream effects of AIDS. This assertion clearly warrants further research.

One indication of the connection between poor governance and HIV is the clear pattern of association between income inequality as measured by the Gini coefficient and HIV prevalence across countries in sub-Saharan Africa—countries with greater inequality have higher HIV prevalence (Figure 2.9.1—using HIV prevalence and economic data from 2006) [6]. However, some of the countries with the highest inequality and HIV prevalence, such as Botswana, South Africa, and Namibia,

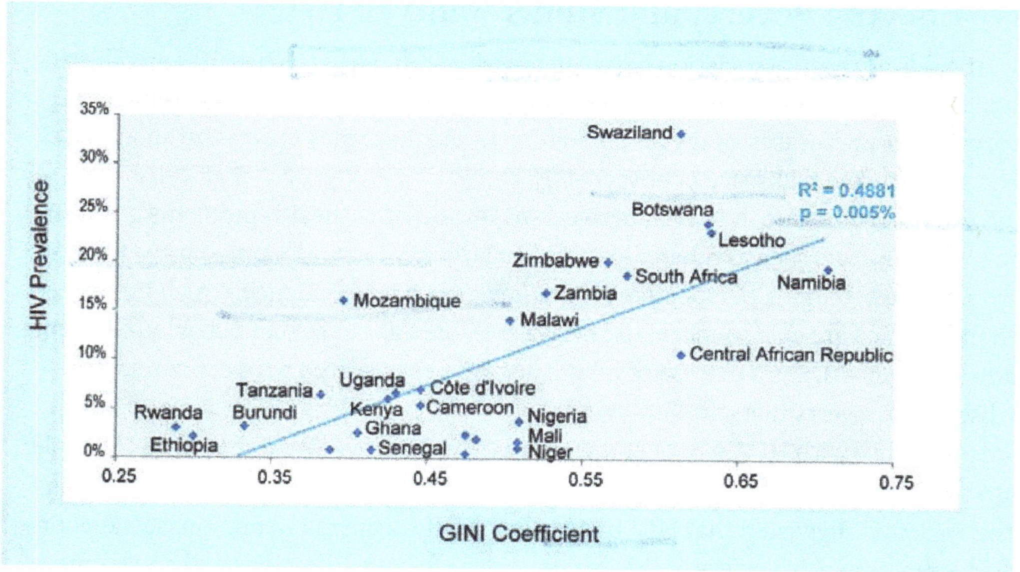

FIGURE 2.9.1 *HIV Prevalence and Income Inequality in Africa*

The GINI coefficient has a value between 0 and 1, representing the extremes of income distribution. A zero value corresponds to the situation where everyone in the population has exactly the same income, whereas a value of 1 would correspond to extreme concentration of income in one person. A high value indicates a more unequal income distribution.

Note that Figure 2.9.1 uses data from only one year and therefore cannot show any dynamic relationship between changes in income inequality (which are slow), and changes in HIV prevalence.

have low levels of domestic corruption as measured by the regional corruption perceptions index published by Transparency International (http://www.transparency.org/policy_research/surveys_indices/cpi), and are regarded as having reasonably good governance. Meanwhile, some countries that have high levels of corruption according to this index, such as Kenya and Côte d'Ivoire, have lower—but still very significant—HIV prevalence, suggesting that inequality is a stronger predictor of HIV prevalence than poor governance. One possible consequence of this apparent association between inequality and HIV is that economic growth that is not pro-poor and that leads to greater income inequality may even fuel the HIV epidemic.

This result also appears to be applicable to gender income inequality—at household level and more generally. Where women's economic and social safety is largely dependent on their partners' occupations and status, they have little choice in determining their own sexual safety [7]. A study in Kenya found that higher gender inequality between young women and adult men is significantly and strongly correlated to positive HIV status (K. Beegle, unpublished data).

Gender inequality is one of many injustices fuelling the epidemic. The spread of HIV is disproportionately high among many groups that experience discrimination and suffer from a lack of human rights protection. This includes groups that have been marginalized socially, culturally, and often economically, such as injection drug users, sex workers, migrants, and men who have sex with men. Women's susceptibility to HIV is further enhanced in members of marginalized or migrant populations: research in Vietnam, for example, revealed that women migrant workers were twice as likely as other women to become HIV positive [8].

The "Downstream Effects": The Impact of AIDS on Poverty and Development

The economic impacts of AIDS are proportionately greater for poor households, and AIDS can be expected to increase both poverty and income inequality. At the same time, AIDS has a significant impact on the aggregate economy of high-prevalence countries.

AIDS kills people in the prime of their working and parenting lives, with a devastating effect on the lives and livelihoods of affected households. Incomes shrink when employed household members become sick or die, and resources are further depleted by medical and funeral-related costs. The impact on poor households is clearly disproportionate, with many struggling to meet demands for treatment and care. (For a comprehensive survey of literature on HIV impacts, see [9].) For example, in India, the financial burden on households living with HIV was 82% of income in the poorest quintile and just over 20% among the richest quintile [10]. The very poor struggle to afford even heavily subsidized antiretroviral treatment. This struggle is particularly acute for women. Although more than half of all adults living with HIV in Zambia are women, when the monthly cost for HIV treatment was reduced from US $64 to US $8 as a result of funding from the Global Fund to Fight AIDS, Tuberculosis and Malaria, many more men than women showed up for treatment. In one rural town, of the 40 adults taking antiretroviral drugs, only three were women. Moreover, even if drugs are free, poor families may have insufficient resources to meet basic nutrition needs or the costs of travel to health clinics for care [11].

We can thus expect AIDS to impede efforts to reduce poverty. In high-prevalence countries such as Botswana, estimates have projected that the number of households living in poverty will increase at a rate that is 0.5% higher per year than if there were no AIDS [12]. A smaller effect can be expected in lower-prevalence countries, but the number of households living in poverty is likely to increase by at least 0.1%–0.5% per year.

The epidemic is dramatically increasing the numbers of orphans, particularly in high-prevalence countries. More than 15 million children worldwide have been orphaned by AIDS—over 12 million of them in sub-Saharan Africa, overwhelming the capacity of social networks and traditional patterns of intergenerational dependency, and creating an uneducated, unsocialized, and often uncared-for generation [4].

Companies in high-prevalence countries can also expect AIDS to decrease productivity and increase costs for recruitment and training, with the magnitude of these effects depending on the employment conditions and benefits offered by the company, the HIV prevalence in the workforce, and the skill levels of the employees most affected. A study in Africa has found widely varying HIV-related costs from 0.5%–10% of the total labour costs—which in some sectors would constitute a very significant proportion of company profit (see the examples in Table 2.9.1 [J. Simon et al., unpublished data]).

TABLE 2.9.1 HIV Prevalence by Wealth Quintile in Eight African Countries (Percentage of Adult Population)

Country	Gender	1	2	3	4	(Wealthiest) 5
Burkina Faso	Men	1.4	2.9	1.3	0.4	2.7
	Women	0.9	1.1	1.5	1.7	3.4
Ghana	Men	1.4	1.5	2.0	1.4	1.1
	Women	1.4	2.7	4.0	3.0	2.4
Cameroon	Men	1.4	2.2	4.7	5.3	5.3
	Women	3.1	4.1	8.1	9.4	8.0
Uganda	Men	4.0	4.2	5.1	5.9	5.5
	Women	4.8	6.6	6.7	7.0	11.0
Kenya	Men	3.4	4.2	2.2	4.3	7.3
	Women	3.9	8.5	7.1	9.7	12.2
Tanzania	Men	4.1	4.3	4.3	7.7	9.5
	Women	2.8	4.7	6.8	10.9	11.4
Malawi	Men	4.4	4.6	12.1	11.7	14.9
	Women	10.9	10.3	12.7	14.6	18.0
Lesotho	Men	18.3	16.8	23.7	21.6	14.8
	Women	19.6	27.9	25.5	27.3	28.9

Government and the public sector are similarly affected by increases in employment costs, but also experience the results of a falling revenue base (to the extent that economic growth is affected), and increased demands for health and other public services related to the epidemic.

At a national level, the macroeconomic impact is expected to be relatively small when compared to that of other factors related to the global economic environment and the quality of economic management in affected countries. Most estimates making use of standard economic models in high-prevalence countries indicate a reduction of about 0.5%–1.5% in the gross domestic product (GDP) growth rate over a 10 to 20-year time frame compared to the situation without AIDS (for a useful summary, see [13]). The impact of tuberculosis—many cases of which are linked to HIV—has been estimated to be $1.4–$2.8 billion per annum, slightly less than half of the AIDS estimates [14], while the impact of malaria has been estimated to be in the same range as AIDS—as much as 1.3% of GDP growth in highly affected countries [15]. This level of impact is significant, therefore, but not catastrophic. Impact in lower-prevalence countries can be expected to be correspondingly lower.

TABLE 2.9.2 HIV-Related Labor Costs

Sector	Country	Number of Workers in Sector	Estimated HIV Prevalence (% of Adult Population)	Cost per AIDS Death or Retirement (Multiple of Annual Compensation)	Aggregate Annual Costs (% of Labor Cost)
Retail	South Africa	500	10.50	0.7	0.50
Agribusiness	South Africa	700	23.70	1.1	0.70
	Uganda	500	5.60	1.9	1.20
	Kenya	22,000	10.00	1.1	1.00
	Zambia	1,200	28.50	0.9	1.30
	South Africa	1,300	14.00	1.2	1.10
	Uganda	300	14.40	1.2	1.90
	Ethiopia	1,500	5.30	0.9	0.60
	Ethiopia	1,500	6.20	1.8	0.60
Media	South Africa	3,600	10.20	1.3	1.30
Utility	South Africa	>25,000	11.70	4.7	2.20
Mining	South Africa	600	23.60	1.4	2.40
	Botswana	500	29.00	4.4	8.40
Tourism	Zambia	350	36.80	3.6	10.80

Some researchers have drawn attention to the longer term potential for progressive weakening of human capital, and the lost transmission of knowledge and skills between generations. This is of particular concern given the increasing recognition that AIDS is a long-term phenomenon for which long-term strategies are required.

long term AIDS impact → weaken human capital
lose knowledge/skills between generation

Responding to the Interactions between AIDS and Poverty

Understanding both upstream and downstream interactions between AIDS and poverty is critical to understanding local and global epidemiological trends and patterns. Such an understanding is, in turn, vital to the development and implementation of effective strategies to prevent and treat HIV.

Growing awareness of the economic aspects of the epidemic has helped catalyze greater political action on AIDS in recent years. For example, AIDS is the only health issue ever to become the subject of a United Nations Security Council debate or a Special Session of the UN General Assembly. It has been featured regularly at G8 meetings and regional summits in Africa, the Caribbean, and elsewhere. In more than 40 countries, National AIDS Programmes are led by the President, Vice-President, or Prime Minister.

Political action has fuelled financial investment. Global expenditure on AIDS in low- and middle-income countries increased from $250 million in 1996 to an expected $10 billion in 2007.

We are now beginning to see a return on this investment. Fewer people are becoming infected with HIV in almost all East African countries, in the Caribbean, in Cambodia, and in southern India. Almost 2.5 million people are now on antiretroviral therapy in developing countries—up from 100,000 five years ago. To build on this progress and ensure that it is sustainable, however, six elements are key.

First, AIDS money has the most impact when strategies are based on the concept of "know and act on your epidemic". UNAIDS' *Practical Guidelines for Intensifying HIV Prevention* [16] provide practical guidance to tailor national HIV prevention responses so that they respond to the epidemic dynamics and social context of the country and reach populations who remain most vulnerable to HIV infection. For example, economic growth and the growth of trade between neighbouring countries can be expected to lead to increased mobility, particularly of transport workers, which is known to increase vulnerability to HIV in the absence of tailored prevention efforts. In parts of Asia, mobile men who have unprotected sex with sex workers are a key factor in spreading HIV [17].

Second, a growing number of small-scale activities indicate the value of combining HIV programmes with poverty reduction initiatives. In Malawi, non-governmental organizations integrate HIV prevention into village banking programmes for women, and combine AIDS education with the provision of microfinance to groups of women through community banking programmes [18]. In Northern Thailand, the Population and Community Development Association's Positive Partnership Project offers loans to partnerships consisting of a person living with HIV and a "buddy" (often a friend or family member who is not living with HIV) to set up small business ventures [19]. The challenge now, however, is to make the shift from small-scale projects to large-scale programmes.

Third, the provision of HIV treatment can help prevent poverty—and indirectly contribute to HIV prevention as well—by helping to break down stigma. A study in Kenya observed a rapid improvement in labour productivity among tea pickers in 12 months after starting antiretroviral treatment [20]. Such findings highlight the economic importance of ensuring that the poor have access to HIV treatment and prevention services. This access requires action in four key areas: increased investment in antiretroviral treatment—by both national and international funders; a reduction in the cost of antiretroviral drugs; improved HIV service delivery systems; and better services for the poor.

Fourth, development plans (whether they concern the development of productive sectors or the provision of social safety nets) must "pass the AIDS test". Development initiatives must contribute to AIDS prevention and treatment in the communities they work in. The World Bank–supported Chad/Cameroon Pipeline Project, for example, supports HIV workplace interventions along the pipeline route—both for workers and for affected communities [21]. Social protection programmes must also include specific measures to address the economic and social needs of households that are directly affected by AIDS.

Fifth, both poverty reduction programmes and AIDS strategies must reduce vulnerability to HIV—particularly for women and young people. Doing so involves protecting human rights and tackling issues around social marginalization and stigma. The link between poverty, gender inequality, and HIV has prompted many institutions to talk about integrating gender and AIDS into development and poverty reduction strategies, but far more action is required [22]. One obvious step is to ensure that domestic legislation is consistent with international human rights norms, and that it is effective in protecting women's rights within marriage, securing their right to own and inherit property, ensuring equality in the workplace, and strengthening laws against domestic violence.

Sixth, addressing AIDS in the world's poorest countries and communities depends on increased and sustained international support, driven by high-level political will. Although it is ultimately the responsibility of all states to provide HIV prevention and treatment for all citizens, and to mitigate the impact of AIDS on the poor, many countries require international support to live up to these responsibilities, and are likely to do so for some time to come. Failure by donors to prioritise the provision of such support is likely to undermine the effectiveness of current and future efforts, and could also lead to the unravelling of progress already made.

Conclusion

AIDS, it has been said, is exceptional [23] in terms of its threat to humanity, and its complexity. The relationship between AIDS and poverty is just one example of that complexity, having more to do with inequality than poverty per se.

Another example of complexity is that the relationship between socioeconomic status and HIV varies considerably from country to country, reflecting differences in culture and traditions. Effective actions to tackle AIDS must directly address these specific factors—the inequalities—that drive HIV transmission in different contexts, and must overcome the obstacles to accessing treatment in different groups. [6].

Complex problems famously require complex solutions. In this case, it is crucial to place AIDS squarely at the centre of all socio-economic development, and provide long-term, high-level domestic and international investment in HIV prevention and treatment in the world's poorest countries.

References

1. afrol News (2002 October 4) WHO calls HIV/ AIDS 'Disease of Poverty.' Available: http://www.afrol.com/Categories/Health/health026_aids_poverty.htm. Accessed 19 September 2007.
2. Mishra V, Bignami-Van Assche S, Greener R, Vaessen M, Hong R, et al. (2007) HIV infection does not disproportionately affect the poorer in sub-Saharan Africa. AIDS (supplement). In press.

3. Kalichman SC, Simbayi LC, Kagee A, Toefy Y, Cain D, et al. (2006) Association of poverty, substance use, and HIV transmission risk behaviors in three South African communities. Soc Sci Med 62: 1641–1649.
4. Barnett T, Whiteside A (2006) AIDS in the twenty-first century: Disease and globalization. 2nd edition. New York: Palgrave Macmillan. 416 p.
5. Sen A (2000) Development as freedom. New York: Oxford University Press.
6. Gillespie S, Kadiyala S, Greener R (2007) Is poverty or wealth driving HIV transmission? AIDS (supplement). In press.
7. Go VF, Sethulakshmi CJ, Bentley ME, Sivaram S, Srikrishnan AK, et al. (2003) When HIV-prevention messages and gender norms clash: The impact of domestic violence on women's HIV risk in slums of Chennai, India. AIDS Behav 7: 263–272.
8. Asian Development Bank (2005) Gender Network News. Special issue: Perspectives on gender and HIV/AIDS. Available: http://www.adb.org/Documents/Periodicals/GNN/newsletter-13.pdf. Accessed 19 September 2007.
9. Gillespie S, Kadiyala S (2005) HIV/AIDS and food and nutrition security: From evidence to action. International Food Policy Research Institute. Available: http://www.ifpri.org/pubs/fpreview/pv07/pv07.pdf. Accessed 19 September 2007.
10. Asian Development Bank, UNAIDS (2004) The impact of HIV/AIDS on poverty in Cambodia, India, Thailand, and Vietnam. Available: http://www.adb.org/Documents/Reports/Asia-Pacific/APO-HIV.pdf. Accessed 19 September 2007.
11. UNAIDS, United Nations Population Fund, United Nations Development Fund for Women (2004) Women and HIV/AIDS: Confronting the crisis. Available: http://www.unfpa.org/hiv/women/. Accessed 19 September 2007.
12. Greener R (2004) Chapter 5: The macroeconomics of HIV/AIDS. In: Haacker M, editor. The impact of HIV/AIDS on poverty and inequality. International Monetary Fund. Available: http://www.imf.org/external/ pubs/ft/AIDS/eng/index.htm. Accessed 19 September 2007.
13. Haacker M (2004) Chapter 2: HIV/AIDS: The impact on the social fabric and the economy. In: Haacker M, editor. The impact of HIV/ AIDS on poverty and inequality. International Monetary Fund. Available: http://www.imf.org/external/pubs/ft/AIDS/eng/index.htm. Accessed 19 September 2007.
14. Grimard F, Harling G (2004) The impact of tuberculosis on economic growth. Department of Economics, McGill University. Available: http://neumann.hec.ca/neudc2004/fp/grimard_franque_aout_27.pdf. Accessed 19 September 2007.
15. Gallup JL, Sachs JD (2001) The economic burden of malaria. Am J Trop Med Hyg 64S: 85–96.
16. UNAIDS (2006) Practical guidelines for intensifying HIV prevention: Towards universal access. Available: http://data.unaids.org/pub/Manual/2007/20070306_Prevention_Guidelines_Towards_Universal_Access_en.pdf. Accessed 19 September 2007.
17. Rao P (2007) Plenary speech at VIII International Congress on AIDS in Asia and the Pacific (ICAAP), Colombo. Available: http://www.unaids.org/en/MediaCentre/PressMaterials/FeatureStory/20070820_ICAAP2007.asp. Accessed 19 September 2007.
18. Global Coalition on Women and AIDS (2006) Economic security for women fights AIDS. Available: http://data.unaids.org/pub/BriefingNote/2006/20060308_BN_GCWA_en.pdf. Accessed 19 September 2007.
19. Population and Community Development Association (2007) Available: http://www.pda.or.th/eng/. Accessed 19 September 2007.

20. Simon J, Larson B, Fox M, Rosen S, Bii M,et al. (2007) Early effects of antiretroviral therapy on work performance: Results from a cohort study of Kenyan agricultural workers. Center for International Health and Development, Boston University School of Public Health. Available: http://www.hivimplementers.org/agenda/pdf/E1/E1%20Simon%20abstract%20811.ppt.pdf. Accessed 26 September 2007.
21. Zewdie D (2000) The World Bank perspective on AIDS. 13th International AIDS Conference; 11 July 2000; Durban, South Africa. Available: http://lnweb18.worldbank.org/AFR/afr.nsf/General/F0986E1B4CD360608525691A004B69CC?OpenDocument. Accessed 19 September 2007.
22. Smith MK (2002) Gender, poverty and intergenerational vulnerability to HIV/AIDS. Available: http://www.oxfam.org.nz/imgs/whatwedo/hivaids/gendervuln.pdf. Accessed 19 September 2007.
23. Piot P (2005) Why AIDS is exceptional. Speech at the London School of Economics. Available: http://www.lse.ac.uk/collections/pressAndInformationOffice/newsAndEvents/archives/2005/Peter_Piot.htm. Accessed 19 September 2007.

Section III

United States

3.1

The HIV/AIDS Epidemic in the United States

The Basics

Kaiser Family Foundation

Key Facts

- The first cases of what would later become known as AIDS were reported in the United States in June of 1981.[1] Today, there are more than 1.1 million people living with HIV and more than 700,000 people with AIDS have died since the beginning of the epidemic.[2,3,4]
- HIV continues to have a disproportionate impact on certain populations, particularly racial and ethnic minorities and gay and bisexual men and other men who have sex with men.[5,6]
- HIV testing is important for both treatment and prevention efforts. Yet, 15% of those infected with HIV are unaware they are infected.[7]
- Antiretroviral therapy (ART) has substantially reduced AIDS-related morbidity and mortality and improved long-term outcomes for people with HIV. Treatment guidelines recommend initiating treatment as soon as one is diagnosed with HIV.[8] According to the U.S. Centers for Disease Control and Prevention (CDC), when an individual living with HIV is on antiretroviral therapy and the level of HIV in their body is undetectable, there is "effectively no risk" of sexual transmission.[9] Still, many people with HIV are not in care, on treatment, or have their virus under control.[10]
- Numerous federal and local government departments and agencies are involved in the domestic HIV/AIDS response, which together provide disease surveillance, prevention, care, support services, and health insurance coverage. Additionally, the private sector and community-based organizations, provide services for people with HIV and those at risk for HIV.

Box 3.1.1: Key Snapshot of the U.S. Epidemic Today

- Number of new HIV infections: **38,500**
- Number of people living with HIV: **1.1+ million**
- Percent of people infected with HIV who don't know it: **15%**
- Percent of people with HIV who are virally suppressed: **51%**

Know

Overview

- As people are living longer with the disease, new infections continue to occur, and diagnoses surpass deaths each year, more people are living with HIV than ever before.[11,12]
- There have been some promising trends, as the number of new HIV infections declined 8% between 2010 and 2015. Still, 38,500 people were newly infected with HIV in the U.S. in 2015, and infections have increased among some populations.[13]
- HIV-related mortality rates, which rose steadily through the 1980s and peaked in 1995, have declined significantly; the age-adjusted HIV death rate has dropped by more than 80% since its peak.[14] This is largely due to ART, but also to decreasing HIV incidence after the 1980s. Still, more 6,000 people died of HIV/AIDS in 2016.[15] While HIV is not a leading cause of death for Americans overall, it remains a leading cause of death for certain age groups –in 2016, HIV was the 9th leading cause of death for those ages 25–34, and for those ages 35–44.[16]
- HIV transmission patterns have shifted over time. In 2017, most newly diagnosed cases of HIV occurred through male-to-male sexual contact (66%).[17] An additional 3% of diagnoses occurred among gay and bisexual men with a history of injection drug use.[18] Diagnoses attributable to injection drug use alone have declined significantly over time and accounted for 6% of new diagnoses in 2017.[19,20] Transmission through heterosexual sex now accounts for more cases than at the beginning of the epidemic—24% of new diagnoses in 2017—but diagnoses attributable to heterosexual sex have declined 16% between 2012 and 2017.[21,22]
- HIV testing is important for both treatment and prevention efforts and rapid testing is now much more widely available. Yet, as of 2016 15% of those infected with HIV are unaware they are infected, and 38% of infections resulted from individuals who did not know they had HIV.[23] Knowledge of HIV status is important because individuals with HIV can engage in care and treatment to achieve optimal health outcomes and can take steps to prevent transmission. Routine HIV testing is recommended for all people ages 13–64,[24] and several recent policies have expanded health insurance coverage of HIV testing.[25]
- Current U.S. HIV treatment guidelines recommend initiating ART as soon as one is diagnosed with HIV,[26] and new research (including the Strategic Timing of Antiretroviral Treatment study or START) has underscored the importance of starting treatment early.[27] Engaging in treatment early and consistently affords individuals with HIV the best possible care outcomes.
- Further, recent research has confirmed the preventive benefits of treatment; when an individual with HIV is consistently engaged with antiretroviral therapy and the level of HIV in their body is undetectable, there is effectively no risk of sexual transmission.[28]
- However, looking across the spectrum from HIV diagnosis to viral suppression reveals missed opportunities for addressing the epidemic. According to the Centers for Disease Control and Prevention (CDC), while many people with HIV are diagnosed (86%), far fewer receive medical care (63%), and fewer still are virally suppressed (51%).[29] Viral suppression is greater among those who are in medical care.[30]

Impact Across the Country

- Although HIV has been reported in all 50 states, the District of Columbia, and U.S. dependencies, the impact of the epidemic is not uniformly distributed.
- Ten states accounted for about two-thirds (64%) of HIV diagnoses among adults and adolescents in 2017 (Table 3.1.1). Regionally, the South accounted for about half of HIV diagnoses in 2017.[31]
- Rates of HIV diagnoses per 100,000 provide a different measure of the epidemic's impact, since they reflect the concentration of diagnoses after accounting for differences in population size across states. The District of Columbia has the highest rate in the nation, compared to states, nearly 4 times the national rate (Table 3.1.1).[32,33] Eight of the top 10 states by rate are in the South.[34,35]
- New HIV diagnoses are concentrated primarily in large U.S. metropolitan areas (80% in 2017), with Miami, Orlando, and Atlanta topping the list of the areas most heavily burdened.[36]

Impact on Racial and Ethnic Minorities

- Racial and ethnic minorities have been disproportionately affected by HIV/AIDS since the beginning of the epidemic, and represent the majority of new HIV diagnoses, people living with HIV disease, and deaths among people with HIV.[37,38]

TABLE 3.1.1 Top Ten States/Areas by Number and Rate of New HIV Diagnoses (Adults and Adolescents), 2017

State	New HIV Diagnoses, Number (%)	State/Area	New HIV Diagnoses, per 100,000
Florida	4,800 (12%)	District of Columbia	46.3
California	4,500 (12%)	Georgia	24.9
Texas	4,364 (11%)	Florida	22.9
New York	2,772 (7%)	Louisiana	22.1
Georgia	2,595 (7%)	Maryland	17.0
North Carolina	1,315 (3%)	Nevada	16.5
Illinois	1,265 (3%)	Texas	15.4
New Jersey	1,109 (3%)	Mississippi	14.3
Pennsylvania	1,094 (3%)	South Carolina	14.3
Louisiana	1,033 (3%)	New York	14.0
Subtotal	**27,847 (72%)**	—	—
U.S. Total	**38,739 (100%)**	**U.S. Rate**	**11.8**

Notes: Mississippi's new HIV diagnosis rate for 2017 was 14.34, and South Carolina's new HIV diagnosis rate for 2017 was 14.29. Table includes data on HIV diagnoses among adults and adolescents and reflects data from U.S. dependent areas.

Source: CDC. *HIV Surveillance Report, Diagnoses of HIV Infection in the United States and Dependent Areas, 2017*, Vol. 29; November 2018. HIV diagnosis data are estimates from 50 states, the District of Columbia, and 6 U.S. dependent areas. Estimates for 2017 are preliminary and are not included in trend calculations.

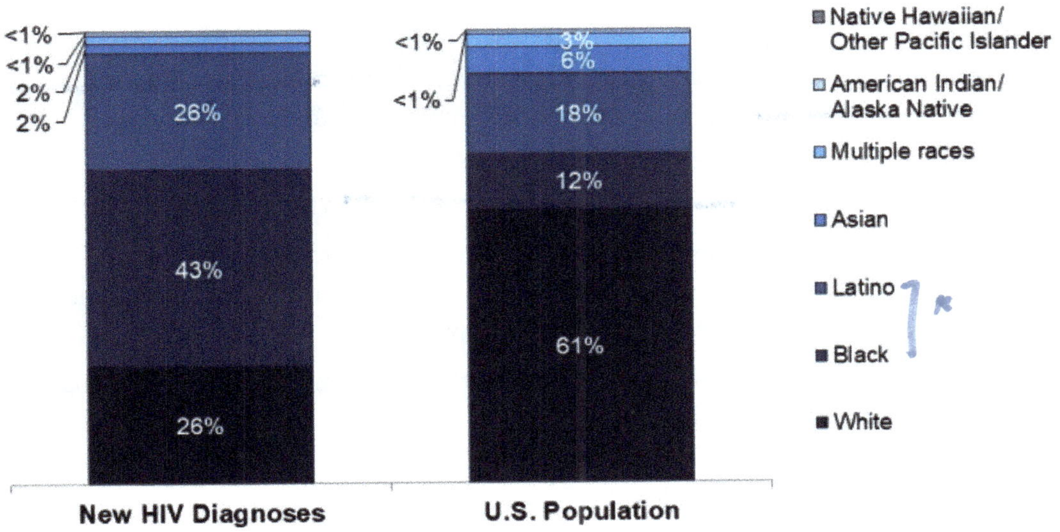

SOURCES: CDC. *HIV Surveillance Report, Diagnoses of HIV Infection in the United States and Dependent Areas, 2017*, Vol. 29; November 2018. HIV diagnosis data are preliminary estimates from 50 states, the District of Columbia, and 6 U.S. dependent areas. KFF. State Health Facts; accessed January 2019.

FIGURE 3.1.1 New HIV Diagnoses & U.S. Population, by Race/Ethnicity, 2017

- Blacks and Latinos account for a disproportionate share of new HIV diagnoses, relative to their size in the U.S. population (see Figure 3.1.1).[39,40] Blacks also account for more people living with HIV than any other racial group—an estimated 468,800 of the more than 1.1 million people living with HIV in the U.S. are black.[41]
- Blacks also have the highest rate of new HIV diagnoses, followed by Latinos –in 2017, the rate of new HIV diagnoses per 100,000 for Blacks (41.1) was about 8 times that of whites (5.1); Latinos (16.1) had a rate 3 times that of whites.[42]
- Blacks accounted for close to half (43%) of deaths among people with an HIV diagnosis in 2016.[43]
- Survival after an AIDS diagnosis is lower for Blacks than for most other racial/ethnic groups, and Blacks have had the highest age-adjusted death rate due to HIV disease throughout most of the epidemic.[44,45] HIV ranks higher as a cause of death for Blacks and Latinos, compared with whites[46] Further, HIV was the 5th leading cause of death for Black women ages 35–44 in 2016.[47]

Impact on Women

- More than 256,500 women are living with HIV in the U.S.[48]
- Between 2010 and 2015, HIV incidence among women decreased 21%.[49]
- Women of color are particularly affected, and in 2017, Black women accounted for 6 in 10 (59%) of new HIV diagnoses among women; white women accounted for 20% and Latinas accounted for 16%.[50]

Impact on Young People

- Teens and young adults continue to be at risk, with those under 35 accounting for 56% of new HIV diagnoses in 2017 (those ages 13–24 accounted for 21% and those ages 25–34 accounted for 35%). Most young people are infected sexually.[52]
- Among young people, gay and bisexual men and minorities have been particularly affected.[53]
- Perinatal HIV transmission, from an HIV-infected mother to her baby, has declined significantly in the U.S., largely due to increased testing efforts among pregnant women and ART which can prevent mother-to-child transmission.[54,55,56]
- A recent survey of young adults (18–30) found that HIV remains a concern for young people, especially for young people of color.[57]

Impact on Gay and Bisexual Men

- While estimates show that gay and bisexual men comprise only about 2% of the U.S. population,[58] male-to-male sexual contact accounts for most new HIV infections (68% in 2015, with an additional 3% occurring in gay and bisexual men with a history of injection drug use) and most people living with HIV (56% in 2015, with an additional 5% occurring in gay and bisexual men with a history of injection drug use).[59,60,61]
- Annual new infections among gay and bisexual men overall and among Black gay and bisexual men have remained stable in recent years. However, there have been increases among certain groups of gay and bisexual men, including Latinos and young males 25–34.[62]
- Blacks accounted for the largest number of new diagnoses (10,069) among gay and bisexual men in 2017, followed by whites (7,607).[63] Additionally, according to a recent study, Black gay and bisexual men were found to be at a much higher risk of being diagnosed with HIV during their lifetimes compared with Latino and white gay and bisexual men.[64] Young Black gay and bisexual men are at particular risk –Black gay and bisexual men ages 20–29 accounted for 52% of new diagnoses.[65]
- A study in 20 major U.S. cities found that about 1 in 5 (22%) men who have sex with men is living with HIV, and, of those, 1 in 4 are unaware of their infection.[66] Prevalence among Blacks was higher (36%) and awareness of infection was lower (67%), compared with men who have sex with men in the study overall.[67]

[...]

Endnotes

1. CDC. *MMWR*, Vol. 30, No. 21; June 1981.
2. CDC. Supplemental Surveillance Report. Estimated HIV Incidence and Prevalence in the United States 2010–2015 (https://www.cdc.gov/hiv/pdf/library/reports/surveillance/cdc-hivsurveillance-supplemental-report-vol-23-1.pdf). Vol 23. No. 1. 2018.
3. CDC. *HIV Surveillance Report,* Diagnoses of HIV Infection in the United States and Dependent Areas, 2017 (https://www.cdc.gov/hiv/pdf/library/reports/surveillance/cdc-hivsurveillance-report-2017-vol-29.pdf),

Vol. 29; November 2018. HIV diagnosis data are estimates from 50 states, the District of Columbia, and 6 U.S. dependent areas. Estimates for 2017 are preliminary and are not included in trend calculations.
4. CDC. *HIV Surveillance Supplemental Report,* Monitoring Selected National HIV Prevention and Care Objectives by Using HIV Surveillance Data (https://www.cdc.gov/hiv/pdf/library/reports/surveillance/cdc-hiv-surveillance-supplemental-reportvol-23-4.pdf), Vol. 23, No. 4; June 2018.
5. CDC. *HIV Surveillance Report,* Diagnoses of HIV Infection in the United States and Dependent Areas, 2017 (https://www.cdc.gov/hiv/pdf/library/reports/surveillance/cdc-hivsurveillance-report-2017-vol-29.pdf), Vol. 29; November 2018. HIV diagnosis data are estimates from 50 states, the District of Columbia, and 6 U.S. dependent areas. Estimates for 2017 are preliminary and are not included in trend calculations.
6. CDC. *HIV Surveillance Supplemental Report,* Monitoring Selected National HIV Prevention and Care Objectives by Using HIV Surveillance Data (https://www.cdc.gov/hiv/pdf/library/reports/surveillance/cdc-hiv-surveillance-supplemental-reportvol-23-4.pdf), Vol. 23, No. 4; June 2018.
7. CDC. Supplemental Surveillance Report. Estimated HIV Incidence and Prevalence in the United States 2010–2015 (https://www.cdc.gov/hiv/pdf/library/reports/surveillance/cdc-hivsurveillance-supplemental-report-vol-23-1.pdf). Vol 23. No. 1. 2018.
8. DHHS. Guidelines for the Use of Antiretroviral Agents in Adults and Adolescents Living with HIV (https://aidsinfo.nih.gov/guidelines/html/1/adult-and-adolescent-treatmentguidelines/0); updated October 2018.
9. CDC. HIV Treatment as Prevention (http://www.cdc.gov/hiv/research/biomedicalresearch/tap/index.html); updated November 2018.
10. CDC. *HIV Surveillance Supplemental Report,* Monitoring Selected National HIV Prevention and Care Objectives by Using HIV Surveillance Data (https://www.cdc.gov/hiv/pdf/library/reports/surveillance/cdc-hiv-surveillance-supplemental-reportvol-23-4.pdf), Vol. 23, No. 4; June 2018.
11. CDC. *HIV Surveillance Supplemental Report,* Monitoring Selected National HIV Prevention and Care Objectives by Using HIV Surveillance Data (https://www.cdc.gov/hiv/pdf/library/reports/surveillance/cdc-hiv-surveillance-supplemental-reportvol-23-4.pdf), Vol. 23, No. 4; June 2018.
12. CDC. *HIV Surveillance Report,* Diagnoses of HIV Infection in the United States and Dependent Areas, 2017 (https://www.cdc.gov/hiv/pdf/library/reports/surveillance/cdc-hivsurveillance-report-2017-vol-29.pdf), Vol. 29; November 2018. HIV diagnosis data are estimates from 50 states, the District of Columbia, and 6 U.S. dependent areas. Estimates for 2017 are preliminary and are not included in trend calculations.
13. CDC. Supplemental Surveillance Report. Estimated HIV Incidence and Prevalence in the United States 2010–2015 (https://www.cdc.gov/hiv/pdf/library/reports/surveillance/cdc-hivsurveillance-supplemental-report-vol-23-1.pdf). Vol 23. No. 1. 2018.
14. CDC. NCHS. Health, United States, 2017 (http://www.cdc.gov/nchs/hus/); September 2018.
15. CDC. NCHS. Deaths: Leading Causes for 2016 (http://www.cdc.gov/nchs/nvss/deaths.htm); November 2018.
16. CDC. NCHS. Deaths: Leading Causes for 2016 (http://www.cdc.gov/nchs/nvss/deaths.htm); November 2018.
17. CDC. *HIV Surveillance Report,* Diagnoses of HIV Infection in the United States and Dependent Areas, 2017 (https://www.cdc.gov/hiv/pdf/library/reports/surveillance/cdc-hivsurveillance-report-2017-vol-29.pdf), Vol. 29; November 2018. HIV diagnosis data are estimates from 50 states, the District of Columbia, and 6 U.S. dependent areas. Estimates for 2017 are preliminary and are not included in trend calculations.

18. CDC. *HIV Surveillance Report,* Diagnoses of HIV Infection in the United States and Dependent Areas, 2017 (https://www.cdc.gov/hiv/pdf/library/reports/surveillance/cdc-hivsurveillance-report-2017-vol-29.pdf), Vol. 29; November 2018. HIV diagnosis data are estimates from 50 states, the District of Columbia, and 6 U.S. dependent areas. Estimates for 2017 are preliminary and are not included in trend calculations.
19. CDC. HIV Surveillance—Epidemiology of HIV Infection (through 2017) (https://www.cdc.gov/hiv/library/slideSets/index.html); November 2018.
20. CDC. *HIV Surveillance Report,* Diagnoses of HIV Infection in the United States and Dependent Areas, 2017 (https://www.cdc.gov/hiv/pdf/library/reports/surveillance/cdc-hivsurveillance-report-2017-vol-29.pdf), Vol. 29; November 2018. HIV diagnosis data are estimates from 50 states, the District of Columbia, and 6 U.S. dependent areas. Estimates for 2017 are preliminary and are not included in trend calculations.
21. CDC. HIV Surveillance—Epidemiology of HIV Infection (through 2017) (https://www.cdc.gov/hiv/library/slideSets/index.html); November 2018.
22. CDC. *HIV Surveillance Report,* Diagnoses of HIV Infection in the United States and Dependent Areas, 2017 (https://www.cdc.gov/hiv/pdf/library/reports/surveillance/cdc-hivsurveillance-report-2017-vol-29.pdf), Vol. 29; November 2018. HIV diagnosis data are estimates from 50 states, the District of Columbia, and 6 U.S. dependent areas. Estimates for 2017 are preliminary and are not included in trend calculations.
23. CDC. *MMWR,* Vol. 68, No. 11; March 2019.
24. CDC. *MMWR,* Vol. 55, No. RR14; September 2006.
25. KFF. HIV Testing in the United States (https://www.k.org/hivaids/fact-sheet/hiv-testing-in-theunited-states/); June 2018.
26. DHHS. Guidelines for the Use of Antiretroviral Agents in HIV-1-Infected Adults and Adolescents (https://aidsinfo.nih.gov/guidelines/html/1/adult-and-adolescent-treatmentguidelines/0); updated October 2018.
27. AIDS*info,* Statement by the HHS Panel on Antiretroviral Guidelines for Adults and Adolescents Regarding Results from the START and TEMPRANO Trials (https://aidsinfo.nih.gov/news/1592/statement-from-adult-arv-guideline-panel---start-and-tempranotrials); July 2015.
28. CDC. HIV Treatment as Prevention (http://www.cdc.gov/hiv/research/biomedicalresearch/tap/index.html); updated November 2018.
29. CDC. Supplemental Surveillance Report. Estimated HIV Incidence and Prevalence in the United States 2010–2015 (https://www.cdc.gov/hiv/pdf/library/reports/surveillance/cdc-hivsurveillance-supplemental-report-vol-23-1.pdf). Vol 23. No. 1. 2018.; CDC. Selected National HIV Prevention and Care Outcomes (2015, 2016) (https://www.cdc.gov/hiv/library/slidesets/index.html).
30. Bradley H et al. Increased HIV viral suppression among US adults receiving medical care, 2009–2013 (http://www.croiconference.org/sessions/increased-hiv-viral-suppression-amongus-adults-receiving-medical-care-2009-2013), Conference on Retroviruses and Opportunistic Infections (CROI), Boston, abstract 53; 2016.
31. CDC. *HIV Surveillance Report,* Diagnoses of HIV Infection in the United States and Dependent Areas, 2017 (https://www.cdc.gov/hiv/pdf/library/reports/surveillance/cdc-hivsurveillance-report-2017-vol-29.pdf), Vol. 29; November 2018. HIV diagnosis data are estimates from 50 states, the District of Columbia, and 6 U.S. dependent areas. Estimates for 2017 are preliminary and are not included in trend calculations.
32. CDC. Atlas Plus. See: https://gis.cdc.gov/grasp/nchhstpatlas/main.html CDC. *HIV Surveillance Report,* Diagnoses of HIV Infection in the United States and Dependent Areas, 2017 (https://www.cdc.gov/hiv/pdf/library/reports/surveillance/cdc-hiv-surveillance-report-2017-vol-29.pdf), Vol. 29; November 2018.

HIV diagnosis data are estimates from 50 states, the District of Columbia, and 6 U.S. dependent areas. Estimates for 2017 are preliminary and are not included in trend calculations.
33. U.S. Census Bureau. Quick Facts: 2017 Population Estimates (https://www.census.gov/quickfacts/fact/table/US/PST045218). July 2017.
34. CDC. Atlas Plus. See: https://gis.cdc.gov/grasp/nchhstpatlas/main.html . CDC. *HIV Surveillance Report,* Diagnoses of HIV Infection in the United States and Dependent Areas, 2017 (https://www.cdc.gov/hiv/pdf/library/reports/surveillance/cdc-hiv-surveillance-report-2017-vol-29.pdf), Vol. 29; November 2018. HIV diagnosis data are estimates from 50 states, the District of Columbia, and 6 U.S. dependent areas. Estimates for 2017 are preliminary and are not included in trend calculations.
35. U.S. Census Bureau. Quick Facts: 2017 Population Estimates (https://www.census.gov/quickfacts/fact/table/US/PST045218). July 2017.
36. CDC. *HIV Surveillance Report,* Diagnoses of HIV Infection in the United States and Dependent Areas, 2017 (https://www.cdc.gov/hiv/pdf/library/reports/surveillance/cdc-hivsurveillance-report-2017-vol-29.pdf), Vol. 29; November 2018. HIV diagnosis data are estimates from 50 states, the District of Columbia, and 6 U.S. dependent areas. Estimates for 2017 are preliminary and are not included in trend calculations.
37. CDC. *HIV Surveillance Report,* Diagnoses of HIV Infection in the United States and Dependent Areas, 2017 (https://www.cdc.gov/hiv/pdf/library/reports/surveillance/cdc-hivsurveillance-report-2017-vol-29.pdf), Vol. 29; November 2018. HIV diagnosis data are estimates from 50 states, the District of Columbia, and 6 U.S. dependent areas. Estimates for 2017 are preliminary and are not included in trend calculations.
38. CDC. *HIV Surveillance Supplemental Report,* Monitoring Selected National HIV Prevention and Care Objectives by Using HIV Surveillance Data (https://www.cdc.gov/hiv/pdf/library/reports/surveillance/cdc-hiv-surveillance-supplemental-report-vol-23-4.pdf), Vol. 23, No. 4; June 2018.
39. CDC. *HIV Surveillance Report,* Diagnoses of HIV Infection in the United States and Dependent Areas, 2017 (https://www.cdc.gov/hiv/pdf/library/reports/surveillance/cdc-hivsurveillance-report-2017-vol-29.pdf), Vol. 29; November 2018. HIV diagnosis data are estimates from 50 states, the District of Columbia, and 6 U.S. dependent areas. Estimates for 2017 are preliminary and are not included in trend calculations.
40. KFF. State Health Facts; accessed December 2018.
41. CDC. Supplemental Surveillance Report. Estimated HIV Incidence and Prevalence in the United States 2010–2015 (https://www.cdc.gov/hiv/pdf/library/reports/surveillance/cdc-hivsurveillance-supplemental-report-vol-23-1.pdf). Vol 23. No. 1. 2018.
42. CDC. *HIV Surveillance Report,* Diagnoses of HIV Infection in the United States and Dependent Areas, 2017 (https://www.cdc.gov/hiv/pdf/library/reports/surveillance/cdc-hivsurveillance-report-2017-vol-29.pdf), Vol. 29; November 2018. HIV diagnosis data are estimates from 50 states, the District of Columbia, and 6 U.S. dependent areas. Estimates for 2017 are preliminary and are not included in trend calculations.
43. CDC. *HIV Surveillance Report,* Diagnoses of HIV Infection in the United States and Dependent Areas, 2017 (https://www.cdc.gov/hiv/pdf/library/reports/surveillance/cdc-hivsurveillance-report-2017-vol-29.pdf), Vol. 29; November 2018. HIV diagnosis data are estimates from 50 states, the District of Columbia, and 6 U.S. dependent areas. Estimates for 2017 are preliminary and are not included in trend calculations.
44. CDC. *HIV Surveillance Report,* Diagnoses of HIV Infection in the United States and Dependent Areas, 2017 (https://www.cdc.gov/hiv/pdf/library/reports/surveillance/cdc-hivsurveillance-report-2017-vol-29.pdf),

Vol. 29; November 2018. HIV diagnosis data are estimates from 50 states, the District of Columbia, and 6 U.S. dependent areas. Estimates for 2017 are preliminary and are not included in trend calculations.
45. CDC. NCHS. Health, United States, 2016 (http://www.cdc.gov/nchs/hus/); September 2018.
46. CDC. NCHS. Deaths: Leading Causes for 2016 (http://www.cdc.gov/nchs/nvss/deaths.htm); July 2018.
47. CDC. NCHS. Deaths: Leading Causes for 2016 (http://www.cdc.gov/nchs/nvss/deaths.htm); July 2018.
48. CDC. Supplemental Surveillance Report. Estimated HIV Incidence and Prevalence in the United States 2010–2015 (https://www.cdc.gov/hiv/pdf/library/reports/surveillance/cdc-hivsurveillance-supplemental-report-vol-23-1.pdf). Vol 23. No. 1. 2018.
49. CDC. Supplemental Surveillance Report. Estimated HIV Incidence and Prevalence in the United States 2010–2015 (https://www.cdc.gov/hiv/pdf/library/reports/surveillance/cdc-hivsurveillance-supplemental-report-vol-23-1.pdf). Vol 23. No. 1. 2018.
50. CDC. *HIV Surveillance Report,* Diagnoses of HIV Infection in the United States and Dependent Areas, 2017 (https://www.cdc.gov/hiv/pdf/library/reports/surveillance/cdc-hivsurveillance-report-2017-vol-29.pdf), Vol. 29; November 2018. HIV diagnosis data are estimates from 50 states, the District of Columbia, and 6 U.S. dependent areas. Estimates for 2017 are preliminary and are not included in trend calculations.
51. CDC. *HIV Surveillance Report,* Diagnoses of HIV Infection in the United States and Dependent Areas, 2017 (https://www.cdc.gov/hiv/pdf/library/reports/surveillance/cdc-hivsurveillance-report-2017-vol-29.pdf), Vol. 29; November 2018. HIV diagnosis data are estimates from 50 states, the District of Columbia, and 6 U.S. dependent areas. Estimates for 2017 are preliminary and are not included in trend calculations.
52. CDC. Slide Set: HIV Surveillance –Adolescents and Young Adults (https://www.cdc.gov/hiv/library/slideSets/index.html) (through 2017).
53. CDC. Slide Set: HIV Surveillance –Adolescents and Young Adults (https://www.cdc.gov/hiv/library/slideSets/index.html) (through 2017).
54. CDC. *HIV Surveillance Supplemental Report,* Monitoring Selected National HIV Prevention and Care Objectives by Using HIV Surveillance Data (https://www.cdc.gov/hiv/pdf/library/reports/surveillance/cdc-hiv-surveillance-supplemental-reportvol-23-4.pdf), Vol. 23, No. 4; June 2018.
55. Nesheim S et al. "A Framework for Elimination of Perinatal Transmission of HIV in the United States." *Pediatrics,* Vol. 130, No. 4; September 2012.
56. Whitmore SK et al. "Correlates of Mother-to-Child Transmission of HIV in the United States and Puerto Rico." *Pediatrics,* Vol. 129, No. 1; January 2012.
57. KFF. National Survey of Young Adults on HIV/AIDS (https://www.greaterthan.org/press-release-national-survey-of-young-adults-on-hivaids/); November 2017.
58. KFF analysis of CDC data.
59. CDC. HIV in the United States: At a Glance; (http://www.cdc.gov/hiv/statistics/basics/ataglance.html) December 2018.
60. CDC. Supplemental Surveillance Report. Estimated HIV Incidence and Prevalence in the United States 2010–2015 (https://www.cdc.gov/hiv/pdf/library/reports/surveillance/cdc-hivsurveillance-supplemental-report-vol-23-1.pdf). Vol 23. No. 1. 2018.
61. CDC. *HIV Surveillance Supplemental Report,* Monitoring Selected National HIV Prevention and Care Objectives by Using HIV Surveillance Data (https://www.cdc.gov/hiv/pdf/library/reports/surveillance/cdc-hiv-surveillance-supplemental-reportvol-23-4.pdf), Vol. 23, No. 4; June 2018.

62. CDC. Supplemental Surveillance Report. Estimated HIV Incidence and Prevalence in the United States 2010–2015 (https://www.cdc.gov/hiv/pdf/library/reports/surveillance/cdc-hivsurveillance-supplemental-report-vol-23-1.pdf). Vol 23. No. 1. 2018.
63. CDC. *HIV Surveillance Report,* Diagnoses of HIV Infection in the United States and Dependent Areas, 2017 (https://www.cdc.gov/hiv/pdf/library/reports/surveillance/cdc-hivsurveillance-report-2017-vol-29.pdf), Vol. 29; November 2018. HIV diagnosis data are estimates from 50 states, the District of Columbia, and 6 U.S. dependent areas. Estimates for 2017 are preliminary and are not included in trend calculations.
64. CDC. Lifetime Risk of HIV Diagnosis (http://www.cdc.gov/nchhstp/newsroom/2016/croi-pressrelease-risk.html); February 2016.
65. CDC. *HIV Surveillance Report,* Diagnoses of HIV Infection in the United States and Dependent Areas, 2017 (https://www.cdc.gov/hiv/pdf/library/reports/surveillance/cdc-hivsurveillance-report-2017-vol-29.pdf), Vol. 29; November 2018. HIV diagnosis data are estimates from 50 states, the District of Columbia, and 6 U.S. dependent areas. Estimates for 2017 are preliminary and are not included in trend calculations.
66. CDC. HIV Surveillance Special Report, HIV Infection Risk, Prevention, and Testing Behaviors among Men Who Have Sex With Men. National HIV Behavioral Surveillance, 20 U.S. Cities, 2014 (http://www.cdc.gov/hiv/pdf/library/reports/surveillance/cdchiv-hssr-nhbs-msm-2014.pdf), No. 15; January 2016.
67. CDC. HIV Surveillance Special Report, HIV Infection Risk, Prevention, and Testing Behaviors among Men Who Have Sex With Men. National HIV Behavioral Surveillance, 20 U.S. Cities, 2014 (http://www.cdc.gov/hiv/pdf/library/reports/surveillance/cdchiv-hssr-nhbs-msm-2014.pdf), No. 15; January 2016.

3.2

HIV in the United States and Dependent Areas

U.S. Center for Disease Control and Prevention, January 2019

Of the 37,968 NEW HIV DIAGNOSES in the US and dependent areas* in 2018:

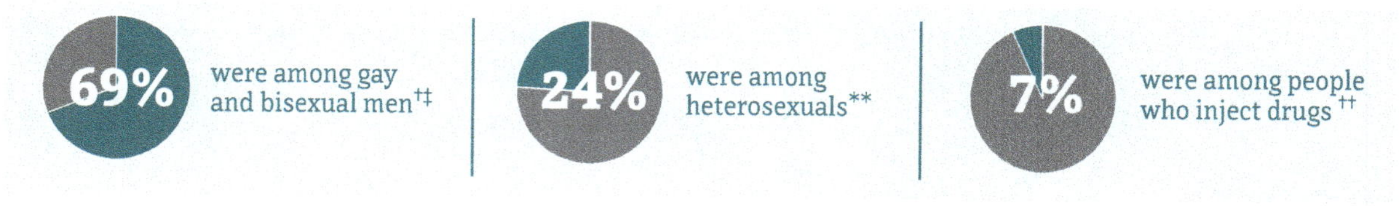

Gay and bisexual men are the population most affected by HIV.

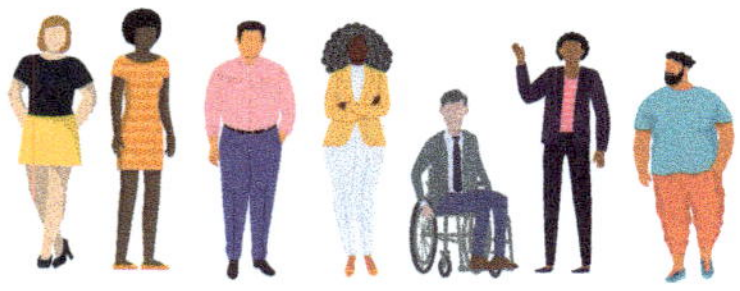

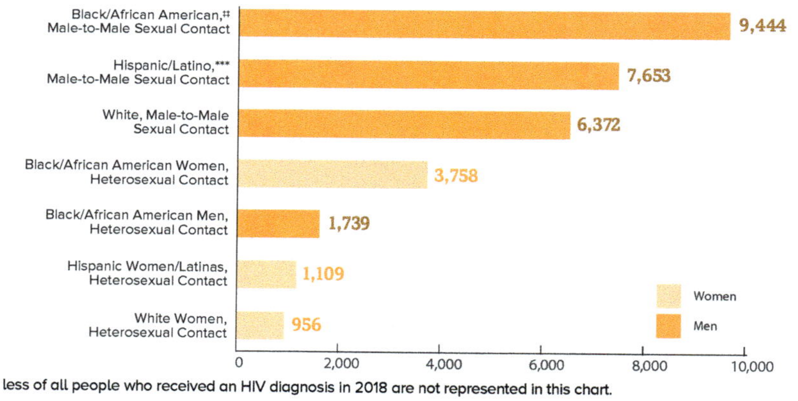

Subpopulations representing 2% or less of all people who received an HIV diagnosis in 2018 are not represented in this chart.

---

* American Samoa, Guam, the Northern Mariana Islands, Puerto Rico, the Republic of Palau, and the US Virgin Islands.
† Includes infections attributed to male-to-male sexual contact *and* injection drug use (men who reported both risk factors).
‡ This fact sheet uses the term *gay and bisexual men* to represent gay, bisexual, and other men who reported male-to-male sexual contact.
** Does not include heterosexuals who reported injection drug use.
†† Does not include infections attributed to male-to-male sexual contact *and* injection drug use (men who reported both risk factors).
‡‡ *Black* refers to people having origins in any of the black racial groups of Africa. *African American* is a term often used for Americans of African descent with ancestry in North America.
*** Hispanics/Latinos can be of any race.

For more information about HIV surveillance data, read the "Technical Notes" in the HIV surveillance reports at www.cdc.gov/hiv/library/reports/hiv-surveillance.html.

Source: https://www.cdc.gov/hiv/pdf/statistics/overview/cdc-hiv-us-ataglance.pdf.

There are also differences in HIV diagnoses by age. People aged 13 to 34 made up more than half of all new HIV diagnoses in 2018.

The number of new HIV diagnoses was highest among people aged 25 to 34.

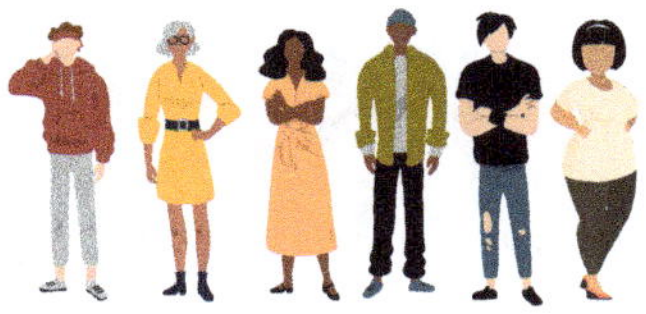

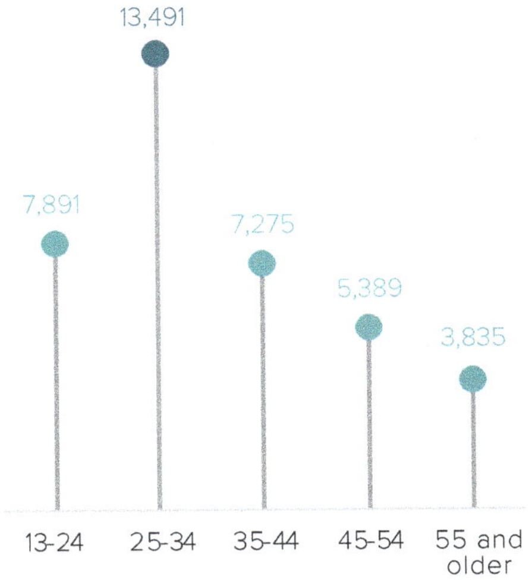

From 2014 to 2018, HIV diagnoses decreased 7% among adults and adolescents overall. However, annual HIV diagnoses have increased among some groups.

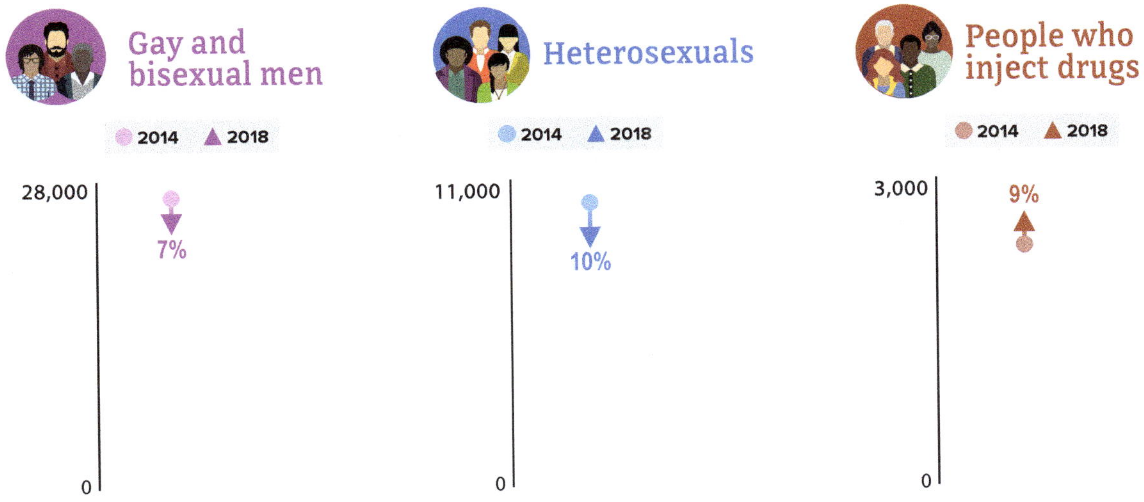

Not all people with HIV are getting the care and treatment they need.

At the end of 2018, an estimated **1.2 MILLION AMERICANS** had HIV. †††

6 in 7 knew they had the virus.

††† In 50 states and the District of Columbia.

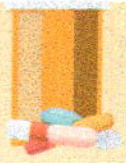

It is important for people to know their HIV status so they can take medicine to treat HIV if they have the virus. Taking HIV medicine every day can make the viral load undetectable. People who get and keep an undetectable viral load (or stay virally suppressed) can live a long and healthy life. They also have effectively no risk of transmitting HIV to HIV-negative sex partners.

Although more than half of adults and adolescents with HIV are virally suppressed, more work is needed to increase these rates. For every **100 adults and adolescents with HIV in 2018:**

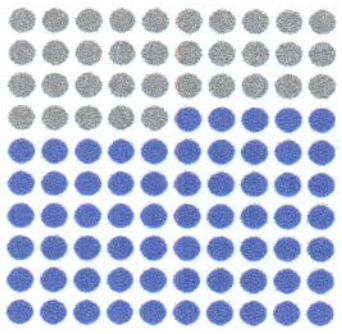

65 received some HIV care

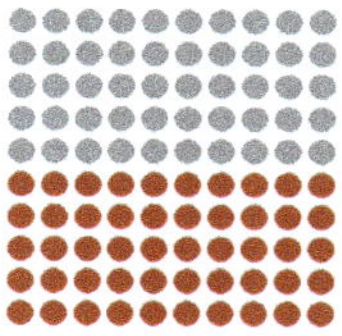

50 were retained in care

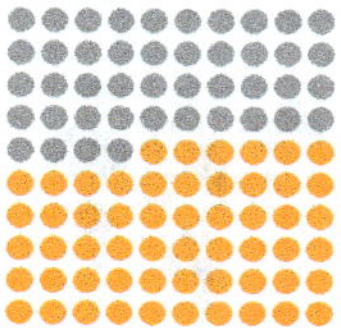

56 were virally suppressed

3.3

New HIV Diagnoses in the U.S. by Transmission Category, 2018

U.S. Center for Disease Control and Prevention

[...]

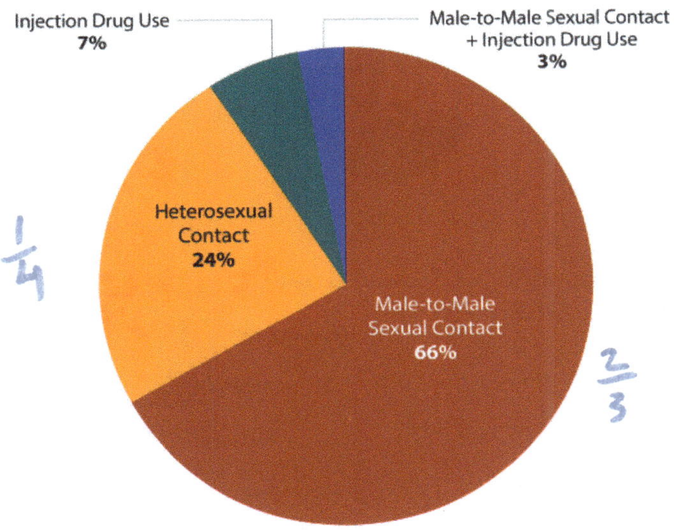

New HIV Diagnoses in the US and Dependent Areas by Transmission Category, 2018

[...]

Source: https://www.cdc.gov/hiv/basics/statistics.html.

3.4

HIV and Gay and Bisexual Men

U.S. Center for Disease Control and Prevention, 2017

Of the 37,968 NEW HIV DIAGNOSES in the US and dependent areas* in 2018, 69% were among gay and bisexual men.†‡

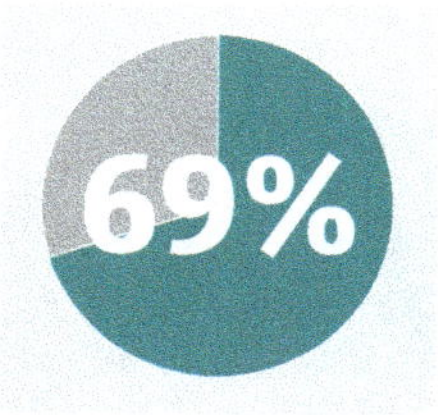

Among gay and bisexual men who received an HIV diagnosis in 2018, racial and ethnic disparities continue to exist.

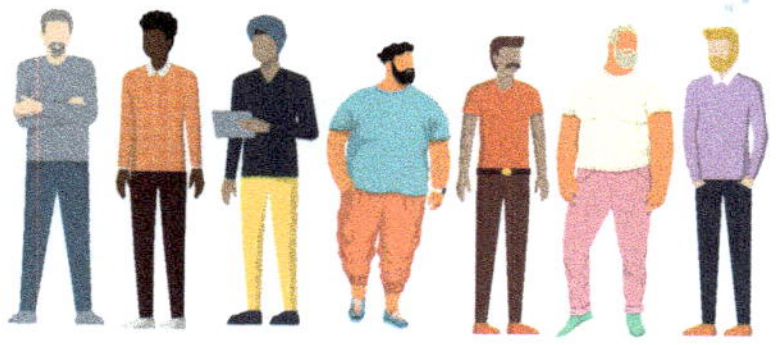

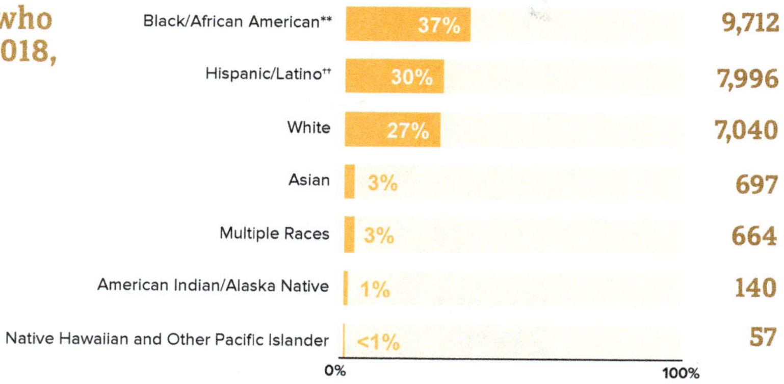

---

* American Samoa, Guam, the Northern Mariana Islands, Puerto Rico, the Republic of Palau, and the US Virgin Islands.
† This fact sheet uses the term *gay and bisexual men* to represent gay, bisexual, and other men who reported male-to-male sexual contact aged 13 and older.
‡ Includes infections attributed to male-to-male sexual contact *and* injection drug use (men who reported both risk factors).
** *Black* refers to people having origins in any of the black racial groups of Africa. *African American* is a term often used for Americans of African descent with ancestry in North America.
†† Hispanics/Latinos can be of any race.

For more information about HIV surveillance data and how it is used, read the "Technical Notes" in the HIV surveillance reports at www.cdc.gov/hiv/library/reports/hiv-surveillance.html

Source: https://www.cdc.gov/hiv/group/msm/index.html.

From 2014 to 2018, HIV diagnoses decreased 7% among gay and bisexual men overall.

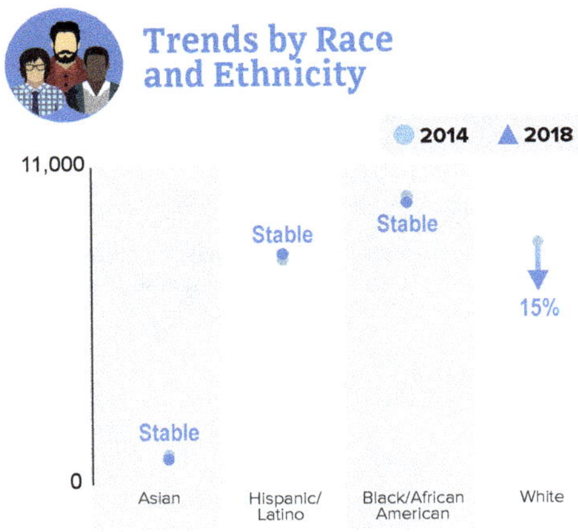

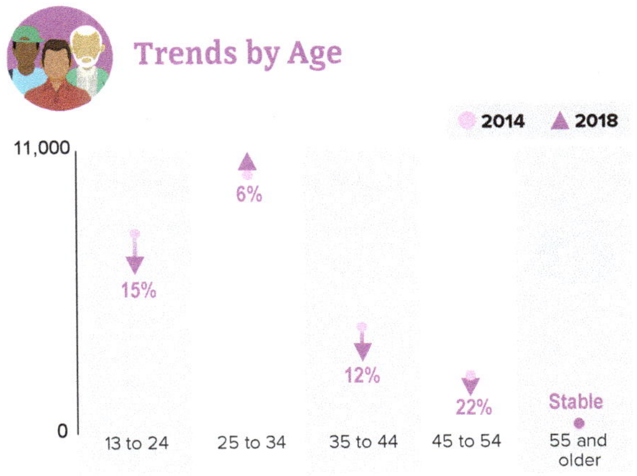

Subpopulations representing 2% or less of HIV diagnoses among gay and bisexual men are not reflected in this chart.

Gay and bisexual men who don't know they have HIV can't get the care and treatment they need to stay healthy.

At the end of 2018, an estimated **1.2 MILLION AMERICANS** had HIV.‡‡ Of those, 740,400 were gay and bisexual men.

5 in 6

gay and bisexual men knew they had the virus.***

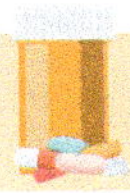

It is important for gay and bisexual men to know their HIV status so they can take medicine to treat HIV if they have the virus. Taking HIV medicine every day can make the viral load undetectable. People who get and keep an undetectable viral load (or stay virally suppressed) can live a long and healthy life. They also have effectively no risk of transmitting HIV to HIV-negative sex partners.

Compared to all people with HIV, gay and bisexual men have about the same viral suppression rates. For every **100 gay and bisexual men with HIV** in 2018:‡‡

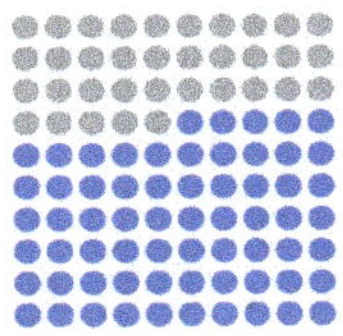

65 received some HIV care

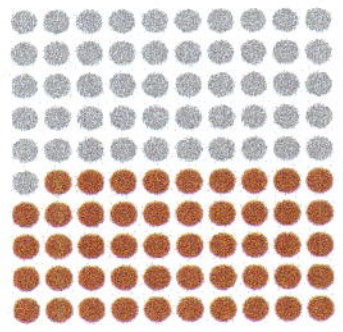

49 were retained in care

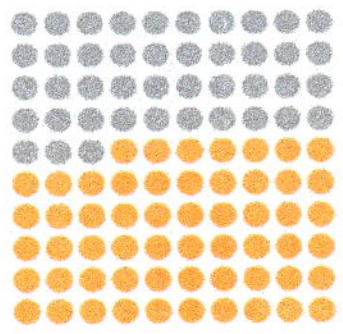

57 were virally suppressed

For comparison, for every **100 people overall** with HIV, **65 received some HIV care**, **50 were retained in care**, and **56 were virally suppressed**.

---

‡‡ In 50 states and the District of Columbia.

*** Includes infections attributed to male-to-male sexual contact *only*. Among men with HIV infection attributed to male-to-male sexual contact *and* injection drug use, 12 in 13 knew they had HIV.

There are several challenges that place some gay and bisexual men at higher risk for HIV.

Lack of Awareness of HIV Status

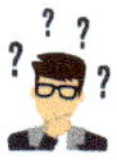

People who don't know they have HIV can't get the care they need and may pass HIV to others without knowing it.

Increased Risk for Other STDs

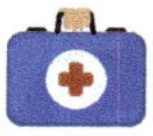

Having another sexually transmitted disease (STD) can greatly increase the chance of getting or transmitting HIV.

Sexual Behaviors

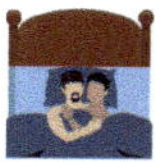

Some factors put gay and bisexual men at higher risk for HIV, including having anal sex with someone who has HIV without using protection (like condoms or medicine to prevent or treat HIV).

Stigma, Homophobia, and Discrimination

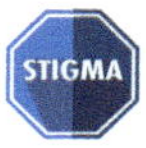

Stigma, homophobia, and discrimination may affect whether gay and bisexual men seek or receive high-quality health services.

3.5

HIV and African American People

U.S. Center for Disease Control and Prevention, 2017

Black/African American* people made up 42% (16,002)[‡] of the 37,968 NEW HIV DIAGNOSES in the US and dependent areas[†] in 2018.

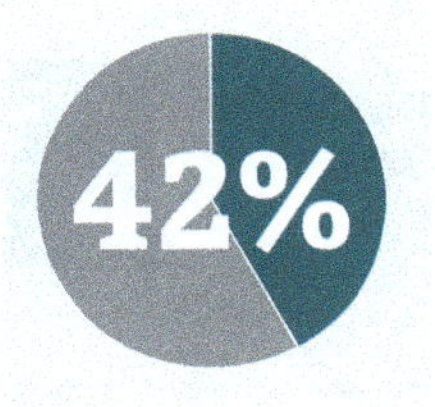

Among Black/African American people, most new HIV diagnoses were among men.

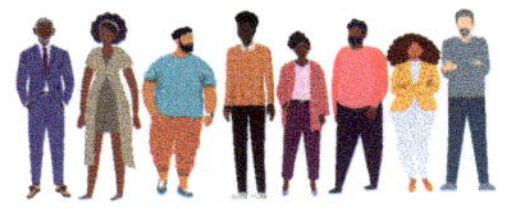

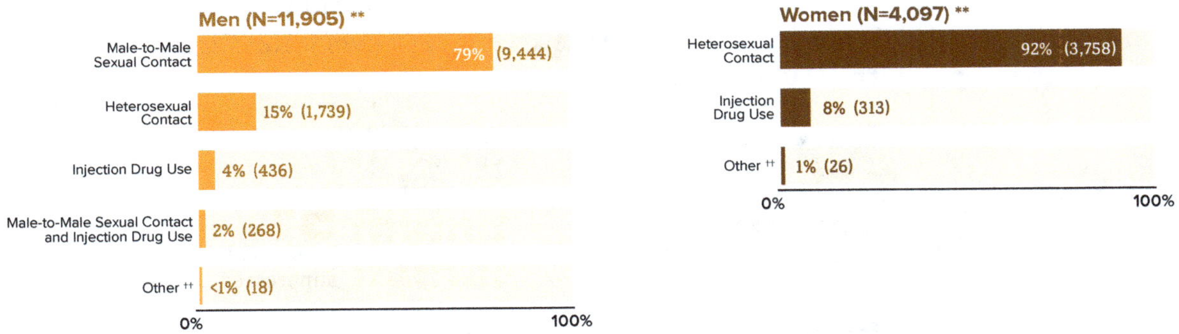

---

* *Black* refers to people having origins in any of the Black racial groups of Africa. *African American* is a term often used for people of African descent with ancestry in North America. This fact sheet uses *African American*, unless referencing surveillance data.

† Adult and adolescent Black/African American people aged 13 and older.

‡ American Samoa, Guam, the Northern Mariana Islands, Puerto Rico, the Republic of Palau, and the US Virgin Islands.

** Based on sex assigned at birth and includes transgender people.

†† Includes perinatal exposure, blood transfusion, hemophilia, and risk factors not reported or not identified.

For more information about HIV surveillance data, read the "Technical Notes" in the HIV surveillance reports at www.cdc.gov/hiv/library/reports/hiv-surveillance.html.

Source: https://www.cdc.gov/hiv/group/racialethnic/africanamericans/index.html.

Good progress has been made with reducing HIV diagnoses among most age groups, with HIV diagnoses decreasing 7% among Black/African American people overall from 2014 to 2018.

Trends by Sex

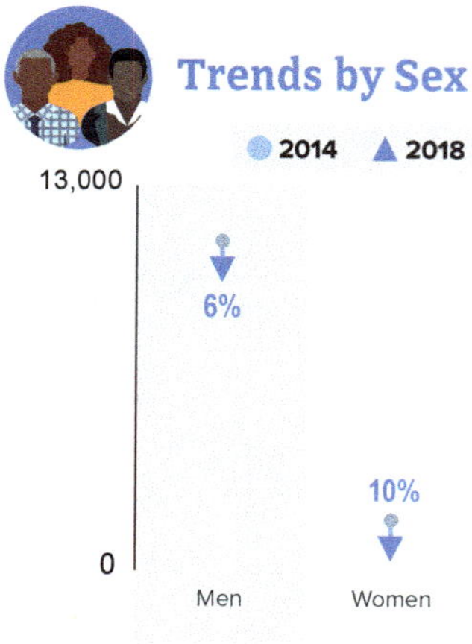

Trends by Age ‡‡

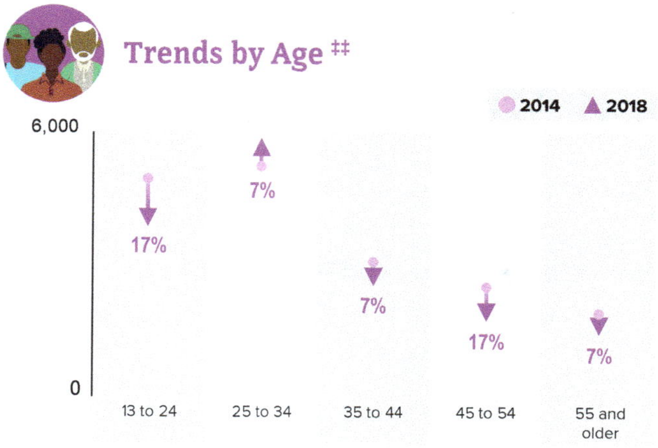

Black/African American people who don't know they have HIV can't get the care and treatment they need to stay healthy.

At the end of 2018, an estimated **1.2 MILLION PEOPLE** had HIV. Of those, 482,900 were among Black/African American people. ***

6 in 7
Black/African American people knew they had the virus.

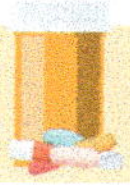

It is important for Black/African American people to know their HIV status so they can take medicine to treat HIV if they have the virus. Taking HIV medicine every day can make the viral load undetectable. People who get and keep an undetectable viral load (or remain virally suppressed) can stay healthy for many years and have effectively no risk of transmitting HIV to their sex partners.

Compared to all people with HIV, Black/African American people have lower viral suppression rates. More work is needed to increase these rates. For **every 100 Black/African American people with HIV in 2018**

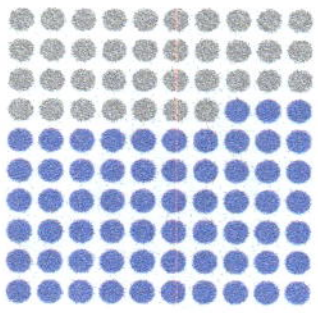

63 received some HIV care

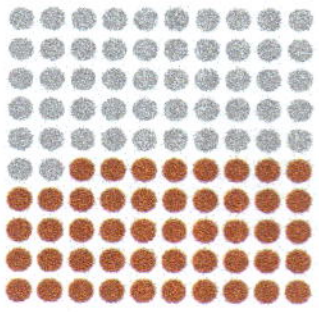

48 were retained in care

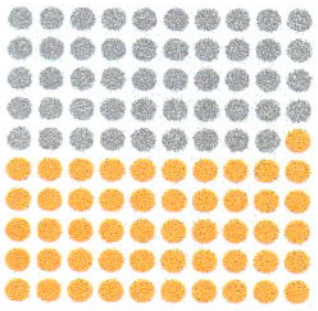

51 were virally suppressed

For comparison, for every **100 people overall** with HIV, **65 received some HIV care**, **50 were retained in care**, and **56 were virally suppressed**.

‡‡ Does not include *perinatal* and *other* transmission categories.
*** In 50 states and the District of Columbia.

There are several challenges that place some African American people at higher risk for HIV.

Knowledge of HIV Status

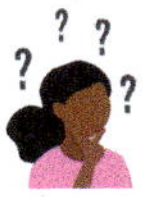

Some African American people don't know their HIV status. People who don't know they have HIV can't get the care they need and may pass HIV to others without knowing it.

Sexually Transmitted Diseases (STDs)

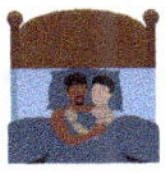

African American people have higher rates of some STDs. Having another STD can increase a person's chance of getting or transmitting HIV.

Racism, HIV Stigma, and Homophobia

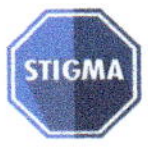

Racism, HIV stigma, and homophobia can negatively impact risk-taking behaviors, knowledge of HIV status, HIV care, and other needed services for many African American people.

Social and Economic Issues

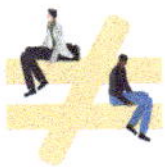

African American people experiencing poverty may find it harder to get HIV prevention and care services.

3.6

HIV and Women

U.S. Center for Disease Control and Prevention, March 2019

There were 37,968 NEW HIV DIAGNOSES in the US and dependent areas in 2018.* Of those, 19% (7,190) were among women.†‡

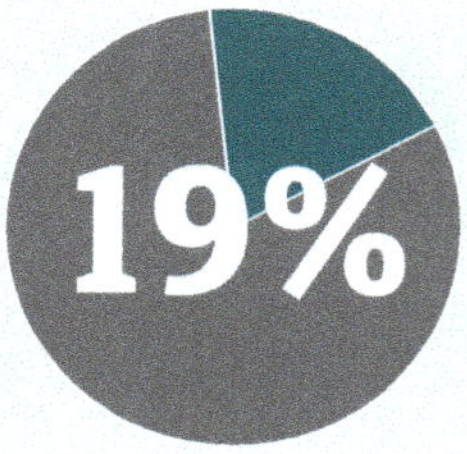

Most new HIV diagnoses among women were attributed to heterosexual contact.

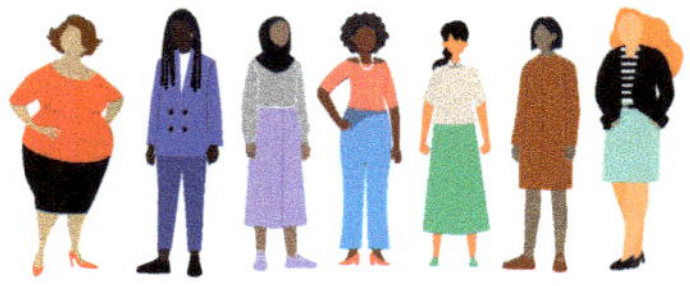

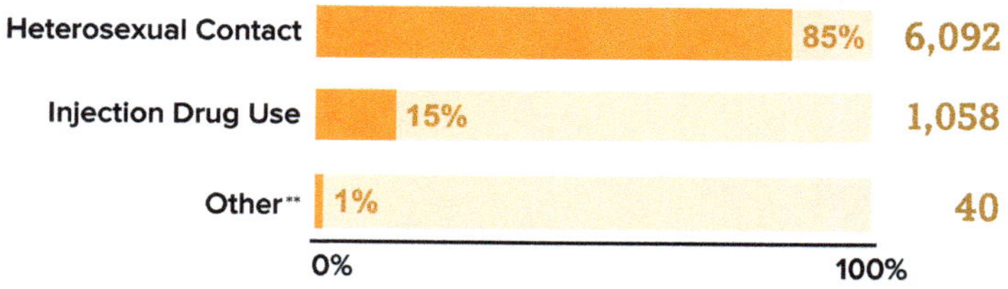

Total may exceed 100% due to rounding.

* American Samoa, Guam, the Northern Mariana Islands, Puerto Rico, the Republic of Palau, and the US Virgin Islands.
† Adult and adolescent women aged 13 and older.
‡ Based on sex assigned at birth and includes transgender people.
** Includes perinatal exposure, blood transfusion, hemophilia, and risk factors not reported or not identified.

For more information about HIV surveillance data, read the "Technical Notes" in the HIV surveillance reports at www.cdc.gov/hiv/library/reports/hiv-surveillance.html.

Source: https://www.cdc.gov/hiv/group/gender/women/index.html.

HIV diagnoses decreased 7% among women overall from 2014 to 2018. Although trends varied for different groups of women, HIV diagnoses declined for groups most affected by HIV, including Black/African American†† women and women aged 25 to 34.

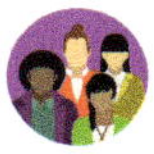

Trends by Race/Ethnicity

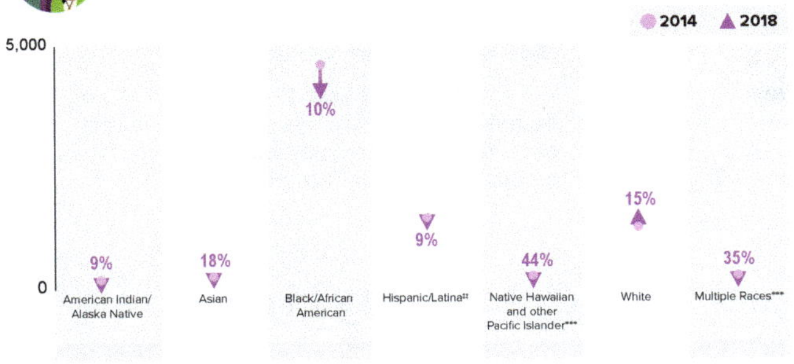

Trends by Age

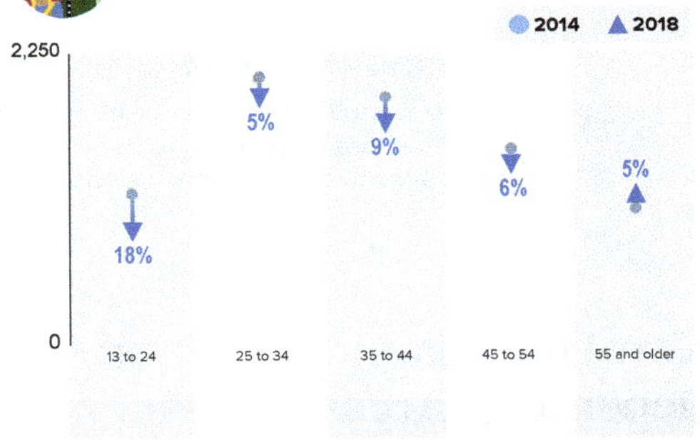

Women who don't know they have HIV can't get the care and treatment they need to stay healthy.

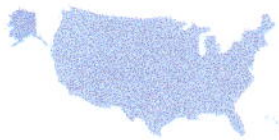

In 2018, an estimated **1,173,900 PEOPLE** had HIV.††† **Of those, 261,800 were women.‡‡‡**

For every 100 people with HIV

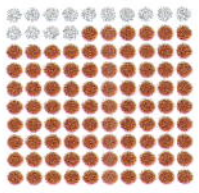

86 knew their HIV status.

For every 100 women with HIV

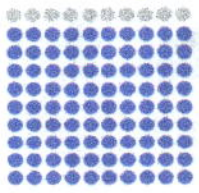

90 knew their HIV status.

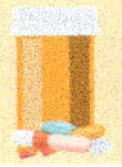

It is important for women to know their HIV status so they can take medicine to treat HIV if they have the virus. Taking HIV medicine every day can make the viral load undetectable. People who get and keep an undetectable viral load (or remain virally suppressed) can stay healthy for many years and have effectively no risk of transmitting HIV to their sex partners.

Compared to all people with diagnosed HIV, women have lower viral suppression rates. More work is needed to increase these rates. **For every 100 women with diagnosed HIV in 2018:** ****

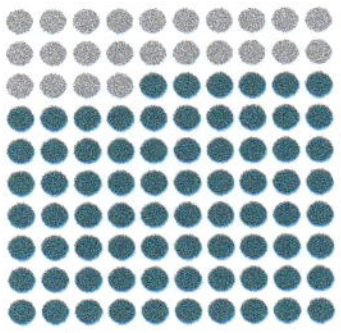

76 received some HIV care

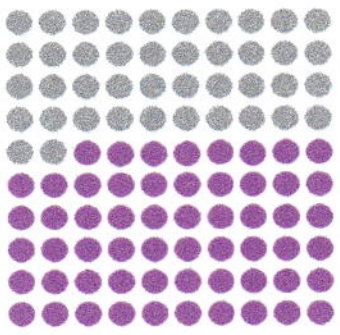

58 were retained in care

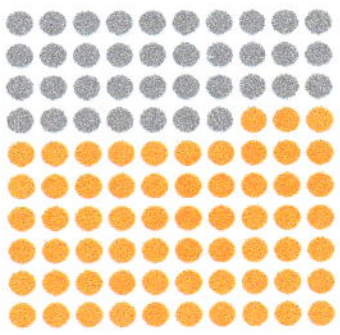

63 were virally suppressed

For comparison, for every **100 people overall** with diagnosed HIV, **76 received some care**, **58 were retained in care**, and **65 were virally suppressed**.

---

†† *Black* refers to people having origins in any of the Black racial groups of Africa. *African American* is a term often used for people of African descent with ancestry in North America.

‡‡ Hispanic/Latina women can be of any race.

*** Changes in subpopulations with fewer HIV diagnoses can lead to a large percentage increase or decrease.

††† In 50 states and the District of Columbia.

‡‡‡ Based on sex assigned at birth.

**** In 41 states and the District of Columbia.

There are several challenges that place some women at higher risk for HIV.

Racism, Discrimination, and HIV Stigma

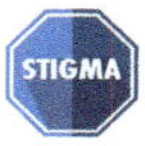

Racism, discrimination, and stigma may affect whether some women seek or receive high-quality health services.

Risk of Exposure

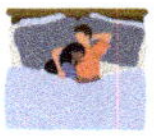

Because receptive sex is riskier than insertive sex, women are more likely to get HIV during vaginal or anal sex than their sex partner.

Unaware of Partner's Risk Factors

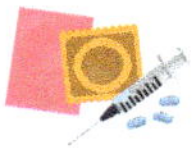

Some women don't know their male partner's risk factors for HIV (such as injection drug use or having sex with men) and may not use a condom or medicine to prevent HIV.

Intimate Partner Violence (IPV)

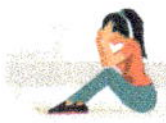

Women who have been exposed to IPV may be more likely to engage in risky behaviors or be forced to have sex without a condom or medicines to prevent or treat HIV.

New HIV Diagnoses Among Women by Race/Ethnicity in the US and Dependent Areas, 2018*

Black/African American women continueto be disproportionately affected by HIV.

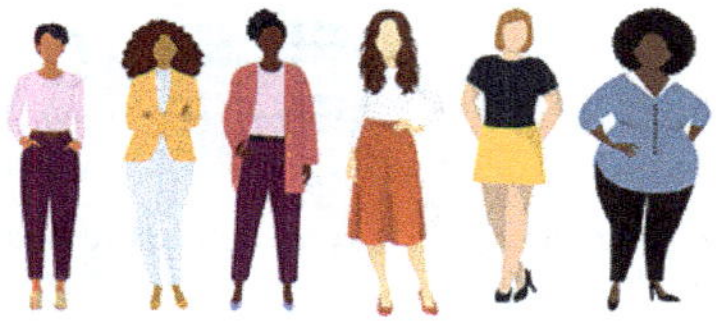

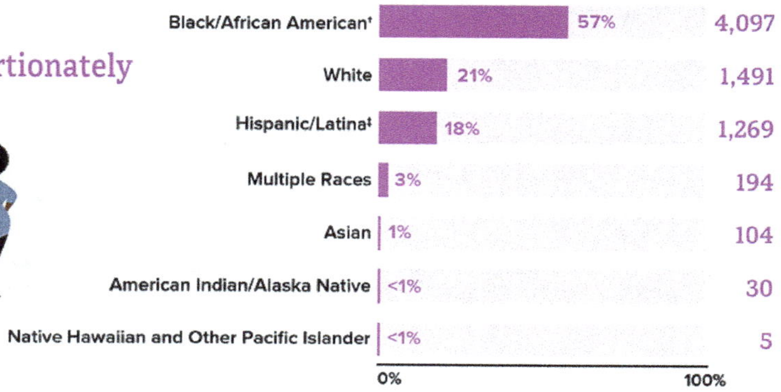

* Based on sex assigned at birth and includes transgender people.
† *Black* refers to people having origins in any of the Black racial groups of Africa. *African American* is a term often used for people of African decent wtih ancestry in North America.
‡ Hispanic/Latina women can be of any race.

3.7

HIV and Youth

U.S. Center for Disease Control and Prevention, April 2019

Of the 37,832 NEW HIV DIAGNOSES in the US and dependent areas* in 2018, 21% were among youth.†

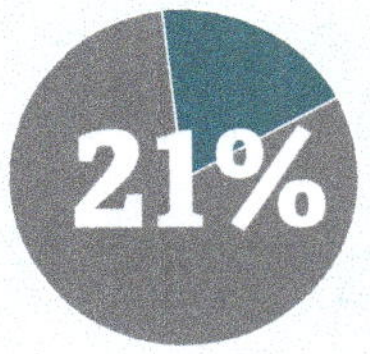

Most new HIV diagnoses among youth were among young gay and bisexual men. ‡ **

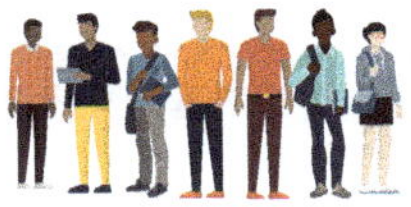

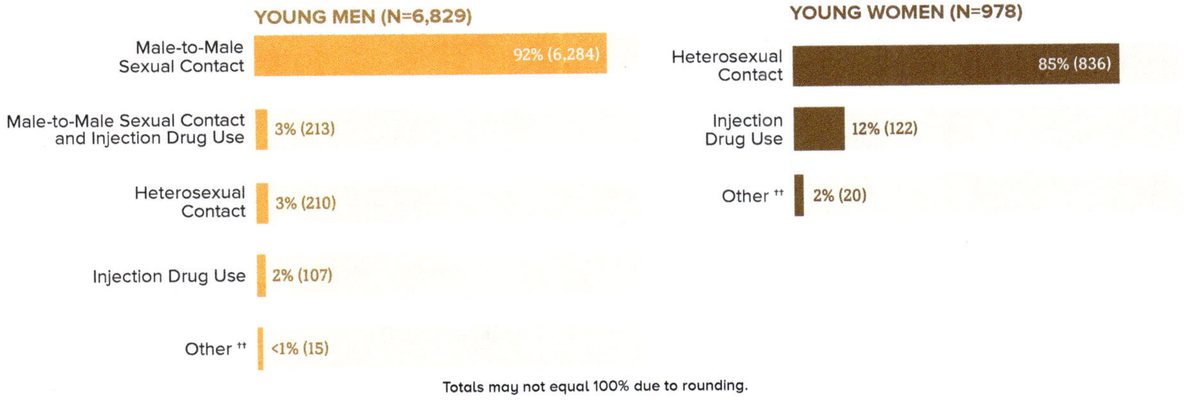

---

* American Samoa, Guam, the Northern Mariana Islands, Puerto Rico, the Republic of Palau, and the US Virgin Islands.
† Persons aged 13 to 24 are referred to as *youth* or *young* in this fact sheet.
‡ This fact sheet uses the term *gay and bisexual men* to represent gay, bisexual, and other men who have sex with men.
** Includes infections attributed to male-to-male sexual contact *and* injection drug use (men who reported both risk factors).
†† Includes hemophilia, blood transfusion, perinatal exposure, and risk factors not reported or not identified.

For more information about HIV surveillance data, read the "Technical Notes" in the HIV surveillance reports at www.cdc.gov/hiv/library/reports/hiv-surveillance.html.

Source: https://www.cdc.gov/hiv/group/age/youth/index.html.

HIV diagnoses declined 10% among youth overall from 2010 to 2017.‡‡ Although trends varied for different groups of youth, HIV diagnoses declined for groups most affected by HIV, including young black/African American gay and bisexual men.***

Trends by Sex

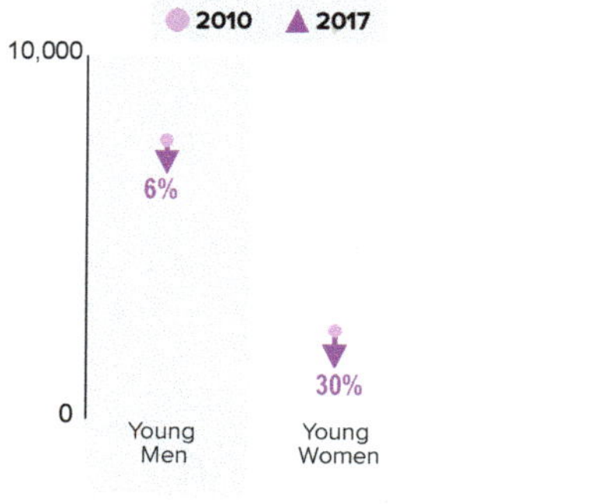

Trends for Young Gay and Bisexual Men by Race and Ethnicity

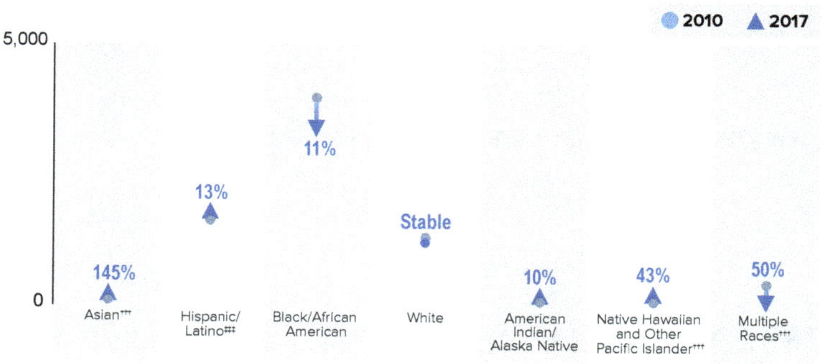

Youth who don't know they have HIV cannot get the care and treatment they need to stay healthy.

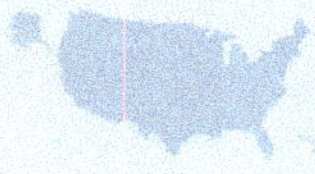

At the end of 2016, an estimated 1.1 MILLION PEOPLE had HIV.‡ Of those, 50,900 were young people.

Nearly 4 in 7 youth knew they had the virus.

Youth were the least likely to be aware of their infection compared to any other age group. It is important for youth to know their HIV status so they can take medicine to treat HIV if they have the virus. Taking HIV medicine every day can make the viral load undetectable. Youth who get and keep an undetectable viral load (or stay virally suppressed) have effectively no risk of transmitting HIV to HIV-negative sex partners.

Compared to all people with HIV, youth have the lowest rates of viral suppression. For every 100 youth with HIV: ‡‡

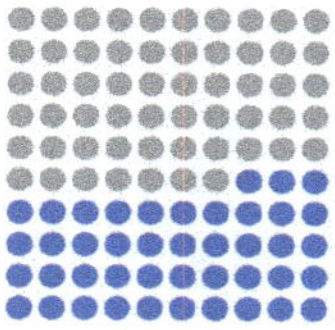

43 received some HIV care

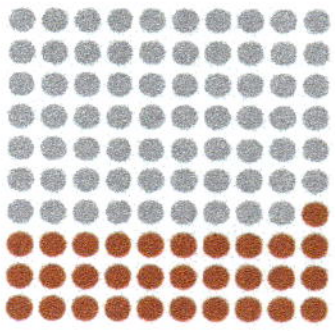

31 were retained in care

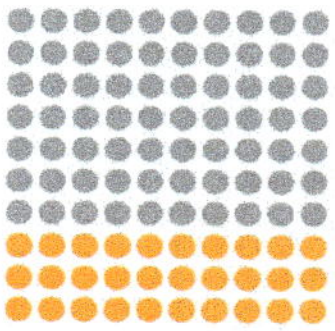

30 were virally suppressed

For comparison, for every **100 people overall** with HIV, **64 received some HIV care**, **49 were retained in care**, and **53 were virally suppressed**.

---

‡‡ In 50 states and the District of Columbia.

*** *Black* refers to people having origins in any of the black racial groups of Africa. *African American* is a term often used for Americans of African descent with ancestry in North America.

††† Changes in subpopulations with fewer HIV diagnoses can lead to a large percentage increase or decrease.

‡‡‡ Hispanics/Latinos can be of any race.

Several challenges make it difficult for youth to access the tools they need to reduce their risk or get treatment and care if they have HIV.

Low Rates of HIV Testing

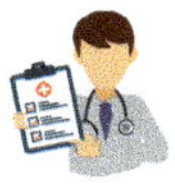

HIV testing rates among high school students are low. People who do not know they have HIV cannot take advantage of HIV care and treatment and may unknowingly transmit HIV to others.

Low Rates of PrEP Use

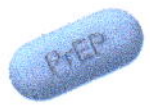

Young people are less likely than adults to use medicine to prevent HIV. Barriers include cost, access, perceived stigma, and privacy concerns.

Socioeconomic Challenges

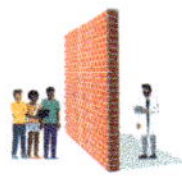

Among people with HIV, young people are more likely than older people to be living in households with low income levels, to have been recently homeless, recently incarcerated, or uninsured. These factors pose barriers to achieving viral suppression.

High Rates of Other STDs

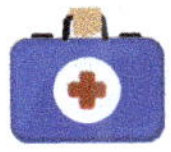

Some of the highest STD rates are among youth aged 20 to 24. Having another STD can greatly increase the chance of getting or transmitting HIV.

3.8

The Scarlet Virus

Ila Mulasi, M.D.

SHE WAS A LARGE WOMAN WITH an easy grin and open demeanor; her threadbare jacket was often askew but always meticulously clean. It was easy to envision her on the front stoops of Baltimore row houses, chatting with neighbors as they numbed their sorrows with hits of speedball, shots in paper bags. She had never left the city limits, had no passport, and often struggled to keep her ID in hand long enough to pick up her monthly disability check. It was impossible not to be drawn into her story, as she leaned over the desk in the cramped exam room, sharing her fears tentatively.

"I'd heard about it, but I never could've thought I'd get the bug," she confided as we reviewed her HIV risk factors. Ms. M. had been "careful," never sharing needles and infrequently having unprotected sex, but somewhere along the way the virus had found its window. For months, maybe years, Ms. M. had unknowingly been a vector for transmission. Without malice, how many others had she exposed? Her face crumpled at the sudden realization. An oral screening swab in the emergency department had marked her as HIV-positive, and she found her way to our clinic. Now she was seated across from me on a worn chair, hallway voices filtering into the room. We talked about labs and medications, adherence issues, things that get in the way of care. "I got this, Doc," she grinned, finding her footing after a few sessions of education and support, reassuring me, "I can do this."

And she did. Ms. M. diligently kept her appointments, adhered to her complex anti-retroviral regimen, regularly had labs drawn. She was popular with everyone—phlebotomists, front-desk staff, social workers, nurses. Confident in her ability to manage her HIV, Ms. M. was one of my rare patients who required little intervention; our appointments seemed more companionable than medical, like visits with an old friend. She informally counseled other patients in the waiting room, reassuring them that they, too, would persevere through this devastating illness, comforting peers who often remained closeted and defamed even as we entered the 21st century. When her stage III uterine prolapse was discovered on a routine gynecologic exam, Ms. M. was unperturbed, saying, "I thought that's how it was supposed to be." Given her years spent on the streets and the torments of living with addiction, a prolapsed uterus probably wasn't as problematic for her as it seemed to us.

Then we were confronted by the stark summary of an annual screening mammogram: "poorly defined spiculated mass lesion most compatible with malignancy, accompanying suspect nodal disease."

Ms. M. had undergone regular screenings, but even with suppressed viral loads, HIV-positive people remain at increased risk for cancer-specific mortality and morbidity.[1] A visceral fear gripped the clinical team, but oncology referrals were made, mastectomy scheduled, radiation oncology consulted. Ms. M. did well at first, tolerating chemotherapy with her usual aplomb, reassuring us again of her tenacity. Quelled as we were by her poise and nonchalance, we were taken aback when surveillance imaging revealed cerebral metastases. In what seemed like an instant, her performance status declined, and suddenly it was clear she could no longer manage at home, even with help from her large, supportive family. Discussions about end-of-life care began again, and Ms. M. reiterated her wishes: comfort and dignity above all else, especially since her days were clearly numbered. A local inpatient hospice unit deemed her symptom burden intractable and transitioned her care; it was there that I saw her last.

The muted pastels of the unit set it apart from the austere surgical floors. The staff seemed centered, focused, and quietly efficient as they attended to their wards. Families had ample sitting options, and myriad efforts at creating a homelike environment were evident. I wandered into Ms. M.'s room, peeking in first to see whether she was up to having visitors. Her bed was oriented toward a sun-filled window, its ledge littered with cards, plants, and foods from well-wishers. At her bedside was her daughter, quietly keeping watch.

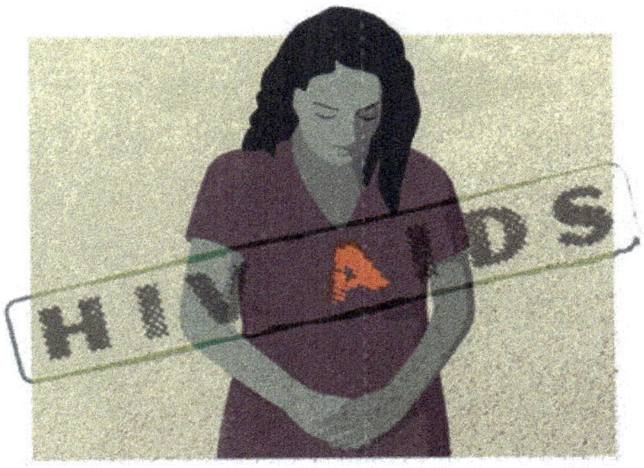

Ms. M. brightened when she spotted me, summoning me to her side with surprising vigor. She pulled me close, surreptitiously watching her daughter, urgently whispering, "She doesn't know—don't say anything—she doesn't know." It took me a minute to comprehend what she was trying to communicate, but then it dawned on me: Ms. M. had never told her daughter about her HIV status.

We talked about how she was doing, the wonderful hospice nurses and aides, the weather starting to warm up. Ms. M. shared family pictures, proud of her grandkids, wistful about what might have been. She confided that she'd been given more than she thought she deserved, that she was ready to meet her maker. Her daughter chimed in now and again, but it was clear that this was goodbye. Ms. M. settled back in the bedsheets, comforted, and offered quietly, "They think it's just the breast cancer—nothing else."

She died 11 days later. They say she didn't suffer and met her end with the same grace and acceptance with which she'd lived her life, but I remained haunted by the burden she carried to her grave. This gregarious, confident woman, a "model patient" who had counseled her peers to be honest and candid as they sought care, who had reassured so many others that they would be okay, that she was living proof of that—she had never shared her status with her daughter (or, as I would later learn, any of her family). HIV was still so immense an anguish that one of the most open and free-spirited patients I knew never felt absolved enough to share her status with her loved ones.

The burden of being stigmatized affects every aspect of our patients' capacity to function, to engage in good health care, to adhere to medications, and to participate fully in their own lives as parents, siblings, partners, friends, and employees. According to the Centers for Disease Control and

Prevention, in 2015, approximately 1.1 million people in the United States were living with HIV, and about 15% of them were unaware of their status.[2] Although the overall incidence of HIV transmission declined by about 10% between 2010 and 2014, the rate of transmission among men who have sex with men remains high and has actually increased, particularly in the black and Latino communities.[3,4] The stigma associated with HIV persists, and despite our substantial medical advances in managing this illness, as recently as October 2017, Betty Price, a physician, Georgia state legislator, and the wife of former Secretary of Health and Human Services Tom Price, suggested that quarantining HIV-positive people might curtail spread of the virus.[5]

Stigma associated with illness is not new. Mental illness, cancer, sexually transmitted diseases, and tuberculosis, among others, still carry an aura of dishonor. As our world becomes smaller and more accessible through social media and technological advances, it simultaneously seems to become narrower and tighter. As human beings, we are inherently attuned to people with whom we share common features, history, or experience. As clinicians, we are obliged to remain transparent, empathetic, and compassionate to a broad cross section of humanity, even when that means reaching outside our comfort zones. Though we may occasionally feel overwhelmed by the number of patients we see and the complexities of their troubles (medical and otherwise), we are compelled to remain vigilant about the trials and hardships each patient faces while moving through this world.

I regret that the stigma of Ms. M.'s illness followed her to the grave. I endeavor to honor her life and the lessons she taught me, as, even in my busiest clinics, I strive to sit down and make space for each patient's voice and concerns. By creating this small sanctuary, I hope I am opening the door for patients, for people, to be able to begin to address the burdens that weigh on them. And I hope that eventually such interactions will enable a greater kind of healing—one that goes beyond the prescription pad.

The patient's initial and other identifying characteristics have been changed to protect her privacy.

Disclosure forms provided by the author are available at NEJM.org.

From the Departments of Internal Medicine, Palliative Medicine, and Family and Community Medicine, University of Maryland Medical Center, Baltimore.

Notes

1. Coghill A.E., Shiels M.S., Suneja G., Engels E.A. Elevated cancer-specific mortality among HIV-infected patients in the United States. J Clin Oncol 2015; 33: 2376–83.
2. Dailey A.F., Hoots B.E., Hall HI, et al. Vital signs: human immunodeficiency virus testing and diagnosis delays—United States. MMWR Morb Mortal Wkly Rep 2017; 66: 1300–6.
3. Singh S., Song R., Johnson A.S., et al. HIV incidence, prevalence, and undiagnosed infections in men who have sex with men. Presented at the Conference on Retroviruses and Opportunistic Infections, Seattle, February 14, 2017.
4. Centers for Disease Control and Prevention. Diagnoses of HIV infection in the United States and dependent areas, 2016: HIV surveillance report. November 2017 (https://www.cdc.gov/hiv/pdf/library/reports/surveillance/cdc-hiv-surveillance-report-2016-vol-28.pdf).
5. Tinker B. Georgia lawmaker: can people with HIV be 'legally' quarantined? CNN. October 22, 2017 (https://www.cnn.com/2017/10/20/health/betty-price-hiv-aids-quarantine/index.html).

3.9

'We're in a Mess.' Why Florida Is Struggling with an Unusually Severe HIV/AIDS Problem

Jon Cohen

IN FLORIDA—IT'S A TUESDAY AFTERNOON IN April, and doctors at the adult HIV/AIDS clinic at Jackson Memorial Hospital in Miami face their usual onslaught of patients. There's the young, recently diagnosed gay man from Venezuela here for his first appointment. An older gay man who emigrated from Colombia and has been treated at the clinic for 18 years. A 37-year-old Massachusetts native who is battling a heroin addiction, has a drug-related heart condition, and has done time for selling sex. Rounding out the queue are an undocumented grandmother from the Dominican Republic, a mentally challenged and occasionally homeless African-American woman, and an elderly Haitian woman in a wheelchair.

The mosaic of patients represents the major drivers of HIV's spread and the communities hard hit by AIDS in the United States. And it helps explain why in 2016, Miami had the highest new infection rate per capita of any U.S. city: 47 per 100,000 people, according to the Centers for Disease Control and Prevention (CDC). That's more than twice as many as San Francisco, New York City, or Los Angeles.

"Miami is the epicenter of the epicenter of HIV/AIDS in the United States," says Mario Stevenson, a virologist with a thick Scottish brogue who heads the infectious disease department at the University of Miami (UM) Miller School of Medicine, which shares a campus with Jackson Memorial. "There's no abatement in our upward slope."

The rest of the state isn't faring much better. Fort Lauderdale, Orlando, and Jacksonville also made the list of top 10 U.S. cities for rate of new HIV diagnoses. And more HIV infections progress to AIDS here than in any other state, in part because many infected people who start taking antiretroviral (ARV) drugs don't stick with them.

Stevenson, who specializes in HIV cure research, left Massachusetts for Florida in 2010. Since then, he has reached beyond probing how HIV hides in chromosomes to also addressing why the virus still infects and sickens so many people walking the streets outside his lab. "Stemming the tide is going to need more than just working at the bench doing molecular biology," says Stevenson, who has pushed UM to bring together affected communities, legislators, and the Florida Department of Health (DOH) to better coordinate the response to their epidemic. "We're saying, 'Hey, guys, we're in a mess.'"

As Florida's HIV/AIDS caseload keeps growing, more leaders are calling for change. Stevenson helped spearhead a task force that last year issued a report called Getting to Zero for Miami. The report built on the treatment-as-prevention principle of the international Ending AIDS movement: Infected people rarely transmit the virus or develop AIDS if they know their status and take ARVs. The report urged Miami to strengthen its testing and treatment efforts—as has happened in San Francisco, New York state, and Vancouver, Canada—and it promoted a proven prevention strategy called pre-exposure prophylaxis (PrEP): giving ARVs to uninfected people who are at high risk. At the state level, the same agenda is at the heart of DOH's plan to eliminate HIV transmission and AIDS deaths, which it has rolled out, albeit slowly, over the past few years.

Florida has made some progress, but Stevenson knows the path ahead will be rough. He and others complain that state officials have turned away federal funding for prevention and care, limited sex education, and generally downplayed the problem. The reformers say that in addition to politics, they must tiptoe around cultural minefields, slash through excessive bureaucracy, and tackle the stigma that compromises HIV/AIDS efforts everywhere.

The push for reform also faces indifference, especially among state and local legislators. For them, other illnesses—heart disease, cancer, diabetes, and Alzheimer's, each of which takes more lives—often eclipse the need for HIV/AIDS resources, Stevenson says. And the epidemic can feel like old news. "Everyone recognizes the problem, but when it comes time on the microphone to say, 'This is what we're doing with HIV,' there's a disconnect," he says. "We know how to address the issue. We know how to fix it. We just have to get up to speed."

Why is HIV spreading rapidly across the Sunshine State, famous for its tropical weather, wide beaches, the Everglades, and amusement parks? The stream of visitors and transplants drawn to those attractions is one piece of the puzzle. More than 100 million tourists visit Florida each year, some lured by the party-hearty, bacchanalian reputation of Miami, Key West, and other beach towns. Since the AIDS epidemic surfaced in 1981, the state's population has doubled to nearly 21 million people, many of them immigrants from Latin America or the Caribbean—and in several of the island nations in the region, HIV is substantially more prevalent than in the United States. Florida is also in the deep South, which, because of a surge of HIV infections among black and Latino men who have sex with men (MSM), is home today to nearly half the estimated 1.1 million people living with HIV in the country.

According to DOH modeling estimates, Florida in 2016 had 135,986 HIV-infected people, just behind California and New York. But 21,214 of those people—15%—did not know their status, and that fuels the state's high transmission rate. "A significant fraction of the new infections come from people who don't even know they have HIV," says Michael Kolber, clinical director of UM's HIV/AIDS program.

Florida's complex demographics magnify the challenge of reaching that 15%. A campaign that might prompt a Haitian immigrant to seek testing differs from what's needed to reach Latinos, blacks, MSM, heterosexuals, drug users, the homeless, or the mentally ill. Urban and rural communities also have vastly different lifestyles and testing options. "It's such a diverse state from the Panhandle to Key West that it's almost like different countries," says Jeffrey Beal, medical director of DOH's HIV/AIDS section, based in Fort Myers.

Many doctors, especially in rural areas, still don't routinely test for HIV, and some are slow to offer infected people treatment. "There's been a lack of attention on the part of my fellow physicians—I have to be very honest about that," says Beal, who began his career in Oklahoma at the start of the AIDS epidemic and burned out from watching so many patients die. He even quit practicing medicine for a year and moved to Florida to become a housing developer with his partner before the shortcomings of the state's HIV/AIDS care in rural areas led him back to the clinic.

At the same time, not enough people seek out testing, further undermining the promise of treatment as prevention. Some fear being ostracized if they're infected: Florida falls in the country's Bible Belt, which CDC notes suffers from "homophobia and transphobia, racism, and general discomfort with public discussion of sexuality." In conservative Clewiston, a few hours' drive north of Miami, Timothy Dean, who is openly gay and has his HIV-positive status tattooed on his arm, sees doctors at the nearby county health department. But he knows several local, infected people who avoid it.

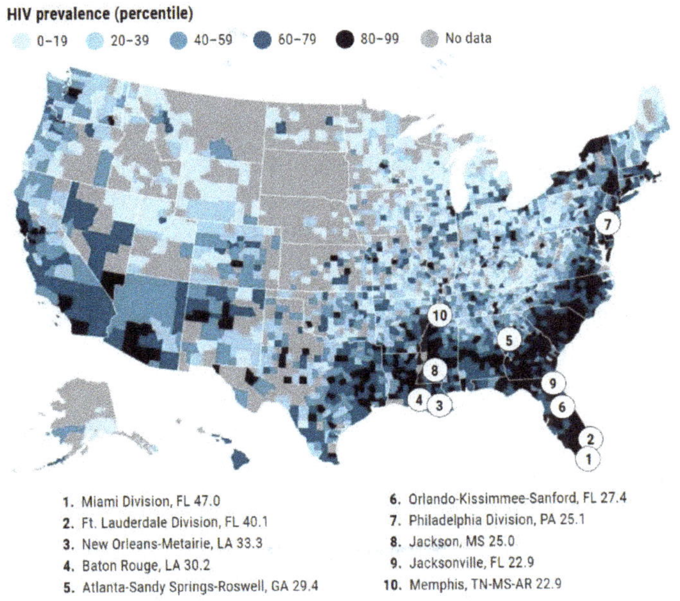

(GRAPHIC) J. YOU/*SCIENCE*; (DATA) AIDSVU, FLORIDA DEPARTMENT OF HEALTH

"This town is very tight-knit, and rumors can start," says Dean, who works for DOH to connect HIV-infected people to care. "Your children may not want nothing to do with you because they find out that you're positive." And Clewiston, a sparsely populated community built around growing and processing sugar cane, has no public transportation, so Dean says seeking care outside of town simply isn't a realistic option for some.

Complacency, rather than fear, is the issue for other groups, such as immigrants from the many countries where HIV is relatively uncommon. MSM from Latin America, for example, may not realize that moving to Florida could boost their risk of infection, says UM HIV/AIDS clinician Susanne Doblecki-Lewis. "The idea that the same behavior can have different consequences in different locations is a little bit difficult to process," Doblecki-Lewis says.

Other public health measures also have lagged here. Needle and syringe exchanges that now are in 32 other states—they were endorsed by the U.S. National Commission on AIDS in 1991—only became legal here in 2016. "We were decades late," says UM clinician Hansel Tookes, who, while still a med student at the school, led a 4-year lobbying campaign that persuaded legislators to change the law.

Similarly, Florida has been slow to promote PrEP, unlike many other locales. Florida Surgeon General Celeste Philip mandated in December 2017 that all 67 county health departments offer PrEP at no cost by the end of 2018. On a smaller scale, UM has a mobile clinic named Gamechanger that will start driving around Miami in the next few months, offering both HIV testing and PrEP.

When people test positive, Florida's system routinely links them to care. But the system falls short at keeping them there. Nearly one in three people are, in medical jargon, "lost to follow-up" for reasons such as transportation difficulties, stigma concerns, relocation, lack of social support, substance abuse, and poverty. In New York City, by contrast, which had nearly 90,000 people who knew their positive status in 2016, 88% were retained in care. As a consequence, only about half of the HIV-infected people here are fully suppressing the virus with ARVs, compared with 76% in New York City. Florida's shortfall has two steep costs: People are more likely to spread the virus to others, and they have a greater risk of developing AIDS themselves.

"This is Dr. Suzie, the doctor of the Haitian community!" announces the host of "Radio Coin," a talk show on WLQY-AM in Miami that caters to the city's large Haitian population. Suzie Armas, who runs Miami's New Health Community Center in a neighborhood known as Little Haiti, takes to the microphone like a preacher at the pulpit. In a mix of Creole and English, she urges listeners to come to her clinic, regardless of whether they have insurance or legal immigration status, and receive a free HIV test.

"If you become positive, next step is to seek treatment," says Armas, a physician's assistant who was a licensed doctor in Haiti and Mexico. "We will take care of you."

Haitian immigrants have one of Florida's highest new infection rates for people born in other countries, and Armas wants to make sure that people with the virus stay on treatment. But that takes a special effort with clients such as Chimens Point du Jour, 57, who worked as a high school administrator in Haiti but speaks limited English and tested positive for HIV in 2016 during a routine checkup at Armas's clinic. Because of language issues, most newspaper articles or public health campaigns have little impact on people like him, Armas notes, and many other Haitians are uneducated, even illiterate. "But every Haitian living in the U.S. listens to some type of radio station," she says. That makes "Radio Coin" a potent tool.

For Point du Jour, another draw is that the clinic offers him free transportation to appointments. "Bél bagay!" he says, which roughly translates to "This place is awesome!"

The center's program for Haitians is but one small-scale attempt to help HIV-infected Floridians stay in care. Another is the Infectious Disease Elimination Act, known as IDEA Exchange, which Tookes and his team began in December 2016. IDEA Exchange offers Miami drug users clean needles, HIV tests, and referrals to rehab and treatment. The exchange also has a mobile unit that travels to the city's drug hot spots.

Shortly after the IDEA Exchange van rolls into Miami's Overtown neighborhood early one April morning, a steady stream of clients shows up. Natasha Dixon, 33, was diagnosed with HIV last year at the van. "I can barely take care of myself," says Dixon, who brings along a kitten that the IDEA Exchange staff later agrees to adopt. A sometimes homeless mother of three, Dixon ran out of ARV pills when she left town to visit her mom. Tookes sees that Dixon urgently needs care and tells her they'll arrange a clinic visit and restart her on the drugs, along with helping her find a place to live. "I want to get my life back together," Dixon says. "This is crazy."

But the Florida health system's bureaucracy works against that sense of urgency. A few weeks later, when Dixon visits Tookes at his clinic, he says he cannot prescribe ARVs to her. Regulations stipulate that she first visit the county health department, meet with a case manager, and then enroll in the federally funded AIDS Drug Assistance Program before receiving treatment. Tookes attributes the breakdown to DOH policies, as well as Florida's decision to not accept the federal government's offer of "expanded" Medicaid, which makes it easier for low-income, younger people to receive care.

"There literally should be a conveyor belt, with a red carpet, to move her from the mobile unit into clinic with me sitting there smiling to welcome her into care," Tookes says. "She made a major first step by coming to see us at clinic, but the barriers within our system are almost insurmountable." Instead, after more than 6 weeks had passed, Dixon still was not back on medication.

Beal says his team recognizes that Florida must revamp its response. He's particularly buoyed by DOH's recent moves. The department has begun to use some new federal money and repurpose state funds to find patients lost to follow-up, make HIV testing a routine part of care, promote PrEP, and immediately offer newly infected people a free, 30-day supply of ARVs while they clear insurance hurdles.

Change is underway. Aside from the new PrEP mandate from the state surgeon general, HIV testing is becoming more routine after a law change that simplifies the consent process. "Disease intervention specialists" at DOH have begun to comb through databases to find and then contact people lost to follow-up. And even Tookes, who is sharply critical of the system in Florida, was heartened in late May when DOH started a new project with IDEA Exchange to rapidly offer treatment to people his team diagnoses.

It's early days. But once those barriers are knocked down, Beal says, "No one can really look me in the face in the state of Florida and say, 'I can't get the medicines I need.'" He does not expect to see an immediate decline in new infections. But, he says, "Hopefully, by 2019, we will."

Section IV

Global Impact

4.1

The Global HIV/AIDS Epidemic

Kaiser Family Foundation

Key Facts

- HIV, the virus that causes AIDS (acquired immunodeficiency syndrome), is one of the world's most serious health and development challenges. Approximately 38 million people are currently living with HIV, and tens of millions of people have died of AIDS-related causes since the beginning of the epidemic.
- Many people living with HIV or at risk for HIV infection do not have access to prevention, treatment, and care, and there is still no cure.
- In recent decades, major global efforts have been mounted to address the epidemic, and despite challenges, significant progress has been made in addressing HIV.

[...]

Global Response

HIV, the virus that causes AIDS (see box), has become one of the world's most serious health and development challenges since the first cases were reported in 1981. Approximately 76 million people have become infected with HIV since the start of the epidemic.[1] Today, there are approximately 38 million people currently living with HIV, and tens of millions of people have died of AIDS-related causes since the beginning of the epidemic.[2]

[...]

Over the past two decades, in particular, major global efforts have been mounted to address the epidemic, and significant progress has been made. The number of people newly infected with HIV, especially children, and the number of AIDS-related deaths have declined over the years, and the number of people with HIV receiving treatment increased to 25.4 million in 2019.[3]

Still, remaining challenges continue to complicate HIV control efforts. Many people living with HIV or at risk for HIV infection do not have access to prevention, treatment, and care, and there is still no cure. HIV primarily affects those in their most productive years, and it not only affects the health of individuals, but also impacts households, communities, and the development and economic growth of nations. Many of the countries hardest hit by HIV also face serious challenges due to other infectious diseases, food insecurity, and additional global health and development problems. In addition, as COVID-19 continues to spread globally, its detrimental effects on the HIV/AIDS response in low- and middle-income countries have already been seen, including disruptions in access to antiretroviral medicines and preventive services.[4] While the full impact of COVID-19 on HIV services and progress remains to be seen, it is estimated that such interruptions could result in many more additional HIV-related deaths.[5]

Latest Estimates[6]

- Global prevalence among adults (the percent of people ages 15–49 who are infected) has leveled since 2001 and was 0.7% in 2019 (see Figure 4.1.1.).
- There were **38 million** people living with HIV in 2019 (see Table 4.1.1.), up from 30.7 million in 2010, the result of continuing new infections and people living longer with HIV. Of the people living with HIV in 2018, 36.2 million were adults and 1.8 million were children under age 15.
- Although HIV testing capacity has increased over time, enabling more people to learn their HIV status, about **one in five** people with HIV (19%) are still unaware they are infected.
- Although there have been significant declines in new infections since the mid-1990s, there were still about **1.7 million** new infections in 2019, or about 5,000 new infections per day.

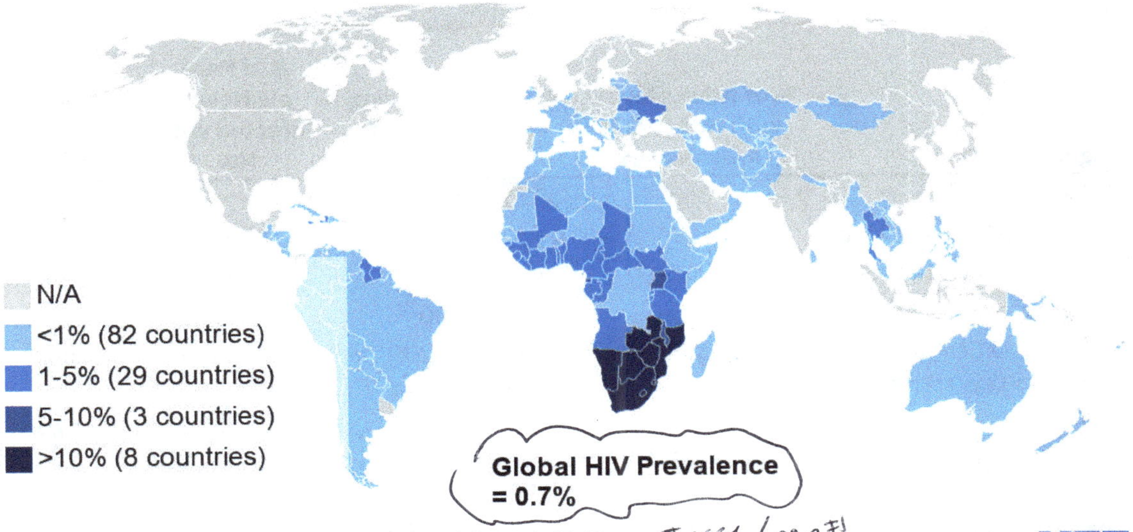

NOTE: Data are estimates. Prevalence includes adults ages 15-49
SOURCE: KFF, based on UNAIDS, AIDSInfo, Accessed December 2020.

FIGURE 4.1.1 Adult HIV Prevalence, 2020

Recent data show that while progress has been made, that progress is unequal within and between countries.[7] Furthermore, the pace of decline varies by age group, sex, and region.

- HIV remains a leading cause of death worldwide and the leading cause of death globally among women of reproductive age.[8] However, AIDS-related deaths have declined, due in part to antiretroviral treatment (ART) scale-up. **690,000** people died of AIDS in 2019, a 37% decrease from 1.1 million in 2010 and a 59% decrease from the peak of 1.7 million in 2004.

Affected Areas

Sub-Saharan Africa,[9] with more than two-thirds of all people living with HIV globally, is the hardest hit region in the world, followed by Asia and the Pacific (see Table 4.1.1). The Caribbean as well as Eastern Europe and Central Asia are also heavily affected.

- **Eastern and Southern Africa.** An estimated 20.7 million people are living with HIV in Eastern and Southern Africa, more than half (54%) of all people living with HIV. Two-thirds of children living with HIV (67%) are found in this region. Despite the significant impact, new infections in the region have declined by 38% since 2010. Almost all of the region's nations have generalized HIV epidemics—that is, their national HIV prevalence is greater than 1%. South Africa has the highest number of people living with HIV in the world (7.5 million). Eswatini (formerly known as Swaziland) has the highest prevalence in the world (27%).
- **Western and Central Africa.** An estimated 4.9 million people are living with HIV in Western and Central Africa. New HIV infections among adults declined by 25% between 2010 and 2019. Women and girls account for 58% of the estimated 240,000 new HIV infections in the region. Another issue facing the region is coverage of antiretroviral therapy for pregnant women, which has been declining in recent years (from 62% in 2016 to 58% in 2019).

TABLE 4.1.1 Snapshot of Global Epidemic Today, by Region

Region	% of Adults Living with HIV (Adult Prevalence)	# of People Living with HIV (% of Global Total)	# of People Newly Infected with HIV	# of AIDS-Related Deaths
Global, Total	0.7%	38.0 million (100%)	1.7 million	690,000
Eastern and Southern Africa	6.7%	20.7 million (54%)	730,000	300,000
Western and Central Africa	1.4%	4.9 million (13%)	240,000	140,000
Asia and the Pacific	0.2%	5.8 million (15%)	300,000	160,000
Western and Central Europe and North America	0.2%	2.2 million (6%)	65,000	12,000
Latin America	0.4%	2.1 million (6%)	120,000	37,000
Eastern Europe and Central Asia	0.9%	1.7 million (4%)	170,000	35,000
The Caribbean	1.1%	330,000 (<1%)	13,000	6,900
Middle East and North Africa	<0.1%	240,000 (<1%)	20,000	8,000

Notes: Reflects 2019 data.

Sources: UNAIDS. AIDSinfo *website; accessed July 2020. UNAIDS.* Core Epidemiology Slides; *July 2020.*

- **Asia and the Pacific.** An estimated 5.8 million people are living with HIV in Asia and the Pacific. The region's annual number of new HIV infections declined by 12% since 2010. However, trends vary from country to country, and the decline in the region may obscure increases in some countries. The region is also home to the two most populous nations in the world—China and India—and even relatively low prevalence translates into large numbers of people.
- **Western and Central Europe and North America.** An estimated 2.2 million people are living with HIV in this region. High coverage of ART plays a key role in the reduction of AIDS-related deaths in the region; since 2010, the number of AIDS-related deaths decreased by 40%. 4 in 5 people living with HIV (81%) are on treatment, and 2 in 3 people living with HIV (67%) are virally suppressed.
- **Latin America.** An estimated 2.1 million people are living with HIV in Latin America. Between 2010 and 2019, new HIV infections increased by 21% while the number of AIDS-related deaths fell by 8% in the region overall. In 2019, 40% of new HIV infections in Latin America occurred in Brazil, which has the greatest number of people living with the disease (920,000) in the region.
- **Eastern Europe and Central Asia.** An estimated 1.7 million people are living with HIV in this region, including 170,000 newly infected in 2019. New HIV infections in the region increased by 72% and AIDS-related deaths increased by 24% between 2010 and 2019. Most of the new infections (99%) in the region are among key populations and their sexual partners, including 48% of infections occurring among people who inject drugs.
- **The Caribbean.** An estimated 330,000 people are living with HIV in the Caribbean. The number of people living with HIV on treatment more than doubled since 2010 (from 68,000 in 2010 to approximately 210,000 in 2019). However, the percentage of people living with HIV who have suppressed viral loads in the region (50%) is below the global average (59%).
- **Middle East and North Africa.** An estimated 240,000 people are living with HIV in the Middle East and North Africa. New infections increased by 25% from 2010 to 2019, while AIDS-related deaths remained stable. Treatment coverage among people living with HIV in this region is 38%, the lowest of any region.

Affected/Vulnerable Populations

- Most HIV infections are transmitted heterosexually, although risk factors vary. In some countries, men who have sex with men, people who inject drugs, sex workers, transgender people, and prisoners are disproportionally affected by HIV.
- Women represent over half (55%) of all adults (15–49 years) living with HIV worldwide, and HIV (along with complications related to pregnancy) is the leading cause of death among women of reproductive age.[10] Gender inequalities, differential access to service, and sexual violence increase women's vulnerability to HIV, and women, especially younger women, are biologically more susceptible to HIV.
- Young people, ages 15–24, account for approximately a third of new HIV infections, and in some areas, young women are disproportionally impacted. In sub-Saharan Africa, among

adults age 15 and older, young women ages 15–24 accounted for 19% of new HIV infections in the region in 2019.

- Globally, children account for 1.8 million people living with HIV; among children, there were 95,000 AIDS-related deaths and 150,000 new infections in 2019. Since 2010, new HIV infections among children have declined by 52%.

HIV & TB

HIV has led to a resurgence of tuberculosis (TB), particularly in Africa, and TB is a leading cause of death for people with HIV worldwide.[11] In 2019, approximately 9% of new TB cases occurred in people living with HIV.[12] However, between 2000 and 2019, TB deaths in people living with HIV declined substantially, largely due to the scale up of joint HIV/TB services. (See the KFF fact sheet on TB.)

Prevention and Treatment[13]

Numerous **prevention** interventions exist to combat HIV, and new tools such as vaccines, are currently being researched.[14]

- Effective prevention strategies include behavior change programs, condoms, HIV testing, blood supply safety, harm reduction efforts for injecting drug users, and male circumcision.
- Additionally, recent research has shown that engagement in HIV treatment not only improves individual health outcomes but also significantly reduces the risk of transmission (referred to as "treatment as prevention" or TasP). Those with undetectable viral loads (known as being virally suppressed) have effectively no risk of transmitting HIV sexually.[15]
- Pre-exposure prophylaxis (PrEP) has also been shown to be an effective HIV prevention strategy in individuals at high risk for HIV infection. In 2015, the World Health Organization (WHO) recommended PrEP as a form of prevention for high-risk individuals in combination with other prevention methods.[16] Further, in 2016, the U.N. Political Declaration on HIV/AIDS stated PrEP research and development should be accelerated.[17]
- Experts recommend that prevention be based on "knowing your epidemic" (tailoring prevention to the local context and epidemiology), using a combination of prevention strategies, bringing programs to scale, and sustaining efforts over time. Access to prevention, however, remains limited, and there have been renewed calls for the strengthening of prevention efforts.[18]

HIV **treatment** includes the use of combination antiretroviral therapy (ART) to attack the virus itself, and medications to prevent and treat the many opportunistic infections that can occur when the immune system is compromised by HIV. In light of recent research findings, WHO released a guideline in 2015 recommending starting HIV treatment earlier in the course of illness.[19]

- Combination ART, first introduced in 1996, has led to dramatic reductions in morbidity and mortality, and access has increased in recent years, rising to 25.4 million people (67% of people living with HIV) in 2019.
- The percentage of pregnant women receiving ART for the prevention of mother-to-child transmission of HIV increased to 85% in 2019, up from 45% in 2010.

- Access to ART among children has more than doubled since 2010, with treatment coverage rising from 18% in 2010 to 53% in 2019.
- Approximately 59% of all people living with HIV are virally suppressed, which means they are likely healthier and less likely to transmit the virus. Viral suppression varies greatly by region, key population, and sex.

Global Goals

[...]

- **UNAIDS targets to end the epidemic by 2030.** On World AIDS Day 2014, UNAIDS set targets aimed at ending the AIDS epidemic by 2030. To achieve this, countries had been working toward reaching the interim "90-90-90" targets—90% of people living with HIV knowing their HIV status; 90% of people who know their HIV positive status on treatment; and 90% of people on treatment with suppressed viral loads—by 2020.[20] However, gains that were achieved in some countries and regions were unequal, and these targets were missed. Based on the 2019 data and trends (the latest data available),[21] 81% of people living with HIV knew their status; among those who knew their status, 82% were accessing treatment; and among those accessing treatment, 88% were virally suppressed.[22] The focus now is on reaching "95-95-95" (or, 95% of people living with HIV knowing their HIV status; 95% of people who know their HIV positive status on treatment; and 95% of people on treatment with suppressed viral loads). Additional interim targets have also been set for 2025, which place a greater emphasis on societal aspects and social services to address the inequalities of HIV.[23]

[...]

Endnotes

1. UNAIDS. *Global HIV & AIDS statistics—2020 fact sheet*, July 2020.
2. UNAIDS. 2020 *Global AIDS Update: Seizing the Moment;* July 2020. UNAIDS. *AIDSinfo website*; accessed July 2020, available at: http://aidsinfo.unaids.org/. UNAIDS. *Core Epidemiology Slides*; July 2020.
3. UNAIDS. 2020 *Global AIDS Update: Seizing the Moment;* July 2020.
4. UNAIDS. *Press release: UNAIDS report on the global AIDS epidemic shows that 2020 targets will not be met because of deeply unequal success; COVID-19 risks blowing HIV progress way off course;* July 2020.
5. UNAIDS. 2020 *Global AIDS Update: Seizing the Moment;* July 2020. UNAIDS. *Press release: UNAIDS report on the global AIDS epidemic shows that 2020 targets will not be met because of deeply unequal success; COVID-19 risks blowing HIV progress way off course;* July 2020. Global Fund. *Results Report* 2020; September 2020. UNAIDS. *COVID-19 and HIV: 1 Moment, 2 Epidemics, 3 Opportunities*, September 2020.
6. UNAIDS. 2020 *Global AIDS Update: Seizing the Moment;* July 2020. UNAIDS. *AIDSinfo website*; accessed July 2020, http://aidsinfo.unaids.org/. UNAIDS. *Core Epidemiology Slides*; July 2020. UNAIDS. *Global HIV & AIDS statistics—2020 fact sheet*; July 2020; UNAIDS. *UNAIDS data 2020, July 2020.*
7. UNAIDS. *Press release: UNAIDS report on the global AIDS epidemic shows that 2020 targets will not be met because of deeply unequal success; COVID-19 risks blowing HIV progress way off course;* July 2020.

8. UNAIDS. *Women and HIV—A spotlight on adolescent girls and young women*, March 2019.
9. Sub-Saharan Africa constitutes as East and Southern Africa and West and Central Africa.
10. UNAIDS. *2020 Global AIDS Update: Seizing the Moment;* July 2020. UNAIDS. *UNAIDS 2016–2021 Strategy*; Aug. 2015.
11. WHO. Tuberculosis, fact sheet, http://www.who.int/mediacentre/factsheets/fs104/en/index.html.
12. WHO. *Global tuberculosis report*; 2020.
13. UNAIDS. *2020 Global AIDS Update: Seizing the Moment;* July 2020. UNAIDS. *AIDSinfo website*; accessed July 2020, http://aidsinfo.unaids.org/. UNAIDS. *Core Epidemiology Slides*; July 2020. UNAIDS. *Global HIV & AIDS statistics—2020 fact sheet*; July 2020; UNAIDS. *UNAIDS data 2020, July 2020.*
14. UNAIDS. 2020 *Global AIDS Update;* July 2020. UNAIDS. *Get on the Fast Track*; 2016. Global HIV Prevention Working Group. *Behavior Change for HIV Prevention: (Re) Considerations for the 21st Century*; Aug. 2008.
15. UNAIDS. *UNAIDS Explainer: Undetectable = untransmittable*; July 2018.
16. WHO. *Guideline on When to Start antiretroviral Therapy and on Pre-Exposure Prophylaxis for HIV*; Sept. 2015. WHO. *WHO expands recommendation on oral pre-exposure prophylaxis of HIV infection (PrEP);* Nov. 2015.
17. United Nations. *Political Declaration on HIV and AIDS: On the Fast-Track to Accelerate the Fight Against HIV and to End the AIDS Epidemic by 2030;* June 8, 2016.
18. UNAIDS. *2020 Global AIDS Update;* July 2020. United Nations. *Reinvigorating the AIDS response to catalyse sustainable development and United Nations reform: Report of the Secretary-General.* June 2017.
19. UNAIDS. *Get on the Fast Track*; 2016. WHO. *Guideline on When to Start antiretroviral Therapy and on Pre-Exposure Prophylaxis for HIV*; September 2015. WHO. *Press Release: NIAID START Trial confirms that immediate treatment of HIV with antiretroviral drugs (ARVs) protects the health of people living with HIV*; May 28, 2015. NIAID. *Starting Antiretroviral Treatment Early Improves Outcomes for HIV-Infected Individuals*; May 27, 2015.
20. These goals and targets were reiterated in the UNAIDS 2016–2021 Strategy, which also aligns with the SDGs. UNAIDS. *Fast-Track: ending the AIDS epidemic by 2030*; 2014. UNAIDS. *UNAIDS 2016–2021 Strategy*; Aug. 2015.
21. UNAIDS. *2020 Global AIDS Update;* July 2020. KFF. *Assessing Global HIV Targets in PEPFAR Countries: A Dashboard*, February 2021.
22. UNAIDS. *Global HIV & AIDS statistics—2020 fact sheet*; July 2020.
23. UNAIDS. *Press Release: UNAIDS calls on countries to step up global action and proposes bold new HIV targets for 2025*; November 26, 2020. UNAIDS. "2025 AIDS Targets," webpage, https://aidstargets2025.unaids.org/#. UNAIDS. *World AIDS Day Report 2020: Prevailing Against Pandemics by Putting People at the Centre*; November 2020.

[...]

4.2

Facts and Figures

HIV and AIDS

UN Women

Prevalence and New Infections

- Globally, in 2016 there were an estimated 17.8 million women living with HIV (15 and older), constituting 52 percent of all adults living with HIV[1].
- Young women and adolescent girls aged 15–24 are particularly affected. Globally, in 2016 there were an estimated 2.4 million adolescent girls and young women living with HIV, that constitute 61 percent of all young people living with HIV (15–24) [2].
- In 2016, of the total estimated 1.7 million new HIV infections among adults (15 and older) globally, 790,000 or 48 percent were among women [3].
- 59 percent of new HIV infections among young persons aged 15–24 in 2016 occurred among adolescent girls and young women [4].
- There are significant regional differences in both the new HIV infections among women and in the proportion of women living with HIV (15 and older) as opposed to men, and the gaps are even more notable among young women (aged 15–24) versus young men:
    - In sub-Saharan Africa, women comprised 56 percent of new infections among adults (15 and older); and the proportion was higher among young women aged 15–24, who made up 67 percent of new infections among young people.
    - In the Caribbean, women represented 45 percent of newly infected adults; while young women aged 15–24 made up 52 percent of new infections.

---

1 UNAIDS, 2017 estimates from the AIDSinfo online database. Additional disaggregations correspond to unpublished estimates for 2016 provided by UNAIDS, obtained from country-specific models of their AIDS epidemics.

2 ibid.

3 ibid.

4 ibid.

- In Eastern Europe and Central Asia, women accounted for 42 percent of new HIV infections; however, among young women aged 15–24, the numbers reached a staggering 57 percent of new infections.
- In the Middle East and North Africa, women comprised 38 percent of newly infected adults; whereas young women aged 15–24 made up 49 percent of new infections.
- In Latin America, women represented 28 percent of those newly infected; while young women aged 15–24 made up 36 percent of new infections.
- In Asia-Pacific, women accounted for 31 percent of new infections; as the numbers reached 39 percent among young women aged 15–24.
- In Western and Central Europe and North America, women comprise 23 percent of new infections; while the numbers were higher for young women aged 15–24, with 31 percent of new infections. [5]

- Specific groups of women are disproportionately affected by HIV. An analysis of studies measuring the pooled prevalence of HIV in 50 countries estimated that, globally, female sex workers are approximately 14 times more likely to be infected than other women of reproductive age [6].
- Based on data reported by 30 countries, the pooled HIV prevalence among women who inject drugs was 13 percent compared with 9 percent among men who inject drugs [7].

Factors that Fuel HIV

- Violence against women and girls increases their risk of acquiring HIV. [8] A study in South Africa found that the association of intimate partner violence and HIV was stronger in the presence of controlling behaviour and high HIV prevalence. [9]
- In some settings up to 45 percent of adolescent girls report that their first sexual experience was forced. [10]

---

5 ibid.

6 Stefan Baral et al. (15 March 2012) "Burden of HIV among female sex workers in low-income and middle-income countries: a systematic review and meta-analysis", *The Lancet Infectious Diseases*, vol. 12, No. 7. p. 542.

7 UNAIDS (2014) *The Gap Report*, p. 175.

8 R. Jewkes et al. (2006) "Factors Associated with HIV Sero-Status in Young Rural South African Women: Connections between Intimate Partner Violence and HIV," International Journal of Epidemiology, 35, p. 1461–1468; R. Jewkes, 2010, "HIV/AIDS. Gender inequities must be addressed in prevention," *Science* 329(5988), p. 145–147; J. Silverman et al., 2008. "Intimate Partner Violence and HIV Infection among Married Indian Women," JAMA 300(6), p. 703–710; R. Stephenson, 2007, "Human Immunodeficiency Virus and Domestic Violence: The Sleeping Giants of Indian Health?" Indian Journal of Medical Sciences, 61(5), p. 251–252; K. L. Dunkle et al., 2004. "Gender-Based Violence, Relationship Power, and Risk of HIV Infection in Women Attending Antenatal Clinics in South Africa," Lancet, 363 (9419), p. 1415–1421; and L. Manfrin-Ledet and D. Porche, 2003. "The State of Science: Violence and HIV Infection in Women," *Journal of the Association of Nurses in AIDS Care*, 14(6), p. 56–68.

9 UNAIDS (2015) World AIDS Day 2015 report *On the Fast-Track to end AIDS by 2030: Focus on Location and Population*, p. 76 ; and Durevall D (2015) "Intimate partner violence and HIV in ten sub-Saharan African countries: what do the Demographic and Health Surveys tell us?" Lancet Glob Health 2015 Volume 3, No. 1: p. e41 Published online 21 November 2014.

10 UNAIDS (2014) *The Gap Report* p. 135.

- Worldwide more than 700 million women alive today were married before their eighteenth birthday. [11] They often have limited access to prevention information and limited power to protect themselves from HIV infection.
- Globally, only 3 in every 10 adolescent girls and young women aged 15–24 years have comprehensive and accurate knowledge about HIV. [12] The lack of information on HIV prevention and the power to use this information in sexual relationships, including in the context of marriage, undermines women's ability to negotiate condom use and engage in safer sex practices.
- Women living with HIV are more likely to experience violence, [13] including violations of their sexual and reproductive rights. [14] Involuntary and coerced sterilization and forced abortion among women living with HIV has been reported in at least 14 countries worldwide. [15]
- Women's access to property and inheritance rights can be critical in preventing HIV. A baseline study conducted in nine countries (Cameroon, Ghana, Kenya, Malawi, Nigeria, Rwanda, United Republic of Tanzania, Uganda, and Zimbabwe) found that stigma associated with HIV-positive status was a significant deterrent to reporting or pursuing property and inheritance rights violations. [16]
- Legal norms directly affect women's risk of acquiring HIV.[17] In many countries where women are most at risk, laws to protect them are weak[18]. A lack of legal rights reinforces the subordinate status of women, especially in relation to women's rights to divorce, to own and inherit property, to enter into contracts, to sue and testify in court, to consent to medical treatment and to open a bank account.[19]
- Discriminatory criminalization laws linked to HIV can disproportionately affect women, as they are more likely to be tested and know their status through antenatal care. [20] HIV-positive mothers are criminals under all of the HIV laws of West and Central Africa, which explicitly or implicitly forbid them from being pregnant or breastfeeding, lest they transmit the virus to the fetus or child.[21]

---

11 UNICEF (2014) *Ending child marriage: progress and prospects.*

12 UNAIDS (2015) World AIDS Day 2015 report *On the Fast-Track to end AIDS by 2030: Focus on Location and Population*, p. 75.

13 WHO and UNAIDS (2010) Addressing violence against women and HIV/AIDS: What works?, p. 33.

14 UNAIDS (2012) *Together We Will End AIDS*, p. 73.

15 UNAIDS (2014) *The Gap Report* p. 127.

16 UN Women (2014) Fact Sheet: Promoting the Legal Empowerment of Women in the Context of HIV/AIDS

17 "Advancing Human Rights and Access to Justice for Women and Girls", *What works for women and girls.*

18 Stella Mukasa and Anne Gathumbi (2008) HIV, Human Rights and Legal Services in Uganda: A Country Assessment, New York, Open Society Institute; Tamar Ezer, Kate Kerr, Kara Major, Aparna Polavarapu and Tina Tolentino (2006) "Child Marriage and Guardianship in Tanzania: Robbing Girls of their Childhood and Infantilizing Women," Georgetown Journal of Gender and Law, 7(357), p. 362; and Tama Ezer, Aisha Glasford, Elizabeth Hollander, Lakeisha Poole, Grant Rabenn and Alexandria Tindall (2007) "International Women's Human Rights Clinic Report: Divorce Reform: Rights Protection in the New Swaziland," *Georgetown Journal of Gender and Law*, 8(883), p. 889.

19 "Advancing Human Rights and Access to Justice for Women and Girls", *What works for women and girls.*

20 International Planned Parenthood Federation, ICW Global, GIZ, UNAIDS and the Global Coalition of Women and AIDS (2011) *Piecing it Together for Women and Girls: The Gender Dimension of HIV-related Stigma—Evidence from Bangladesh, the Dominican Republic and Ethiopia.*

21 Global Commission on HIV and the Law (2012) *Risks, Rights, and Health*, p. 23.

The Response to HIV

- At 46 percent, global coverage of antiretroviral therapy had reached 17 million people at the end of 2015. Gains were greatest in the world's most-affected region, Eastern and Southern Africa.[22]
- Globally, 77 percent of pregnant women have been accessing antiretroviral medicines to prevent mother-to-child transmission of HIV.[23] Still, more than half of the UNAIDS Global Plan's 21 priority countries are failing to meet the needs for family planning among at least 25 percent of all married women.[24]
- Governments increasingly recognize the importance of gender equality in national HIV responses. However, only 57 percent (of 104 reporting countries) included a specific budget.[25]
- The Global Fund to Fight AIDS, Tuberculosis and Malaria increased expenditure benefiting women and girls from 42 percent of its total portfolio in 2013 to approximately 60 percent in 2015. Much of the increase was in the areas of reproductive, maternal, newborn, child and adolescent health.[26]

In 2015, 39.2 percent of the Global Fund Country Coordinating Mechanisms members in implementing countries were women, an increase from 33.9 percent in 2010.[27] These data do not, however, offer an indication of the impact of women's voices in such mechanisms.[28]

---

22 UNAIDS (2016) *Global AIDS Up-date 2016*, p. 1, 3.

23 UNAIDS (2016) Factsheet 2016, p. 8.

24 UNAIDS (2014) *The Gap Report*, p. 42.

25 UNAIDS (2015) Report on the *UNAIDS 2014–2015 results, accountability and budget matrix* (UNAIDS/PCB(32)/13.9), p. 52.

26 See http://www.theglobalfund.org/en/financials and http://www.theglobalfund.org/en/womengirls/

27 See http://www.theglobalfund.org/en/womengirls/

28 UN Secretary-General (23 December 2015) Report of the Secretary-General *Women, the girl child and HIV and AIDS*, p. 10.

Women and Girls and HIV

UNAIDS, 2017

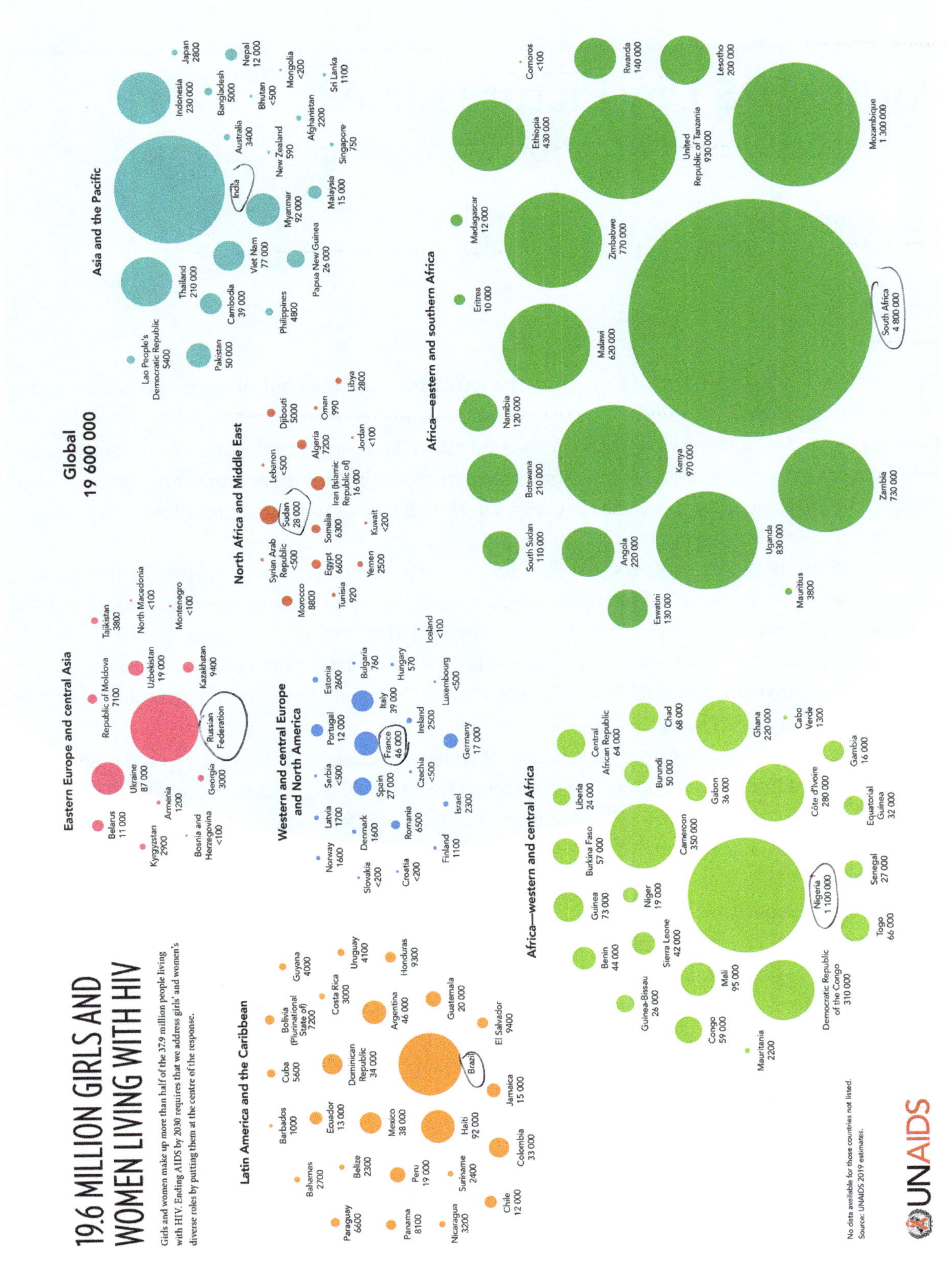

4.4

World AIDS Day Picture Mixed

Researchers Note Major Progress, Looming Challenges

Michael Smith

On world AIDS day 2017, the picture of the pandemic is somewhat brighter—but with some ominous shadows.

On the bright side, more people than ever are on anti-HIV therapy and work continues apace on improving medications and developing new preventive methods, including two important vaccine trials. In the U.S. the CDC reported this week that delays in HIV diagnosis—an important factor in propagation of the virus—are shrinking.

In the shadows, new data suggests that HIV resistance to some drugs is rising rapidly in low- and middle-income countries, which might affect the success of therapy. In many countries, men with HIV are less likely than women to be diagnosed, on therapy, and in control of their virus. And in one developed country, the Russian Federation, the epidemic is expanding, rather than contracting.

The theme of this year's World AIDS Day is "Let's End it" but that's easier said than done, according to three well-known researchers.

"The aspirational slogan ... suggests that the goal of ending the epidemic is in our grasp and hinges only on our collective commitment to do so," argued Steven Deeks, M.D., of the University of California San Francisco, Sharon Lewin, M.D., of the Peter Doherty Institute of Infection and Immunity in Melbourne, Australia, and Linda-Gail Bekker, MBChB, Ph.D., of the Desmond Tutu HIV Centre in Cape Town, South Africa.

"However, the remarkable progress, activism, resources, ingenuity, and sheer fortitude that have brought us this far will be needed in at least equal measure to take us to the end," they concluded in a special HIV issue of *PLoS Medicine*.

That "remarkable progress" includes the largest-ever number of people with HIV who have access to therapy—some 20.9 million people in July, according to the Joint United Nations Programme on HIV/AIDS (UNAIDS). That's about 53% of the estimated 36.7 million people living with HIV around the world.

The latest data from UNAIDS also suggests that the rate of new infections is down and—a reflection, perhaps, of the increasing numbers on treatment—so is AIDS-related mortality.

"The significance of these achievements cannot be overstated," Deeks, Lewin, and Bekker wrote. "In the past three decades, global biomedical and public health programs not only discovered how HIV causes disease and developed effective strategies to prevent and treat the infection, but also built a global public health response that is unprecedented in its scale and effectiveness."

But many gaps remain, including an important "blind spot," according to UNAIDS Executive Director Michel Sidibé, speaking in Ottawa today. "Men are not using services to prevent HIV or to test for HIV and are not accessing treatment on the scale that women are," he said in a statement.

In a report released on World AIDS Day—dubbed "The Blind Spot"—the UN agency said that fewer than half the men living with HIV are on treatment, compared to 60% of women, and there is evidence that they are more likely than women to start therapy late, to interrupt treatment, and to be lost to follow-up.

Health officials have found ways to reach women at risk of HIV—in antenatal clinics, for instance—but have struggled to find similar ways of reaching men, the report says. Some results of that gap:

- Men and boys accounted for about 58% of the estimated 1.0 million AIDS-related deaths in 2016. The imbalance was worse in sub-Saharan Africa, where men and boys accounted for 41% of people living with HIV and 53% of AIDS-related deaths.
- Outside of eastern and southern Africa, 60% of all new HIV infections among adults are among men.
- Men who have sex with men (MSM) are 24 times more likely to catch HIV than men in the general population; HIV prevalence among MSM is 15% or higher in some two dozen countries.
- Some 80% of injection drug users are men and in several countries HIV prevalence among people who inject drugs exceeds 25%.
- In prisons, HIV prevalence is estimated at between 3% and 8%; some 90% of inmates are men.

In general, HIV epidemics grow in marginalized and vulnerable groups that lack society's attention and are often denied access to important healthcare interventions. A current case in point is the Russian Federation, according to Chris Beyrer, M.D., of Johns Hopkins Bloomberg School of Public Health in Baltimore, and colleagues.

While it's difficult to pin down the numbers, the Russian Federation is thought to have the largest number of HIV infected citizens of any country in Europe, Beyrer and colleagues reported in *PLoS Medicine.*

"Actual infections, including those that remain undiagnosed and/or unreported, are doubtless substantially higher," they wrote, and the epidemic in Russia "continues to expand significantly." More than 103,000 new HIV diagnoses were reported in 2016, up 5% from the previous year and AIDS deaths are also rising: 14,631 were reported from January to June 2017, up 13.5% over the previous six months.

Official figures for 2016 suggest that injection drug use accounts for 48.8% of infections, followed by heterosexual sex at 48.7% and homosexual sex at 1.5%, with a handful of perinatal infections.

"These proportions are of uncertain validity, however," Beyrer and colleagues noted. In particular, laws that ban the sharing of information related to homosexuality, as well as official support for stigma towards MSM, are "highly likely to affect these results," they wrote.

The range of interventions that have been shown to reduce the spread of HIV includes opioid agonist substitution therapy (such as methadone), needle and syringe exchanges, HIV treatment as prevention, and pre-exposure prophylaxis (PrEP), among others, they wrote.

But in Russia, "all of these interventions are either not available or are unavailable at the scale necessary to control HIV," they concluded, adding that the Russian epidemic is "a true public health crisis and one that could largely have been avoided."

Another issue that has experts concerned is HIV drug resistance.

Anti-HIV medications attempt to prevent viral replication but the virus, which is highly adaptable, can quickly evolve ways around the drugs unless they are consistently taken as directed—so-called acquired resistance.

Especially worrisome is what is called pretreatment resistance, meaning a new HIV infection is already resistant to some drugs even before the patient has begun therapy.

In an analysis of data from low- and middle-income countries, researchers found that pretreatment resistance to one class of drugs—the non-nucleoside reverse transcriptase inhibitors (NNRTIs)—has been rising sharply.

The issue is particularly important because the NNRTIs are part of most first-line anti-HIV regimens in those countries, according to investigators led by Ravindra Gupta, M.D., of University College London in England.

In a systematic review and meta-regression analysis of 358 datasets, representing 56,044 adults in 63 countries, Gupta and colleagues estimate pretreatment NNRTI resistance in 2016 at about 10% in most regions—11% in southern Africa, 10.1% in eastern Africa, 7.2% in western and central Africa, and 9.4% in Latin America and the Caribbean.

Importantly, they reported online in *The Lancet Infectious Diseases*, the yearly odds of pretreatment resistance have been rising: 23% in southern Africa, 17% in eastern Africa, 17% in western and central Africa, 11% in Latin America and the Caribbean, and 11% in Asia.

"Treatment resistance indicators have turned to red in several countries," increasing the risk that first-line therapy with NNRTIs will no longer be effective, commented Sabine Yerly, Ph.D., and Alexandra Calmy, M.D., Ph.D., both of Geneva University Hospitals and Faculty of Medicine in Switzerland.

Changing the guidelines for first-line therapy will likely reduce the rates of pre-treatment resistance, but by itself will not be enough to prevent its recurrence, they argued in an accompanying commentary.

They argued that different drugs must be used and health authorities must ensure treatment for all people who need it, including those now excluded or disengaged from care, to prevent the emergence of resistance in the first place.

Meanwhile, the National Institute of Allergy and Infectious Diseases reported, just in time for World AIDS Day, that a new vaccine candidate is under test in Africa—the second major trial looking for what is regarded as the keystone of HIV prevention.

The so-called Imbokodo trial, a phase IIb proof-of-concept study, will enroll 2,600 HIV-negative women in sub-Saharan Africa to evaluate both safety and efficacy of the vaccine candidate. Earlier studies have shown it is safe in healthy volunteers.

The vaccine candidate being tested in Imbokodo is based on "mosaic" immunogens—vaccine components designed to induce immune responses against a wide variety of HIV strains.

That's different from the so-called HVTN 072 efficacy trial, which is currently testing a tweaked version of the vaccine regimen tested in the RV144 Thai trial—the only candidate HIV vaccine ever shown to provide some protection against the virus.

That candidate is actually two vaccines—a modified canarypox virus called ALVAC carries the HIV gag, env, and pro genes, while a second vaccine targets the HIV gp120 protein. In its first iteration, that vaccine reduced the risk of HIV infection by about 30%, although with wide confidence intervals; the HVTN investigators are hoping the changes they've made, including an adjuvant and an extra shot, will increase its efficacy.

While all this is going on, other investigators are investigating the potential of what are called "broadly neutralizing antibodies" to prevent HIV, although that work is in the early stages.

Adding an effective vaccine to current prevention strategies would have "potentially transformative benefits" in the fight against HIV, Deeks and colleagues argued.

Section V

Africa

5.1

The Blesser's Curse

How Sugar Daddies and Vaginal Microbes Created the World's Largest HIV Epidemic

Olga Khazan

VULINDLELA, SOUTH AFRICA—MBALI N. WAS JUST 17 when a well-dressed man in his 30s spotted her. She was at a mall in a nearby town, alone, when he called out. He might have been captivated by her almond eyes and soaring cheekbones. Or he might have just seen her for what she was: young and poor.

She tried to ignore him, she told me, but he followed her. They exchanged numbers. By the time she got home, he had called her. He said he wasn't married, and she doesn't know if that was true. They met at a house in a different township; she doesn't know if it belonged to him. Mbali, who is now 24, also doesn't know if he had HIV.

She enjoyed spending time with the man during the day, when they would talk and go to the movies. But she didn't like it when he called at night and demanded to have sex, which happened about six times a month. When she refused him, he beat her. For her trouble, he gave her a cellphone, sweets, and chocolates.

At the time, she had another boyfriend, who was her own age. The older man ordered her to leave the younger boy, and when she refused, he beat her again. Eventually, she grew tired of the abuse and ended the relationship.

Today, Mbali lives with her grandmother in Vulindlela, a verdant rural area near the eastern coast of South Africa, in the humid, hilly province of KwaZulu-Natal. Vulindlela means "open a way" in Zulu, but like many young women here, Mbali faces a lot of closed doors. She graduated high school but didn't have the money for college, so she spends most of her days helping her grandmother with housework and taking care of her 2-year-old son. I asked if her experience with her "blesser," as men who initiate transactional relationships are known here, prompted her to warn her friends against dating older men. She let out an exasperated little laugh.

"No!" she said. "They'll just say I'm so jealous."

Mbali is HIV negative. But 36 percent of the adults in Vulindlela are positive, as are about 60 percent of the women aged 25 to 40. Although HIV infection rates have stabilized globally, hundreds of thousands of South Africans are infected every year; more than 7 million live with the virus in their bodies. And in the midst of this, the largest HIV epidemic in the world, the HIV prevalence among adolescent girls is roughly five times greater than that of boys. By performing genetic analyses on samples of HIV virus in Vulindlela, researchers have concluded that the high rate of infections here—among both sexes—is driven in part by relationships like the one Mbali had when she was 17.

In a country where two-thirds of people under age 25 are unemployed, some poor South African women and teens date older, wealthier men, who provide them with everything from food to hairpieces to school uniforms. In exchange, the men demand discreet, often condom-free sex. At the same time, many of these young women maintain more egalitarian relationships with boys their own age. Some of the sugar daddies, as these men are also sometimes called, infect the girls with HIV. When those teen girls reach adulthood, they find husbands and pass their HIV onto them. Those husbands, in turn, become the next crop of sugar daddies, infecting the next generation of teen girls and perpetuating the cycle.

This cycle of contagion, researchers are finding, is driven not only by economics and culture but also by the human body's own microbes. The reproductive tract is home to a delicate balance of bacteria, some of which appear to keep HIV and other viruses at bay. The grooming practices some South African women use to entice wealthy boyfriends might be upsetting this balance, and increasing their risk of HIV infection.

***

Salim Abdool Karim, the epidemiology professor who is uncovering these connections, has a gray beard and enormous voice. When he was a student, everyone called him *Slim*, Afrikaans for "clever," and the name has stuck. He's of Indian descent, which meant that, under the country's apartheid-era racial code, he was funneled into the country's only medical school for nonwhites at the University of Natal, now known as the University of KwaZulu-Natal, in Durban. It's where he's worked off and on for more than three decades, and it's where he and his wife, the epidemiologist Quarraisha Abdool Karim, run the Center for the AIDS Program of Research in South Africa, or CAPRISA. They spend their days trying to figure out why, exactly, South Africans keep dying of a disease that much of the world has nearly forgotten.

In the early '80s, HIV was still relatively unknown in South Africa. Salim only realized the awful extent of the disease in 1987, when he moved to New York to study public health at Columbia University. It was a terrifying time: Around half a million people in the city had the virus, which was poorly understood. A prostitute who bit a policeman and claimed she had AIDS was walked into the courtroom by officers wearing surgical masks. "You couldn't escape HIV in New York," Salim told me in his office one day in February. In New York, it became clear to the Abdool Karims that HIV was about to ravage southern Africa.

He and Quarraisha returned to Durban and zoomed in on a puzzling trend: While many in the United States still viewed HIV as a gay men's disease, the South Africans with HIV were disproportionately young, heterosexual, and female. Though the disease was still relatively rare, girls were getting HIV five to seven years younger than their male counterparts. That, the Abdool Karims realized, meant young mothers would pass the infection onto their kids. A whole generation of nurses and teachers—the jobs dominated by women—might be wiped out. "Oh, my goodness," Salim thought. "This is a tragedy on a scale that we have yet to even grapple with."

Today, the virus kills more than 100,000 South Africans—roughly the population of Green Bay, Wisconsin—each year. While antiretroviral drugs, widely available for free in South Africa, can halt HIV's erosion of the immune system, there are simply too many South Africans with too high a risk of getting HIV for the country to treat its way out of the problem. Everyone seems to agree: Prevention is key.

In the '90s, the Abdool Karims began studying different substances that had the potential to prevent HIV infection, especially in women. For the most part, they were a bust: When they tested nonoxynol-9, a spermicide, in a small group of truck-stop sex workers, not only did it have no effect on infection rates, but the substance also inflamed the women's vaginas, causing burning and itching.

Their progress improved in 2003, when they began testing a drug called tenofovir, which prevents the virus from replicating and seemed to have few side effects. In 2010, Quarraisha presented the findings of their tenofovir gel study at the International AIDS Conference in Vienna: When women applied the gel to their vaginas before and after sex, she reported, the risk of HIV infection dropped by 39 percent. For the first time, women had a way to reduce their risk of HIV infection that didn't require their partners' permission. It was a rare glimmer of hope in what had become a dismal field, and the conference attendees rewarded Quarraisha with a standing ovation.

The Abdool Karims were elated and proud. But still, they wondered: Why *only* 39 percent?

***

In Vulindlela, women walk alongside dirt roads with babies slung on their backs, and people still answer to the three local *amakhosi*, or Zulu chiefs. Older people smear red clay on their skin to protect it from the sun. Horses and cows roam the streets freely, and outhouses dot the rolling hills. Today, most people live in small, cinder-block houses, but when CAPRISA first began doing research here in 2001, many still dwelled in traditional mud huts.

In the late 1800s, in KwaZulu-Natal and several other areas, the colonial government imposed a tax on every hut "occupied by a native." They exempted "houses of European construction" occupied by residents "conforming to civilized usage." The tax burden forced many Zulus to work in the gold mines, some of which were hundreds of miles away. Miners usually lived in single-sex hostels for much of the year, returning to see their families only every few months. Separated from their wives, the men turned to sex workers, who became vectors of sexually transmitted diseases.

"If you want to create a society in which you wanted a sexually transmitted infection to spread," Salim said, "you couldn't do it better than the way in which the colonialists designed South Africa. They designed it to create family instability."

Though the situation is less extreme now that apartheid has ended, itinerant labor remains common, and many men maintain multiple partners. Men who are able to get good jobs are sought after as patrons and partners by women who aren't.

Salim and his colleagues wanted to pinpoint exactly who was getting HIV in KwaZulu-Natal, and from whom. In 2014, CAPRISA staff collected blood from the residents of nearly 10,000 households in Vulindlela. They looked at the HIV viruses inside the samples and analyzed each virus's genes. They identified clusters in which people had passed the virus to one another.

They found that the girls in their teens and early 20s were getting infected by men who were, on average, about nine years older than they were. When they reached their late 20s, these women were infecting partners of their own age, who often didn't realize it right away. With wandering eyes and high levels of the virus coursing through their blood, some of the men were then infecting the next crop of 16- and 17-year-old girls.

About 40 percent of the men who were passing HIV to younger women had older, female partners at the same time. I wondered aloud to Salim how a society could become so overrun by sugar daddies when the consequences—for women and men—are so severe. What he guessed was this: In many cases, the girls' parents know about the blessers. "Many of them also support the girl's family," he said.

Gethwana Mahlase, a community leader in Vulindlela, told me that the poverty here used to be much worse, and the effects were often fatal. Under apartheid, the country's rural areas had little infrastructure, and the sick had to be carried to the hospital. In the 1980s and '90s, some women Mahlase knew had 16 children. They frequently died in childbirth from conditions like high blood pressure, which women in more affluent nations can typically survive with access to medical care.

Economic conditions have improved somewhat, but many people here and across South Africa are still sorely in need of jobs. Among the legacies of apartheid is one of the highest levels of income inequality on earth. On the beach in Durban, the largest city in KwaZulu-Natal, I saw a thin man pick a plastic bag out of a garbage can and lick off its residue—right next to a watchtower advertising the area as the Bay of Plenty. Many kids have no choice but to attend high schools where 60 students might cram into a classroom. Poor and middle-class families often don't have the means to pay for college and can't get loans.

"Girls here are happy to have a boyfriend from Johannesburg to take them out of poverty," Pamela Gumbi, a scientist at the Vulindlela CAPRISA clinic, told me. In the Valley of a Thousand Hills, a community not far from Vulindlela that looks exactly like its bucolic-sounding name, high schoolers told me local girls were dating the region's big earners: the drivers of minibus taxis.

The blesser trend shapes men's lives, too. In a village north of Vulindlela called KwaMsane, I talked with a group of men who were hanging out by a shipping-container snack store in the middle of the day, eating sugarcane as chickens pecked at the grass nearby. A 33-year-old named Zothani bemoaned the lack of local job opportunities, suggesting that leads to some of the sexual practices researchers and policy makers are trying so desperately to change. "The more time we are not working, the more people are giving birth, giving birth," he said.

Several young men told me that they worry girls won't want to date them unless they are able to buy them things—a modern anxiety layered on top of the Zulu custom of *lobola*, in which suitors pay a bride price of several head of cattle.

Others said they don't mind if their girlfriends have sugar daddies; they think they stand to benefit. "I'm unemployed, so if she has an extra relationship, that money supports me," said Sanele Ndlovu, a 20-year-old construction worker in Vulindlela, who was speaking hypothetically.

Like a few other men I talked to, Ndlovu is even starting to think he should try to find a sugar mama. The women are doing it, so why not? "There's nothing wrong with falling in love with an older woman," he said. "She's cute, she has no husband, so capitalize on the opportunity."

***

Almost as soon as the sugar-daddy trend became widely known in South Africa, it became oversimplified in the media and in popular imagination. There's a perception, among some here, that the women who seek out sugar daddies are vain and irresponsible. They want nice weaves—considered more fashionable than close-cropped natural hair—and clothes that will look stylish on Instagram, the thinking goes. That makes it easy to blame women for the consequences of promiscuity. "You take a decision to say, 'I will take off my clothes'—you just can never say it was a mistake," said the KwaZulu-Natal health minister, Sibongiseni Dhlomo, addressing a tent full of schoolkids in 2016. "Let there be no one who will say they don't know what happened when they fall pregnant ... Therefore, it is up to you to ensure that does not happen."

These stereotypes are reinforced by the rise of websites like BlesserFinder, which tries to connect sugar daddies with those hoping to be "blessed." (BlesserFinder was started by a man, according to news reports.)

My conversations with women who have had transactional sex, or who know those who have, revealed a more complicated picture. For one thing, the women who have blessers aren't very promiscuous. In CAPRISA's Vulindlela study, most people had fewer than five sex partners in their lifetimes. The average American Baby Boomer, by comparison, has had 11.

But the sex they *are* having is very risky. Many of the sugar daddies refuse to wear condoms, saying they "don't want to waste their money on plastic," as one teenager put it to me. Women avoid disclosing their HIV statuses to their sugar daddies out of fear they'll be cut off financially. Since many of the sugar daddies are married, young women meet them at hotels and don't tell their parents where they are, heightening their vulnerability to violence. In Pretoria, a 15-year-old was recently found dead in a pit latrine after telling her friends she had gone to meet an older man. The suspect, a 33-year-old man, had posted on Facebook that he wanted to find a curvy woman to bless.

The idea that women who have blessers are making bad choices also presumes that there are better choices available. I met A., a pretty, dark-skinned 31-year-old, in a cold, dark exam room of a clinic in Durban. She lives in Umlazi, a large township nearby. She calls it a place for "poor people," with too many *tsotsis*—criminals.

A. had a baby at 16 and dropped out of high school. She and the baby's father broke up because he beat her, she says, pointing to scars on her arms. She now has HIV, and when her mother found out she almost made her go to an *inyanga*, a traditional healer. She says no one ever told her about condoms. "We are Zulus. We don't talk about sex," was the attitude at home, she said.

A. is unemployed. For food, cellphone minutes, and things for her daughter, she turns to a new, older man she's dating, who she says "treats me well sometimes." He's married, and she feels bad when his wife calls to chew her out. "I'm dating this married guy because I get whatever I want," she says. Meanwhile, she's also dating a "poor guy, because he's the love of my life."

She's looking for a job as a housekeeper—a profession she likes because sometimes, her employers feed her. "Other jobs you have to bring your own food," she said, "which is not gonna happen because sometimes we have just sleeping food, and in the morning there's no food."

She and the older man, the blesser, don't use condoms, and she hasn't told him that she's HIV positive. Mostly, she's just hoping to start making her own money soon. "Life is not good for someone who is not employed," she said. "You sleep, watch TV, sleep, watch TV."

"Sometimes," she added, "I don't live my life."

At this, her eyes welled up with tears. A nurse standing nearby told me to stop my line of questioning.

***

Up the coast from Vulindlela, closer to the border with Swaziland, there's a poor, sleepy town called Mtubatuba. The most happening place to be is a club called the White House, a small cement building with a large outdoor patio. On a recent warm Friday night, a DJ spun Zulu dance music while groups of men and women stood around tables, drinking, dancing in place, and taking selfies.

It could have been college night anywhere on earth. The bouncer told me many girls here come with nothing and expect guys to buy them drinks all night. The girls might go home with the best-looking or most generous of their benefactors. But this, a practice familiar the world over, is not exactly "blessing."

I approached two 25-year-olds, Nkundu Matha and Thandeka Mathamulo, to ask if women look for blessers here. No, they said, the guys are mainly locals, without blesser-level jobs. If they did meet a blesser, I wondered, how would they react if he asked them to have sex without a condom? "Nice to see you and goodbye," Mathamulo said.

This attitude might help explain the results of a 2014 study of the area by scientists from Harvard University and the Africa Health Research Institute, who found no evidence that having an older male partner increased the risk of HIV infection.

Even though the blesser phenomenon is real, it seems its effects are uneven, and the country's HIV epidemic is shaped by other factors, too. Some of them, researchers are finding, are hidden within the women themselves.

In 2010, when the Abdool Karims got their standing ovation in Vienna, they were nevertheless confounded by the fact that the tenofovir gel didn't fully protect the women from HIV. They decided to investigate whether there was something about a woman's biology that increases her risk of contracting the virus.

In 2015, CAPRISA released a study in which it measured the cytokines—proteins that serve as markers of inflammation—in the vaginas of 889 women. They found that women who had more of these cytokines, and thus more inflammation, were three times more likely to get HIV over a three-year period. But where was this inflammation coming from? To find out, they sequenced the entire vaginal microbiomes of 120 women.

About 1,300 species of bacteria naturally occur in the vagina. A healthy vagina is dominated by a "good" germ called *Lactobacillus*, which, under a microscope, looks like a fistful of rod-shaped Mike and Ikes. It scrubs the genital tract with a mild acid and helps keep the "bad" bacteria to a minimum.

Gynecologists, hoping to dissuade their patients from douching, sometimes liken vaginas to self-cleaning ovens. But really, they are more like gardens that—for the most part, and in most women—weed themselves. Sometimes, though, they get overrun by invasive, pernicious flora. And that is where the trouble begins.

Prevotella bivia, it turned out, was the main source of the inflammation that leads to HIV infection. *Prevotella* is normally found in the gut, but it can migrate into the vagina from the anus. In small numbers, it can be fine. But it can also swarm the place, usurping the *Lactobacillus* and other healthy bacteria like dandelions taking over a rose garden. On *Prevotella*'s surface are lipopolysaccharides, which break off and spark inflammation. If a woman happens to get exposed to HIV during a *Prevotella* inflammation, her risk of infection is much higher.

The CAPRISA scientists decided to test another "bad" bacterium, *Gardnerella vaginalis,* typically associated with bacterial vaginosis, to see if it had an effect on tenofovir. (Bacterial vaginosis, as many women know, can resemble a yeast infection but must be treated with antibiotics.) Salim's colleagues added tenofovir to a culture of *Gardnerella*. Within four hours, about half the tenofovir was gone.

"We were doing these studies and wondering, 'Why is tenofovir not protecting these women?'" Salim said. "It's not protecting them because they've got *Gardnerella*, and the *Gardnerella* is eating up all the tenofovir!"

Today, tenofovir is an integral part of PrEP, or pre-exposure prophylaxis, a pill the South African government has made available for free to sex workers and some university students. Since the pill doesn't travel through the genital tract, PrEP might avoid being eroded by the vaginal microbiome, but the Abdool Karims and their colleagues aren't sure yet.

There's plenty of other evidence, however, that maintaining a healthy, *Lactobacillus*-dominant vaginal microbiome protects against HIV. One meta-analysis of 23 studies from 2008 found bacterial vaginosis was associated with a 60 percent higher risk of HIV infection. Just last month, the researchers at AHRI found an extraordinarily high rate of bacterial vaginosis—42 percent—among women in the region around Mtubatuba, where HIV is also widespread.

Currently, scientists at CAPRISA and elsewhere are studying what exactly causes *Prevotella* and *Gardnerella* to take over the vagina; they have found interesting associations, but no common thread. Women with high levels of *Prevotella* in their vaginas are more likely to be obese, and black and Hispanic women, regardless of nationality, are more likely to experience bacterial vaginosis. European women are more likely to have *Lactobacillus*-dominant vaginas than African women are. (Could this be why there's so much more HIV in Africa than in Europe? Researchers don't know.)

Semen, too, has a microbiome, and it's even less studied than its vaginal counterpart. But semen could be causing some of these vaginal disturbances: Semen contains lots of foreign proteins, and women's bodies become accustomed to those in their regular partner's semen. But if they are exposed to different proteins, say those in their sugar daddy's semen, "your body reacts like crazy," Salim says.

The Depo-Provera shot is the most common form of birth control among poor women here—largely because it's convenient, and because women with unsupportive partners can hide it from them. The problem, according to the CAPRISA scientists, is that Depo contains high amounts of progestin, which tamps down the levels of estrogen in the body. Because *Lactobacillus* flourishes in highly estrogenic environments, Depo may open the door to *Prevotella* and other "bad" bacteria.

Perhaps most damaging to the vaginal microbiome are the practices women use to please their blessers—or even just especially valuable boyfriends. A desirable vagina, many women here believe, is tight and dry. It's common for women to coax their nether regions into this state by stuffing them with various powders, ashes, and even chewing tobacco.

One study published in 2011 found that women who used "powders, creams, herbs, tablets, sticks, stones, leaves, and traditional products" to dry out or tighten their vaginas were 31 percent more likely to contract HIV. CAPRISA is now conducting a study to see if the increased risk is due to inflammation, vaginal-bacteria disturbances, or both.

Before I left CAPRISA, I met with another of its researchers, Sinaye Ngcapu, whose colleagues call him Dr. Healthy Vagina. While Salim and Quarraisha guide all the different facets of CAPRISA's work, Ngcapu strives to decode the vaginal microbiomes of African women. His goal is to design better HIV-prevention tools—ones that don't melt away in microbes' presence.

He grabbed an empty can of Coke Zero on the table to demonstrate why it's important to understand the microbiome if you want to stop HIV. "If you were to understand how this Coca-Cola is made, you will know how to get rid of the sugar that's inside it," he explained.

I paused to ask Ngcapu whether his enthusiasm for the vaginal microbiome ever raises eyebrows—at least among those outside the medical community.

Ngcapu is black, young, and a member of another South African ethnic group, the Xhosa, who live mainly in the country's south. HIV tore through Xhosa communities, too, and until very recently, apartheid kept people like Ngcapu from acquiring the skills necessary to halt that devastation. To him, this battle is personal.

"It's scary when you hear that in certain areas, one out of three women is positive," he said. "As a South African, you have to use South African strategies to answer South African questions. If there will be a cure, it should come here, where HIV is killing our brothers and sisters."

5.2

Why Africa's HIV Crisis Continues to Devastate Young Women

Michael Gerson

MARY, WHO IS 24 BUT LOOKS barely 18, has already experienced more than enough betrayal for any lifetime. Shyly but deliberately, she told of feeling sick at 16 and being diagnosed with HIV. After her mother—her only provider—was sent to prison, an aunt took Mary in, but forced her to sleep in an open-walled shed behind the house. Then she was raped by a boyfriend. "I went home crying and bleeding," she recalled. Mary told no one, fearing she would be turned out on the street. "I kept quiet, by myself." Four months later, she learned she was pregnant.

For the sake of the child—a girl born HIV-free—she took antiretroviral drugs. But then a friend introduced her to a Christian pastor. "He lays his hands on you and says the sickness will go," Mary remembered. "I believed him." She put her medicines down the toilet and stopped treatment for two years.

Last year, Mary got married and initially did not reveal her medical history to her spouse, fearing another rejection. "It is difficult to stand up and say you are positive," Mary explained. "It was my secret." But a counselor persuaded her to be tested again along with her husband. When her test came back positive and his negative, she ran crying from the clinic, convinced she would be abandoned. But her husband followed after her. "He said to me, 'This is not the end of the world.'"

True enough. Yet it is hard to imagine why the world—family, pastor, rapist—should be so relentlessly cruel to such a sweet and gentle young woman. Gentle, but not fragile. Just revealing her status and story to strangers, in a place where stigma is strong, took some of the greatest personal courage I've witnessed. (I traveled to Zambia as part of a task force convened by the Center for Strategic and International Studies to examine issues related to women's and family health.)

Stories like Mary's—in the millions—add up to one of the most urgent health crises of our time. While vast progress has been made in AIDS treatment in sub-Saharan Africa, barely a dent has been made in HIV infection rates among young women (which are significantly higher than among young men). With the youth population of Africa booming (40 percent of Zambians are under 16), a realization is dawning: The AIDS epidemic will be uncontrollable unless the number of infections among young women is rapidly and dramatically reduced.

young women= key population

In Zambia, about 11 percent of women become HIV-positive by age 24. A sad variety of cultural factors are implicated. Gender-based violence. Child marriage (in spite of national laws against it). A male-dominated society means that young women often lack the power to negotiate safer sex or to access health services without the permission of male partners. Extreme poverty can lead young women to engage in transactional sex, but so can the desire for consumer goods that demonstrate status among girls from wealthier backgrounds.

High rates of HIV infection among young women are a medical crisis for which there is no purely medical answer. Norms need to be changed. The empowerment of young women has become an essential health priority. Data from Botswana show that just keeping girls in school decreases the rate of HIV infection by 12 percent each year.

There is now significant focus and funding dedicated to this issue from the Global Fund to Fight AIDS, Tuberculosis and Malaria, and from the President's Emergency Plan for AIDS Relief. The U.S. global AIDS coordinator, Dr. Deborah Birx, has announced an initiative called DREAMS, designed to dramatically reduce new HIV infections in adolescent girls and young women in high-burden "hot spots" in 10 African countries.

Here in Zambia, the target population is 63,000 vulnerable young women in three areas. The theory: Surround them with support and services in every part of their lives. HIV testing and counseling. Contraceptive information and access. One-stop facilities to report gender-based violence and receive care. Financial literacy programs. Educational subsidies. Outreach to religious and traditional leaders. Outreach to young men to challenge destructive gender norms and attitudes (like how someone, at some point, reached Mary's husband).

If this model proves effective, it will need to be quickly brought to scale. Sexism, it turns out, is not only unfair but also unhealthy. To stop an epidemic, young women such as Mary, no longer quiet, must no longer feel alone.

5.3

Rape Has Become a Way of Life in South Africa

Charlene Smith

Police reported this week that they were achieving success in combating most crimes, but not rape. Jackie Selebi, the national police commissioner, said there were 115.3 cases per 100,000 people in 1994, compared with 113.7 in 2003/04. Selebi said rape statistics might be exaggerated because many rape cases were reported on a Friday and Saturday night, only to be withdrawn on a Monday.

It's the withdrawal of cases that bears closer examination, because it says nothing about women lying about rape as the ignorant might believe, but it says everything about a society that fails women and children and is allowing HIV/AIDS to proliferate without check. South Africa has the highest rates of rape in the world, according to Interpol, and the highest incidence of HIV. The National Prosecuting Authority tells us that 50 percent of all cases before South African courts are for rape, except in Durban and M.D.antsane, where it is 60 percent.

Although the Law Reform Commission estimates there are 1.7 million rapes a year, on average only 54,000 rape survivors lay charges each year. Why? It is because rape survivors are treated so badly by so many. Every time a rape survivor does not lay a charge, she allows a rapist or rapists—because 75 percent of rape in South Africa is gang rape—to believe he or they can do it again. And he or they will. Again and again, until a rape survivor does battle with the police, doctors, psychologists and the courts to get the justice she deserves, and to protect the next woman or child.

A Medical Research Council study into conditions for rape survivors in Gauteng in 2002 found that the treatment of survivors by police and medical and court personnel was deplorable. Two researchers were so traumatised by what they witnessed that they had to go for counselling.

The Medical Research Council reported that 26 percent of doctors and nurses who treated rape cases didn't think them a serious medical problem. Yet rape carries the risk of sexually transmitted diseases (STDs), including HIV, a range of other infections, pregnancy and long-term psychological scarring.

Last year the cabinet removed Section 21 from the new Sexual Offences Bill, which would have given post-exposure prophylaxis (PEP, which is medication to prevent HIV) as well as medication to prevent STIs and pregnancy to rape survivors. They left in Section 22, which guarantees medical care for the rapist and undertakes to rehabilitate any alcohol or narcotics addictions he might have.

In other words, the government will help to remove self-inflicted addictions from the criminal, but won't have legislation compelling hospitals to provide women and children with the medication that prevents them from getting criminal-inflicted HIV. Professor Ames Dhai of the University of Natal points out that there are twice as many rape survivors at risk of seroconversion to HIV than there are babies born in South Africa to HIV-positive mothers, yet there are few calls for PEP for rape survivors. She asks: Is it because of residual stigma against those raped?

Just over a month ago a 21-year-old student was forced at knifepoint into an alley off Long Street, Cape Town, and was raped. When she went to Groote Schuur Hospital she, like many rape survivors, found it difficult to use the word rape.

She told the admissions clerk she had been attacked. Because government hospitals do not see the necessity to train staff to be sensitive towards this problem, he told her to see her private doctor. She had to wait until the next morning—and yet the administration of PEP is urgent: to prevent HIV it has to take place less than 72 hours after the first act of penetration or attempted penetration.

Her doctor, being as incompetent as most GPs in dealing with rape survivors—in part because most universities give scant training to medical students on how to deal with rape—made her wait while he tried to figure out what medicines she should take. He finally gave her a prescription for two months of PEP instead of just 28 days.

It took her six hours and eight chemists to find a chemist that stocked anti-retrovirals—she finally sat in the eighth pharmacy, which didn't have the drugs, and refused to move until she was told where she could find them. Only then did a chemist pick up a phone and help her to get access to them. In the country with the world's highest rate of HIV and rape, why do so few pharmacies stock anti-retrovirals, or at the very least three-day PEP starter packs for rape survivors? This failure has nothing to do with the new medical regulations: few were stocking ARVs before.

The young woman's father phoned the police from Johannesburg, and was told that the cameras on Long Street had not picked up anything untoward on that night, so there was no point in laying a charge. Failures like these lead to statistics like these:

- UNAIDS reported last year that in South Africa two-and-a-half times more women are infected than men because many women experience forced sex.
- UNICEF reports that six times more girls than boys in Africa are infected with HIV.
- A Human Sciences Research Council study found a significant cohort of HIV-infected children whose mothers were not HIV-positive. How did they become infected?
- In South Africa, police tell us, 41 percent of those raped are under the age of 12. In Meadowlands, Soweto, police say 90 percent of rape in that community is against children younger than 12.

Superintendent Nico Snyman, head of that police station, says that despite a good arrest rate, only a small percentage of cases get prosecuted because families will accept compensation from the rapist or rapists, and the child is then prevented from testifying. In the case of a young man raped in Wentworth, Durban, three years ago, when he was 14, the thugs who raped him offered his impoverished grandmother R3,000 ($438) to get him to drop the case. She wanted the money, but he refused despite continuing threats.

Investigating officers were changed three times, the prosecutors four times. The victim went for counselling at a well-known child counselling centre, but because he is an orphan and his grandmother unemployed, he couldn't afford bus fare to continue and no one bothered to go to him. Last week the case against the accused was dismissed for lack of evidence. The prosecutor did not add extortion to the charge sheet, nor did she bother to get anyone to testify how the victim took rat poison after the rape and spent a week in Addington Hospital's psychiatric ward because he was so traumatised.

The investigating officer was on leave and did not testify, and no victim impact statement was used. Gangsters got away with the rape of a boy because no one cared, and this was a case the National Prosecuting Authority's Sexual Offences Unit received frequent complaints about.

A nine-year study by Cape Town's Red Cross Children's Hospital, published in the *SA Medical Journal* in December 2002, found that the average age of children raped was three. Research has shown that 40 percent of those raped in South Africa are at risk of becoming HIV-positive if they do not receive PEP.

Experts believe that if post-exposure prophylaxis was given immediately to rape survivors, South Africa could cut new HIV transmission dramatically. Yet little is done to advance this HIV preventive mechanism.

What are the costs of providing PEP? The cost to the government of each HIV test is less than 60c (9¢), according to the department of health. PEP costs it about R60 ($8.66) for 28 days. In other words, to treat 54,000 reported rapes each year would cost the government less than R600,000 ($86,000).

A rape specialist, Dr. Adrienne Wulfsohn, says the hospital costs of treating one rape survivor who contracts HIV is around R600,000 ($86,000) during her shortened life. Better treatment of rape survivors would result in more reporting and would give them the confidence to go through with their cases. What is more, most rapists are involved in other crimes—you jail a rapist and you invariably put away a dangerous criminal responsible for other offences.

South Africans need to become more serious about combating this crime.

Charlene Smith, a journalist, was raped and stabbed in her home in 1999 and has since become an internationally recognised expert on sexual violence and post-exposure prophylaxis

5.4

Nigeria Has More HIV-Infected Babies than Anywhere in the World

It's a Distinction No Country Wants

Jon Cohen

NIGERIA—ON A JANUARY MORNING, 12-YEAR-old Yusuf Adamu slumps in his father's lap, head pressed against his chest. Infected at birth with HIV, he is tiny for his age and has birdlike limbs. He has been feverish for 3 days, which is why his father, Ibrahim, brought him to the pediatric HIV/AIDS clinic at Asokoro District Hospital in Abuja, Nigeria's capital. "He's been losing weight, he is not eating well, he's still taking his drugs, and he's complaining of chest pains and coughing," Ibrahim tells the nurse. Yusuf's records show that at his last blood check 6 months ago, HIV had already ravaged the boy's immune system, even though he was receiving antiretroviral (ARV) drugs. When the doctor, Oma Amadi, examines his mouth, it is filled with white sores from candidiasis, a fungal infection. "The boy has been sick for so long," she says. "I'm going to admit him." When Amadi removes Yusuf's shirt to listen to his chest, the boy winces at the touch of her stethoscope. Amadi suspects Yusuf has tuberculosis, and after x-raying his lungs, the doctors put him in an isolation room.

Yusuf's mother was never tested for HIV before he was born: She received no prenatal care and delivered at home. Yusuf was not tested for the virus until she died of AIDS 3 years later. Ibrahim then learned that he, too, is HIV-positive, as are his two other wives. One ended up transmitting the virus to a second child, now 4.

The entire family receives ARVs, but Yusuf has only had intermittent access to the drugs. Dosing is based on weight, and Yusuf's has fluctuated so much that he has required monthly hospital visits. Ibrahim, a security guard, earns the equivalent of only about $20 a month. The Adamus live 20 kilometers and three bus rides from the hospital. The round trip bus fare costs $2, and Ibrahim has to miss a day of work for each checkup, when he also picks up his son's ARVs. Ibrahim simply can't afford regular treatment for his son. "There is no food at home," Ibrahim says.

HIV infected babies in Nigeria

Yet poverty alone does not explain the root of Yusuf's plight—which hundreds of thousands of other Nigerian children living with HIV now face. At a time when rates of mother-to-child transmission of HIV have plummeted, even in far poorer countries, Nigeria accounted for 37,000 of the world's 160,000 new cases of babies born with HIV in 2016. The most populous country in Africa, Nigeria does have an exceptionally large HIV-infected population of 3.2 million people. But South Africa—the hardest-hit country in the world, with 7.1 million people living with the virus—had only 12,000 newly infected children in 2016. The high infection rate, along with the lack of access to ARVs—coverage is just 30%—helps explain why 24,000 children here died of AIDS in 2016, nearly three times as many as in South Africa.

Mother-to-child transmission is only one part of Nigeria's HIV epidemic. But that route of transmission epitomizes the country's faltering response to the crisis, highlighting major gaps in HIV testing that allow infections to go untreated and the virus to spread. "Nigeria contributes the largest burden of babies born with HIV in the world—it's close to one in every four babies [globally] being born with HIV—and that's really not acceptable," says Sani Aliyu, who heads the National Agency for the Control of AIDS (NACA) in Abuja. And it is a solvable problem—even here. The key is to find and treat the relatively small population of pregnant, HIV-infected women, because those who receive ARVs rarely transmit the virus to their babies. Like most countries, Nigeria has made mother-to-child transmission a priority for more than a decade, and it has seen a reduction in children born with HIV. Still, the country stands out for its slow progress. "What we've realized is that we need to think outside the box," Aliyu says.

A pregnant woman living with HIV has a 15% to 30% chance of transmitting the virus to her baby in utero or at birth, and breastfeeding will infect up to 15% more. In 1994, a study showed that one ARV drug, azidothymidine, cut transmission rates by two-thirds if given to the mother before and after delivery and to the baby for 6 weeks. But few poor countries used that regimen because it was expensive and complex, requiring an intravenous drip of the drug during labor. Five years later, a study in Uganda showed a single dose of another ARV, nevirapine, given to a mother in labor and a baby at birth, could reduce transmission by 50%, which soon became a standard of care. Countries all over the world began aggressive prevention campaigns. Nigeria launched a program in 2002 when it had 54,000 newly infected children, and transmissions began to slowly decline.

Today, the standard of care is to treat all HIV-infected people, including pregnant women, with daily combinations of powerful ARVs. When treatment suppresses the virus in pregnant women and, as an additional safety measure, their newborn babies also receive ARVs for 6 weeks, transmission rates typically plummet to less than 1%. In the developed world and many developing countries, mother-to-child transmission is now rare. But the regimen can't be given if pregnant women don't know whether they are infected.

According to estimates from the Joint United Nations Programme on HIV/AIDS, 21.58% of HIV-infected, pregnant Nigerian women transmitted the virus to their children in 2016. Nigeria's central problem is that some 40% of women give birth at home or in makeshift clinics run by traditional birth attendants, where women are unlikely to get tested. The reasons women do not seek care at more formal health care facilities like Asokoro Hospital are many and overlapping: poverty, fear of stigma and discrimination for simply seeking an HIV test, lack of education, tradition, and husbands wary of health care.

Another barrier is the "formal" fee that the government levies for care at a clinic. Deborah Birx, director of the U.S. President's Emergency Plan for AIDS Relief (PEPFAR) in Washington, D.C., which has invested more than $5 billion in preventing and treating HIV in Nigeria, says the fee "opens the door" for others to tack on more insidious "informal" fees. "If you want to get your lab results back or you want to get your blood drawn, that nurse may charge you," Birx explains. Those fees, she says, "are very hard to police." When one Nigerian state eliminated the formal fee, the number of women who came to clinics for antenatal care doubled, she says.

Muktar Aliyu, an HIV/AIDS researcher at Vanderbilt University in Nashville who is Sani's identical twin, says corruption is a major factor. "It's a big elephant in the room," says Muktar Aliyu, who still conducts studies in his home country. Scams such as informal fees are just part of the problem. The Global Fund to Fight AIDS, Tuberculosis and Malaria in 2016 suspended payment to the country after detecting what it called "systematic embezzlement" by Ministry of Health staff as well as improper auditing.

Conducting large-scale HIV testing is also hard because the virus is dispersed unevenly across the country, with some states having a much lower prevalence than others. In Niger, a state in the central part of the country, it is just 1.7%, according to 2015 estimates. "We'd test 1000, 2000 individuals and we'd get barely 20, 30 positive," Muktar Aliyu says. But Benue, an east-central state that has been hardest hit, has an estimated adult prevalence of 15.4%.

Several people at the front of Nigeria's HIV/AIDS response link the shortcomings to the government's lack of "ownership" of the epidemic. Foreign assistance—mainly from PEPFAR and The Global Fund—pays for nearly the entire HIV/AIDS response. Health Minister Isaac Adewole, an OB-GYN who worked in HIV/AIDS, says the "No. 1 challenge" is for Nigeria to move "from a donor-dependent program to a country-owned program." To give an example of the problem, Muktar Aliyu notes that foreign assistance often focuses on bolstering programs, including testing, at large treatment centers, not the 800 or so smaller clinics spread across the country. "In the next 5 years, at the most, country ownership will come through for HIV programs in Nigeria," Sani Aliyu promises. "It's my job to make sure that money is available."

Since taking over NACA in 2016, Sani Aliyu has made some progress. For the first time, the federal government has been taking steps to prevent mother-to-child transmission, and state governments have devoted up to 1% of their budgets to efforts against HIV/AIDS. President Muhammadu Buhari, who appointed Sani Aliyu, authorized federal funds to pay for 60,000 new HIV-infected people to receive ARVs and vowed to add that same number to the treatment rolls each year. "The program, if successful, will serve as the exit gateway for PEPFAR as future programs acquire national ownership status," Sani Aliyu says.

Perhaps most important, NACA—with $120 million in funding from PEPFAR and The Global Fund—now is working on a massive epidemiologic survey that many hope will bolster the country's efforts. Because HIV testing is so spotty, Birx explains, it's possible that official estimates of Nigeria's number of newly infected children are too high—or too low—and that HIV/AIDS workers target the wrong regions. "Our epidemic data from Nigeria is the weakest of all the countries," Birx says. The nationwide survey of HIV now underway, the largest ever done in the world, should be completed by the end of the year. "I'll be frank: I used to be upset with Nigeria," she says. "Now, I'm just waiting for the data."

Still, no one doubts that children are getting infected far too often. And some innovators are taking action.

On a Sunday morning in mid-January, about 1000 parishioners fill the pews at the St. Vincent de Paul Catholic Church in Aliade, a remote, agricultural area in Benue state. Today, Reverend Emmanuel Dagi is leading celebrations called Baby Shower and Baby Reception, programs tailor-made to steer around the obstacles that keep so many pregnant women here from seeking an HIV test and receiving care.

Near the end of the church service, Dagi asks women who are pregnant or who have recently given birth to come forward for a blessing with their husbands. More than 50 people cluster around the pulpit, some women with large pregnant bellies, others with swaddled babies in their arms. "Defend these mothers and these fathers and their children from every evil," Dagi says. He walks from one end of the pulpit to the other, sprinkling the faithful with holy water.

The priest then asks the expecting couples to attend Baby Shower, where they receive a gift bag and have blood drawn for tests for hepatitis B, sickle cell anemia, and HIV—casually lumped into the mix to sidestep stigma. People with newborns attend a separate celebration, Baby Reception, where they, too, receive gift bags. At the same time, health workers discreetly check with all people who tested HIV positive at earlier services to make sure they've been following proper procedures: taking ARVs for themselves, administering them to their newborns, and bringing the babies in for a blood test at 6 weeks of age, the earliest the virus can reliably and efficiently be detected.

Those celebrations are part of the Healthy Beginning Initiative, funded by the U.S. National Institutes of Health and the Centers for Disease Control and Prevention. It has now expanded to more than 115 churches, some of which also test for malaria, syphilis, and anemia. Led by Echezona Ezeanolue, a pediatrician who works with the Healthy Sunrise Foundation based in Las Vegas, Nevada, the intervention takes advantage of the fact that some 90% of Nigerians regularly attend either church or mosque services. "That was a perfect place to test this," says Ezeanolue, a Nigerian who left the country 20 years ago. (Ezeanolue resigned from the University of Nevada in Las Vegas in March after a prolonged dispute with the school about what it alleged were financial irregularities with the maternal HIV program he ran there. He insists he did nothing wrong.)

Sani Aliyu adds that Baby Shower has another advantage. "The religious leaders don't carry the burden of politicians," he says. "People believe in what they say, and people follow them."

In a study of the project in 40 churches, half of which received the intervention, Baby Shower increased HIV testing in pregnant women from 55% in the control churches to 92%, the researchers reported in the November 2015 issue of The Lancet Global Health. A study published in AIDS and Behavior last year shows that in women's male partners, testing jumped from 38% to 84%. "With Baby Shower, you don't have to go to the hospital for an HIV test—you go to the church and nobody suspects anything," says Amaka Ogidi, coordinator of the project here. A follow-up study is assessing the actual impact on HIV transmission rates to the babies.

Ogidi says she at first had reservations because the idea of a baby shower is a U.S. concept. "We're not used to celebrating pregnancy—we're used to celebrating childbirth," she says. But the intervention has steadily grown in popularity, especially since the Baby Reception component was added. "The program is just like a sweet-smelling perfume," Ogidi says. "You smell it and say, 'Oooh, can I have some for myself?' You see smiles on faces and it's infectious."

The Mama Metta Traditional Clinic and Maternity Home in the Iyana Ipaja neighborhood of Lagos also is introducing prevention of mother-to-child transmission into a familiar setting. The clinic, set on a street wide enough only for foot traffic, resembles a small house. Feyami Temilade, who runs the clinic, is a traditional birth attendant, and she is known as Mama Metta because she becomes something of a second mother to every woman in her care.

This Friday morning, 16 big-bellied women sit on wooden benches in the waiting room. The walls are cluttered with framed certificates from courses Temilade has completed over the past 35 years, awards, fading photos of herself in celebratory garb, calendars, and pregnancy infographics. A poster above Temilade's desk says, "Know Your HIV Status" in English, Yoruba, and Nigerian Pidgin. A certificate next to it notes that she participated in a training workshop for traditional birth attendants run by the Society for Women and AIDS in Africa in—astonishingly—1991.

The women wait their turn for checkups and to fill bottles with two herb concoctions she has prepared. The cost of the visit, says Temilade, who will listen to babies through a metal fetoscope called a Pinard horn, is a mere 200 nairas—about $0.55.

Birth attendants are unregulated in much of Nigeria. But Lagos state, which includes Nigeria's largest city, has a Traditional Medicine Board that accredits and monitors practitioners. Since 2012, the board has offered regular HIV/AIDS training, which includes an internship at a hospital, for Temilade and some 2000 other birth attendants.

Temilade has been in business here so long that two of the women here today were born in the facility, which has a birthing room with two beds. "If you're pregnant, you're eating for two people," Temilade tells the group. She also warns them to avoid high heels and not to sit in the same position for too long. "Come here for HIV tests," she says, explaining that she'll link anyone who tests positive to a hospital.

That's a start, Sani Aliyu says. But, ultimately, he believes, getting women to antenatal clinics in established health facilities will be key to stopping mother-to-child transmission here. "In most cases, at least 80% of them will get tested and commence treatment," he says. One state has experimented with paying incentives to traditional birth attendants to bring pregnant women to formal health care settings.

Pregnant women make up only a fraction of Nigeria's huge HIV-infected population, and Sani Aliyu well recognizes that halting the epidemic here, as in other countries, depends on treating nearly everyone who is living with the virus—not just mothers and babies. "It's going to be a lot of work to put everybody with HIV on treatment," he says. But protecting babies from infection, he says, "should be a low-hanging fruit that can be reached."

Section VI

Russia and China

6.1

Russia's HIV/AIDS Epidemic Is Getting Worse, Not Better

Jon Cohen

In 2015, a dermatologist in Russia's fourth largest city, Yekaterinburg, diagnosed Katia with herpes. "I had no idea what it was," says Katia, who asked that her last name not be used. But because she had suffered repeated illnesses over the preceding 2 years and had an alcoholic ex-boyfriend who simultaneously had other girlfriends, she suspected that something more serious might be wrong. She asked the doctor to give her a referral for an HIV test. "Why?" he asked. "Are you going to marry a foreigner?"

"I persisted and said, 'I'm not leaving here until I get a referral.'"

The day Katia learned the test results, she walked the streets for hours crying, unable to even find her car. The literature she received explained she had the AIDS virus and said the outlook was grim. She read that the virus, if untreated, could kill her in as few as 3 years. Katia, then 30, had a young daughter. Who would raise her? And Katia had to hide her infection from her employer—her father. "If I told my father I had HIV, he wouldn't understand. He'd run away from me. Overall, the attitude here is horrible. When I look at [Western] Europe or the United States, I don't understand why it's so different here."

For Katia, the differences between east and west would soon become far starker.

Since 2015, the World Health Organization (WHO) in Geneva, Switzerland, has recommended treating everyone who tests positive for HIV, but doctors—despite what the literature suggested—assured Katia her immune system hadn't suffered enough damage to warrant antiretrovirals (ARVs). Two years later, Katia was married to a new partner and wanted to have another child. She had read on social media that HIV was a scam by Big Pharma, but that made no sense to her because the government promises free treatment. Other sites said proper treatment would almost eliminate her risk of transmitting the virus to her husband, who was uninfected, or their baby. She went to the AIDS center and requested ARVs. "They told me, 'Don't worry, your level of virus is low, you won't infect your husband, he's in the military and he's strong.'" Finally, in February 2017, after more than 2 months and a battery of tests, the doctors agreed to treat her, and in May, she became pregnant.

In June, the pharmacy ran out of ARVs.

Through social media, Katia contacted an HIV-infected woman, 2000 kilometers away in St. Petersburg, who was part of a "reserve pharmacy"—a network that gathers and redistributes ARVs from people who have either switched treatments or died. The woman told Katia whom to contact in Yekaterinburg. "I asked how much the pills would cost," Katia says. "She was like, 'Are you out of your mind? Just go and get your pills.'"

Almost anywhere in the world, an HIV-infected woman who has an uninfected partner and wants to have a baby would be first in line to receive ARVs. The challenges Katia faced in getting treatment amid Russia's epidemic highlight the country's faltering response, which critics have blasted as misguided, lackadaisical, and downright dismissive. Some federal health officials even question the term epidemic. "This is a very large and very serious epidemic, and certainly one of the few epidemics in the world that continues to get worse rather than get better," says Vinay Saldanha, the Moscow-based regional director for the Joint United Nations Programme on HIV/AIDS (UNAIDS) in Eastern Europe and Central Asia. "This is a public health crisis."

Yet the informal network of HIV-infected people that ultimately supplied Katia with ARVs highlights another, less recognized side of Russia's response. The darker the night, as Fyodor Dostoevsky wrote in *Crime and Punishment*, the brighter the stars. Bold, committed HIV/AIDS advocates in Russia are pushing hard for change—and a few places in the country show signs, albeit modest, of mounting effective responses.

UNAIDS calculates that between 2010 and 2015, Russia accounted for more than 80% of the new HIV infections in the entire Eastern European and the Central Asian region. By Russia's own estimates, the epidemic grew 10% per year during that period, with the new infections roughly split between people who inject drugs and heterosexual transmission. At about the same time, new infections in the rest of Europe and North America dropped by 9%. By the end of 2017, the Russian Ministry of Health estimates, just shy of 1 million people were living with HIV. Even official accounts acknowledge that only one-third of those receive ARVs.

Many people, even within the government, think those estimates understate the epidemic. Vadim Pokrovsky, who heads the Federal Scientific and Methodological Center for Prevention and Control of AIDS in Moscow, an epidemiological surveillance arm that's independent from the Ministry of Health, does battle with the divisions that oversee HIV and tuberculosis (TB). His group estimates that between 1.1 million and 1.4 million Russians are infected with HIV. And Michel Kazatchkine, special adviser to UNAIDS in Eastern Europe and Central Asia, and colleagues concluded in a study published last year that the true number of infected people may be as high as 2 million. They based their number on an estimate by Pokrovsky's team that only half the infected people in Russia knew their HIV status in 2013.

Kazatchkine, who earlier headed The Global Fund to Fight AIDS, Tuberculosis and Malaria, also in

A changing epidemic

The HIV/AIDS epidemic in Russia began in people who inject drugs, but heterosexual transmission has increasingly become a major driver. In small surveys, men who have sex with men have extremely high infection rates, but they rarely are studied.

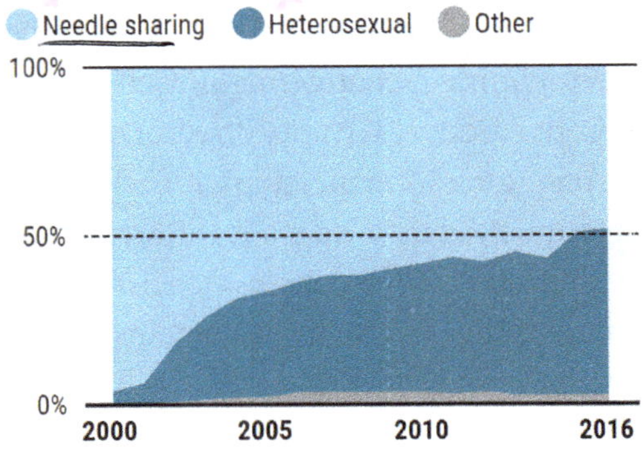

J. YOU/*SCIENCE*

Geneva, says Russia has unnecessarily let a containable epidemic explode. "Having gone through years of AIDS in Europe and then in Africa and everywhere as head of The Global Fund, I just cannot accept that there have been so many missed opportunities," he says.

HIV took off in Russia in the mid-1990s, later than in Western European countries, and at first the spread was limited mainly to heroin users sharing needles and syringes. Even before he took over The Global Fund in 2007, Kazatchkine and others urged the government to use proven "harm reduction" prevention strategies, including needle and syringe exchange programs and opiate substitutes such as methadone. Several nongovernmental organizations (NGOs) started programs for drug users, but the government offered no funding for what it saw as "Western" ideas that went against conservative Russian culture—and to this day opiate substitutes remain outlawed. The government also did little for another highly stigmatized group, men who have sex with men (MSM), who also are at high risk of infection. Since 2013, a "propaganda law" has made posting or discussing information geared toward MSM illegal. They rely on NGOs for many HIV services, as do sex workers.

Compounding the problem, several NGOs left the country starting a decade ago after Russia, emboldened by a strengthening economy, began phasing out The Global Fund's support—which to date has totaled $378 million. "They said, 'We don't need The Global Fund or money from outside; we'll cover everything ourselves,' but they didn't do it," Pokrovsky says. "We not only stopped outreach work, we lost many people working in NGOs because they had no federal support." Other NGOs pulled up stakes after President Vladimir Putin in 2013 enacted a law that forced many of them to register as "foreign agents."

"They basically let the epidemic grow because of lack of prevention and because of very low access to treatment," Kazatchkine says. "In short, they did it all wrong."

No program yet provides ARVs to high-risk uninfected people, a prevention strategy called pre-exposure prophylaxis (PrEP) that has had remarkable success, particularly with MSM in Western Europe, Australia, and the United States. "Who would PrEP be for?" Kazatchkine quips. "There are no MSM."

On top of all those challenges, Russia has a dysfunctional medical system, says Olga Bogolyubova, a psychologist who did HIV/AIDS research in St. Petersburg but, fed up, moved to the United States in 2015. Bogolyubova, who works at Clarkson University in Potsdam, New York, says Russia's broken system vastly complicates attempts to add HIV/AIDS programs for vulnerable populations. "The Russian medical system can be difficult to navigate and abusive even to people who aren't vulnerable," she says, noting long waits to see specialists and short supplies of medicines for many conditions. "A navy admiral recently shot himself because he couldn't get access to cancer care."

Tereza Kasaeva, a deputy director of the Ministry of Health who coordinates the country's HIV/AIDS programs (after meeting with Science in November 2017, she became head of WHO's Global TB Programme), acknowledges that Russia "didn't pay much attention" to the problem until the past 5 years, but she says the current criticism is overblown. "Everybody is talking about the need to avoid stigma," Kasaeva says. "We are against the stigma on the Russian Federation about the situation."

Kasaeva and her colleagues stress that the number of people getting treatment has increased severalfold over the past few years, and they note that they recently completed their first strategic plan to battle the disease. "We understand that now we have a problem and we're trying to solve it," she says. Everyone who requests treatment receives it, she insists, although some "people are trying to hide" and don't request it. Yes, shortages of ARVs occurred in some places last year, but that was only because of speed bumps in a shift away from regional drug purchase and distribution to a more streamlined, cost-effective federally run program.

Kasaeva recognizes that harm reduction programs might slow HIV's spread in the short term, but they don't address underlying problems, she says. "They're very popular and they look so smart and pretty, but in fact if we look into the problem deeply, it's not solving the problem." Harm reduction, "according to the opinion of a huge number of Russian experts," focuses on the symptoms and not the causes of addiction, she says. In contrast, the country's "systematic program of rehabilitation for drug users," she insists, has long-term effectiveness.

Yevgeny Roizman, who until last month was the powerful mayor of Yekaterinburg, has embraced that effort. (Roizman resigned in protest after regional lawmakers voted to end direct election of the mayor.) In 1999 he started a rehab program called City Without Drugs that, at the request of parents, forcibly removed teen addicts from their homes and locked them up while they went through withdrawal, chaining them to their beds at times. Criticism from human rights groups—featured prominently in Western European and U.S. media—and lawsuits ultimately shut the centers, but Roizman offers no apologies. He insists the program helped his region, the Sverdlovsk Oblast, eliminate heroin addiction and slow the spread of HIV. "My goal was to stop youth from using drugs," Roizman says. Although he offers few hard numbers to back his claims that the program worked, he has an abundance of anecdotes, proudly noting that he recently located 22 of the first teens treated at City Without Drugs who now have 38 kids of their own. "They're not doing drugs ever since they got to us," he says.

Roizman sees no need for harm reduction programs for drug users; NGOs that offered needle exchange in Yekaterinburg failed to make a dent, he says. He visited Ukraine, which legalized opiate substitution therapy, to see how it worked. "An army of heroin addicts," he says, was "reconfigured into an army of methadone addicts."

In other ways, however, Roizman's agenda is not entirely at odds with the international HIV/AIDS community, and he has a progressive bent. A published poet who opened a free museum of religious icon painting and sculpture, he strongly supported the opposition to Putin in the March election and is critical of "the main government officials" for not speaking about HIV. Roizman promotes condoms and sex education for teens. And he publicly took an HIV test himself to encourage people to know their status and start treatment if needed. "There are more serious problems and issues that we have to battle, but bearing in mind the dynamics, we do understand that HIV might just steal the future."

A different approach is in view on the banks of the Volga River in Kazan, the capital of the Republic of Tatarstan. Kazan's ornate kremlin (which means "fortress"), replete with both a mosque and a cathedral, dates back to Ivan the Terrible in the 16th century. The city has fanciful buildings of more recent vintage, too: a 30-meter-tall, copper-colored cauldron, a wedding palace built in 2013; and a swank soccer arena that opened the same year and is hosting World Cup games this month. The city is well-heeled, with an unusually large Muslim population for this part of Russia and a long history of independence—which helps explain why it stands out in its HIV/AIDS response.

Kazan in 1999 began aggressive needle and syringe exchange programs and other harm reduction efforts with support from NGOs, the semiautonomous republic itself, and eventually The Global Fund. "We've had a stable epidemic," says Larisa Badrieva, an epidemiologist and researcher there.

"We really reached a lot of people very, very quickly." The city recorded about 1000 new HIV cases in 2001, she says, and that number fell to about 150 in 2008, with little evidence that the virus was spreading to the general population. A relatively high percentage of HIV-infected people in Tatarstan—about 50%—is being treated with ARVs. Yet Badrieva is worried about the future. With the pullout of The Global Fund and with other outside assistance drying up, Badrieva says only one of seven centers in the city dedicated to drug users is still operating, and she is unsure whether it will remain open much longer. "Unless there's a dramatic shift in the drug scene, we'll see an increase of HIV infection across all groups," Badrieva predicts.

Like Kazan, St. Petersburg is often out of step with Moscow and has made solid headway against HIV/AIDS. The most westernized city in the country, St. Petersburg "is kind of an oasis," says Gregory Vergus, who works with an HIV/AIDS NGO called the International Treatment Preparedness Coalition. As a federal city, St. Petersburg directly receives funding from Moscow for HIV prevention, and Vergus says it invests the money wisely, focusing on vulnerable groups. "Most regions spend their HIV prevention money on balloons, songs, and working with grannies," he says.

Saldanha says he's particularly heartened about the latest data from the city. "We're hoping that St. Petersburg has now turned the corner," he says. In 2016, new infections in the city dropped below 2000 people a year for the first time since the epidemic took off, according to the city's AIDS center. Of the 36,000 residents who know they are living with HIV, about half now receive ARVs, and 82% of that group have undetectable levels of virus in their blood, meaning they are adhering to their treatment regimens. "We're doing something right," says Tatiana Vinogradova, deputy director of the St. Petersburg AIDS Center.

St. Petersburg still faces serious challenges, Vinogradova notes. Recent surveys that tested large groups of sex workers and MSM both showed double-digit prevalence of HIV, and only about 5% of the people already knew their status. Many migrants who have HIV also come to the region from former Soviet countries and do not have the proper St. Petersburg registration necessary to receive treatment and care. "It's a big problem, and we have no instruments to do anything about it," she says.

Still, Saldanha says, the fact that "St. Petersburg is finally pulling its head above water" gives him hope for the country as a whole. "It's very much a sign that in contemporary Russia, you can implement evidence-based HIV prevention programs," he says. But St. Petersburg is only one city in a highly populated, geographically expansive country. "They have a treatment coverage level that is half what it is in Zimbabwe," he stresses. "This epidemic is not going to go away on its own."

6.2

Justice Tough to Find for Chinese Patients

Barbara Demick

TIAN XI IS AMONG 1 MILLION Chinese infected by transfusions at government-run hospitals. One million more were infected donating blood. The government has yet to apologize or investigate the coverup.

It was just a small bump on the head, the result of one boy pushing another against a desk. It was such an unremarkable occurrence in a third-grade classroom that it should have been forgotten a day later, buried in the recesses of childhood memory.

Who could have imagined that it would dictate the course of Tian Xi's life and of those around him?

After the incident, the 9-year-old was sent home from school to rest. That night he threw up, so his mother took him to Xincai People's Hospital No. 1, where a young doctor fresh out of medical school diagnosed a mild concussion and recommended a transfusion for a quicker recovery.

His parents collected their savings, the equivalent of six months' salary, to buy four bags of blood. They didn't want their son, a top student who they were sure would be the first in their family to attend a university, to miss too much school.

It was April 1996, and few people in this small city in Henan province had ever heard of HIV/AIDS.

Now 23 years old and weighing only 112 pounds—the result of the early stages of AIDS—Tian is confined to a detention center in Henan province. He is charged with storming uninvited into the offices of the director of the hospital where he was infected with human immunodeficiency virus and sweeping everything off the top of the desk with his arm. A fax machine, computer and water cooler were broken in the Aug. 2 incident. He is to be sentenced soon.

"He just wanted to sit down and talk about what happened to him because of a mistake made by the hospital," said his father, Tian Demin, 53, sitting on a squat metal stool in the single room where he and his wife live off a back alley—the rest of their house has been rented out to raise money for their ailing son.

The room, with tile flooring and a ceiling fan, looks less like a home than a law office stuffed with legal papers, medical reports and many dog-eared petitions that their son has written imploring various government officials for help.

Tian Xi is one of perhaps 1 million Chinese infected with HIV, the virus that causes AIDS, as a result of blood transfusions at government-run hospitals. About 1 million more people were infected through the process of donating blood. Although the cases date back to the 1990s, the Chinese government has yet to offer an apology or investigate a massive coverup that allowed the disease to spread exponentially after it was well known that the blood supply was tainted.

Besides free retroviral drugs, victims have received almost no compensation. When they've tried to file lawsuits, courts have in most cases either rejected their claims or refused to accept the cases. As a result, victims usually petition officials—an archaic system dating back to imperial times in which the aggrieved would travel to the capital to implore the emperor for help.

"It's the worst way of handling things," says Li Xige, 42, a former post office employee from a nearby town in Henan province who received tainted blood during a caesarean section in 1995. The girl she gave birth to died at age 8. She and a younger daughter are sick with AIDS.

Li did get compensation eventually (she is prohibited from disclosing the amount), but only after repeated petitions to President Hu Jintao and Premier Wen Jiabao, a stint in prison, another under house arrest and suicide threats.

"If you don't fight, you'll get nothing," Li said. "It would be better for the government to come up with a plan for all of us who are sick or who lost children."

China's handling of AIDS patients is a case study of a dysfunctional legal system in which victims have no other recourse but to take the fight for justice into their own hands—a lonely, embittered struggle that often puts them and their defenders on the wrong side of Chinese law.

If anything, the political space for AIDS activism has shrunk. Hu Jia, one of the best-known AIDS activists, is serving a 3½-year sentence for "inciting subversion of state power." His wife announced this month that she was closing the charity he'd founded because of constant harassment by police and tax authorities. Several prominent AIDS activists have fled to the United States.

"Ten years ago, we still could research AIDS; now it is extremely difficult," said Wan Yanhai, a former public health official and head of a non-governmental organization who fled in May and now lives in Washington. He believes the heightened sensitivity is because two out of the nine members of the Politburo Standing Committee, Li Changchun and Li Keqiang, served as Communist Party secretaries in Henan province, the epicenter of the scandal.

"These are extremely powerful people who could be held responsible for the blood scandal," Wan said. "That's why so many of us have had to leave China."

The roots of the scandal go back to the mid-1980s, even before there was a term in Chinese for Acquired Immune Deficiency Syndrome. Trying to protect its blood supply against what was considered a decadent Western disease, the Chinese government banned the import of blood products and, in the spirit of Deng Xiaoping's economic liberalization, decided to go into the blood business itself.

By 1992, blood collection stations sprouted throughout the countryside. Poor farmers were encouraged to sell their blood to get rich quick. "Extend your arm. Expose a vein. Make a fist. And it's 50 yuan [$7.50]" was a popular slogan.

The blood stations often extracted the valuable plasma—which could be sold abroad for medication—and then re-injected the donors with leftover blood cells so they'd be able to give blood again without becoming anemic. Before re-injection, the staff often mixed the blood of various donors without screening for disease.

In Zhoukou county, about 60 miles away from where Tian Xi's family lives, a doctor assigned to a blood station noticed a high rate of hepatitis among blood donors in 1994 and warned the Ministry of Health. Then, in 1995, the doctor examined a blood donor, who tested positive for HIV.

"I was very worried. If just one person was infected, everybody was at risk," recalled the doctor, Wang Shuping. On her own initiative, she collected blood samples from 52 donors and had them tested for HIV. Thirteen were positive.

"We've got to close the blood collection stations immediately and inform the donors. People are in big danger," Wang said she told her superiors. The response, she said, was thugs sent to vandalize her clinic.

She fled China in 2002 and now lives in Utah.

Official silence turned mistakes into tragedies that begat more tragedies, as blood donors infected each other when their pooled blood was re-injected. They in turn infected spouses, children and blood recipients.

At the same time, hospitals were encouraging patients to get blood transfusions whether they needed them or not, offering doctors who sold blood commissions of $1 or $2 per bag.

"So many people were selling blood, you needed somebody to buy it," said Tian Xi's mother, Chen Minggui, 48. "We think that's what happened with my son. When he bumped his head, he didn't lose one drop of blood, but in the hospital they gave him a transfusion of four bags."

Tian spent seven days in the hospital recuperating and receiving well-wishers. He was a popular boy; even the mother of the boy who'd pushed him came to visit and offered to help Tian's family pay for the medical treatment. Tian's mother declined the offer.

"Nah. Boys will be boys," she said she told the other mother. "Besides, Tian Xi is going to be fine."

Within a few years, Tian's health deteriorated. He frequently got sore throats and unexplained fevers. He often missed school. He was once among the top 10 students in a class of 2,000, but his ranking fell to the top 300, respectable but not good enough for Tsinghua or Peking universities, the Chinese equivalent of Harvard and Yale, to which he aspired. He lost so much weight that his cheekbones jutted out of a skeletal head.

"Tian Xi is studying too hard. Make sure he eats more," his mother recalled the neighbors telling her.

Despite heavy government censorship, news reports about AIDS among blood donors began appearing in 2000. Tian's parents didn't pay attention: Although of modest means, they didn't associate with the kind of poor villagers who sold their blood to make money. They barely remembered their son's hospitalization. But, in 2004, they received notice from the hospital that everybody who'd had transfusions should get tested for HIV as a precaution.

Tian got his results July 19, 2004. By a strange coincidence, it was the same day the results were released from the gaokao, the all-important test Chinese high schoolers take to apply to university. He'd done well enough to go to a decent, if not top tier, university in Beijing—and he had one of the most dreaded diseases.

"He was crying all the time. He wanted to kill himself," his mother said.

Against all odds, Tian did go to college, studying software engineering in Beijing. Henan authorities initially agreed to some aid—about $1,400 a year to subsidize his education. The university helped him rent a room in a basement off campus in Beijing because it didn't want him in the dormitories. But the assistance stopped in 2009 when he graduated.

Unable to get a job with his poor health, and unable to afford expensive medications for hepatitis C, which he also contracted with the transfusion, he remained in Beijing, bringing his petitions to the Health Ministry, the Supreme Court and any government offices he could approach without being arrested.

Tian's petitions were an irritant to Henan officials, who pressed him to stop his campaign and return home. Finally, on July 23 of this year, Tian received a text message from Xincai county's Communist Party secretary, Gu Gouyin, asking him to come home from Beijing to negotiate a settlement.

"I will help you find a solution to your problems," the message read.

When Tian arrived for an appointment in Xincai, Gu had been called out of town for business. They rescheduled, and again Gu failed to show up.

"He realized it was a trap. Tian Xi had been lured down here because he was embarrassing people by petitioning in Beijing," said his father, who added that his son had only brought a month's supply of his retroviral drugs from Beijing and had initially gone to People's Hospital No. 1 to request medication, which the facility refused to supply.

The family doesn't deny that Tian Xi behaved badly, not only knocking equipment off the director's desk but also showing up repeatedly at the hospital, trying to visit the director at home and vandalizing an office door.

"Tian Xi's case is symbolic. There are so many patients who were just seeking compensation and got into the same kind of trouble because they ran out of legal options," said Liang Xiaojun, Tian's Beijing-based lawyer.

Wan Yanhai, the former health official turned activist, said blood recipients have gotten less compensation than blood donors.

"The blood donors lived in the same villages. They got together and attacked government offices. They became powerful," Wan said. "The blood recipients are scattered all over the country. They are isolated and don't have a group identity."

Even today, many transfusion recipients who might be HIV positive have not been tested and have not been notified that they are at risk.

Wan said tainted blood might have been used for transfusions as late as 2004, and that well over 1 million people could have been infected.

Official statistics, however, are lower. The Health Ministry reported that 740,000 people were living with HIV/AIDS as of the end of 2009, and that 220,000 others had died of the disease.

Section VII

Contemporary History

7.1

AIDS: The Early Years and CDC's Response

James W. Curran, M.D.[1], and Harold W. Jaffe, M.D.[2]

Initial Reports

The *MMWR* description of five cases of *Pneumocystis carinii* pneumonia (PCP) among homosexual men in Los Angeles was the first published report about an illness that would become known as acquired immunodeficiency syndrome (AIDS) (*1*). Appearing 4 months before the first peer-reviewed article (*2*), the timeliness of the report can be credited to the astute clinical skills and public health sensitivity of Dr. Michael Gottlieb and his colleagues at the University of California, Los Angeles, School of Medicine and Cedars-Sinai Hospital, who worked closely with Dr. Wayne Shandera, the CDC Epidemic Intelligence Service (EIS) officer assigned to the Los Angeles County Department of Health Services.

The Parasitic Diseases Division of CDC's Center for Infectious Diseases already had become concerned about other reports of unusual cases of PCP. The Division housed the Parasitic Disease Drug Service, which administered the distribution of pentamidine isethionate for PCP treatment. Because PCP was rare and pentamidine was not yet licensed in the United States, it was available only from CDC. A review of requests for pentamidine had documented that PCP in the United States was almost exclusively limited to patients with cancer or other conditions or treatments known to be associated with severe immunosuppression (*3*). Recent requests for this drug from physicians in New York and California to treat PCP in patients with no known cause of immunodeficiency had sparked the attention of Division staff.

Shortly after the first report, additional cases of other life-threatening opportunistic infections (OIs) and a malignancy, Kaposi sarcoma (KS), were reported (*4*). After learning of these first cases, CDC, under the leadership of its Director, Dr. William Foege, formed a Task Force on Kaposi's Sarcoma and Opportunistic Infections to begin surveillance and conduct epidemiologic investigations. Despite the fiscal constraints at the time, approximately 30 CDC EIS officers and staff participated in the Task Force during the summer of 1981.

The first step for the Task Force was to establish a case definition for surveillance and investigation of the outbreak. The key underlying factor for the disease appeared to be severe suppression of the cellular

1 Rollins School of Public Health, Emory University, Atlanta, Georgia
2 Office of the Director, CDC, Atlanta, Georgia

Curran, J., & Jaffe, H. W. (2011). *MMWR. Supplements.* *60*(4);64–69.

Source: https://www.cdc.gov/mmwr/preview/mmwrhtml/su6004a11.htm.

immune system. The OIs initially reported were life-threatening and often fatal. Although KS was a known but infrequent cancer in the United States, the classical form of the disease was rarely life-threatening and typically occurred among elderly men. Another epidemiologic form of KS was seen among immunosuppressed renal transplant recipients.

To track KS/OI, the surveillance case definition had to emphasize specificity and accuracy of diagnosis. Thus, the original CDC case definition included 1) biopsy-proven KS among persons <60 years of age or biopsy- or culture-proven life-threatening or fatal OIs and 2) no known underlying illness (e.g., cancer or immune deficiency disease) or history of immunosuppressive therapy. This definition was soon adopted both in the United States and worldwide and was used for surveillance in countries where diagnostic capacities were available. The CDC case definition for what came to be called AIDS was modified in 1985 (5), 1987 (6), and 1993 (7). The World Health Organization employed a modified case definition for use in settings with limited diagnostic capacity (usually developing countries).

By the end of 1981, 159 cases of KS and OIs had been reported in the United States, with the earliest cases retrospectively identified in 1978 (8). By month of illness onset, cases demonstrated a clear increase over time (Figure 7.1.1). About half of the reports were for KS alone and 40% for PCP alone; 10% of patients were reported with both KS and PCP. Seventy-five percent of cases were reported from New York City or California, and all but one case were in men. Within 6 months, it was clear that a new, highly concentrated epidemic of life threatening illness was occurring in the United States. The co-occurrence of KS and OIs suggested that the epidemic was one of immunosuppression and that KS or OIs were a consequence of the immunosuppression.

Although the case definition's specificity was crucial for identifying the emerging epidemic, it lacked sensitivity. In fact, the reported KS/OI cases were described as "the tip of the iceberg" of a spectrum of illness being seen by physicians in New York City and California. These illnesses included other cancers (particularly non-Hodgkin lymphoma); thrombocytopenic purpura; and notably, persistent, unexplained generalized lymphadenopathy. Dr. Donna Mildvan and her colleagues in New

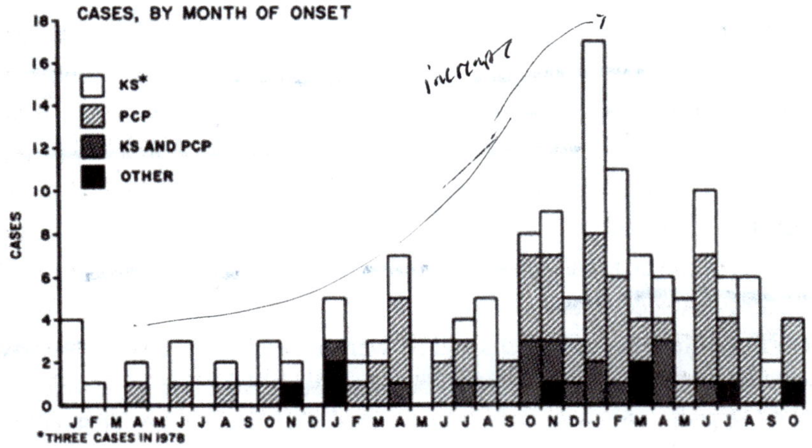

FIGURE 7.1.1 *Incidence of Kaposi's Sarcoma (KS), Pneumocystis carinii Pneumonia (PCP), and other opportunistic infections—United States, 1979–1981*

Source: Epidemiologic aspects of the current outbreak of Kaposi's sarcoma and opportunistic infections. N Engl J Med 1982; 306:248–52. Reprinted with permission.

York City, assisted by EIS officer, Dr. Bess Miller, described 57 cases of unexplained lymphadenopathy among gay men (*9*). At the time, nearly one third of the reported persons with KS had a history of such lymphadenopathy. Since lymphadenopathy and other symptoms often waxed and waned, it was speculated that such findings represented a milder, if much more common, form of the syndrome.

Early in 1982, CDC conducted a national case–control study that included most living patients with KS/OIs reported in the United States. The 50 cases among gay men were compared with control gay men matched by city of residence, race, and age. The studies, led by Drs. Harold Jaffe and Martha Rogers, found that case-patients tended to be much more sexually active than controls and were more likely to have had other sexually transmitted infections (*10,11*).

In early 1982, Dr. David Auerbach, the EIS officer who had replaced Dr. Shandera in Los Angeles, was approached by a member of the local gay community about a possible sexual link between the still rare cases in southern California. In collaboration with Dr. William Darrow of the Task Force, Dr. Auerbach investigated 13 of the first 19 cases reported from Los Angeles and Orange counties and found that nine had reported sexual contact with another person reported with AIDS within 5 years before their onset of symptoms (*12*). Auerbach and Darrow then extended the epidemiologic investigation nationwide to 90 patients (approximately three quarters of reported cases among gay men alive at the time). Forty of the 90 patients in 10 cities were linked by sexual contact with another case-patient (*13*). These findings, along with the results from the case–control study, strongly suggested that the new syndrome was caused by a sexually transmissible infectious agent. Nonetheless, whether because of competing hypotheses or merely denial, many scientists and the public were skeptical of the infectious agent causation theory.

Then, in early summer 1982, an elderly man with severe hemophilia A was reported to have died from PCP. Shortly thereafter, two additional PCP cases were reported among young men with severe hemophilia from separate states. These latter cases were investigated in depth by Dr. Dale Lawrence of the Task Force, who determined that their PCP was accompanied by severe unexplained immunosuppression, and these patients had no history of homosexual contact or needle sharing (*14*). For more than a decade, persons with hemophilia in the United States had received reconstituted lyophilized clotting factor concentrates, derived from human plasma, to prevent the devastating effects of their disease. However, the concentrates were pooled from the plasma of >1,000 donors per lot and were known to transmit hepatitis viruses.

Within the next several months, AIDS cases also were reported among infants (*15–17*), female sex partners of men with, or at high risk for, AIDS (*18,19*), and an infant and adults who had received blood transfusions (*20,21*). Taken together, these cases provided strong evidence that AIDS was caused by an infectious agent that could be transmitted by blood and from mother to child, as well as through homosexual and heterosexual contact.

In the summer of 1982, life-threatening OIs and KS were also reported among 34 Haitian migrants to the United States (*22*). Most were reported to be heterosexual men with no known risk factors who had migrated from Haiti within the past 2 years. Cases of disseminated KS had been recently reported from Port-Au-Prince as well (*23*). These reports indicated an epidemiologically distinct pattern of illness that ultimately would be explained mostly by heterosexual transmission. The reporting of these cases as "Haitian entrants" was accurate and, these authors believe, necessary for public health purposes, but the stigma of "AIDS labeling" added to the already considerable burden for thousands of Haitian migrants fleeing poverty and political persecution (24).

Recommendations for Prevention

During the initial year after the first reports of AIDS, when the term "gay plague" was commonly used, the disease received relatively little attention from the mainstream media, the public, or politicians. By the end of 1982, however, it was clear that others were at risk for the disease, and what had been complacency turned into serious concern, even panic. Many persons caring for AIDS patients were concerned about their own safety and, in some cases, health-care workers refused to provide needed care. To provide guidance for protection of clinicians and laboratory workers managing patients with AIDS and their biologic specimens, CDC issued guidelines in November 1982 that were based on those previously recommended to protect against hepatitis B virus infection (25).

In March 1983, CDC, in conjunction with the Food and Drug Administration and the National Institutes of Health (NIH), issued interagency recommendations for the prevention of AIDS on the basis of the epidemiologic data (Table 7.1.1) (26). These recommendations, which were immediately endorsed by a variety of professional and community organizations, were developed before the cause of the syndrome was discovered and 2 years before antibody testing would be available for diagnostic testing of individuals or screening of blood donations. Yet, even in retrospect, the recommendations appear to have been essentially correct. They illustrate the power of epidemiologic investigation in understanding and preventing new diseases, even in the absence of an identified cause.

The causative retrovirus was described by Drs. Francois Barre-Sinoussi and Luc Montagnier and their colleagues from the French Pasteur Institute in May 1983 (27). Additional proof of causality,

TABLE 7.1.1 Recommendations for prevention of acquired immune deficiency syndrome (AIDS), March 1983

Sexual contact should be avoided with persons known or suspected to have AIDS. Members of high risk groups should be aware that multiple sexual partners increase the probability of developing AIDS.
As a temporary measure, members of groups at increased risk for AIDS should refrain from donating plasma and/or blood. This recommendation includes all individuals belonging to such groups, even though many individuals are at little risk of AIDS. Centers collecting plasma and/ or blood should inform potential donors of this recommendation. The Food and Drug Administration (FDA) is preparing new recommendations for manufacturers of plasma derivatives and for establishments collecting plasma or blood. This is an interim measure to protect recipients of blood products and blood until specific laboratory tests are available.
Studies should be conducted to evaluate screening procedures for their effectiveness in identifying and excluding plasma and blood with a high probability of transmitting AIDS. These procedures should include specific laboratory tests as well as careful histories and physical examinations.
Physicians should adhere strictly to medical indications for transfusions, and autologous blood transfusions are encouraged.
Work should continue toward development of safer blood products for use by hemophilia patients.

Source: CDC. Prevention of acquired immune deficiency syndrome (AIDS): report of inter-agency recommendations. MMWR 1983; 32:101–3.

as well as the demonstration of sustained viral growth in vitro, was reported by Dr. Robert Gallo and colleagues at the U.S. National Cancer Institute, NIH, in 1984 (28). In 2008, Drs. Barre-Sinoussi and Montagnier were awarded the Nobel Prize in medicine for their discovery of human immunodeficiency virus (HIV).

The availability of laboratory reagents and techniques to identify HIV led to rapid scientific advances in understanding the natural history of the infection and AIDS. CDC's Dr. Paul Feorino and colleagues first demonstrated persistent HIV infection among seropositive blood donors who had transmitted HIV many years earlier, indicating that HIV-infected persons can be asymptomatic and viremic for many years and that seropositivity is equivalent to infection and infectivity (29). Dr. Harold Jaffe and colleagues from the San Francisco Health Department and CDC's Hepatitis Division reported a 6-year follow-up of a cohort of gay men originally recruited in 1978 for studies of hepatitis B virus infection in San Francisco (Figure 7.1.2) (30). By analyzing retrospectively obtained specimens, they found that at the time the first few AIDS cases were reported from the cohort in 1981, 30% of the 7,000 men were already infected with HIV. If these data were extrapolated nationally, as many as 200,000–300,000 gay men had already been infected in the United States at the time of the 1981 case reports. Using these natural history data, Dr. Meade Morgan projected that the cumulative incidence of AIDS would reach 270,000 by 1991 (31). These projections provided a wake-up call to those concerned about the future economic and human costs of the epidemic in this country.

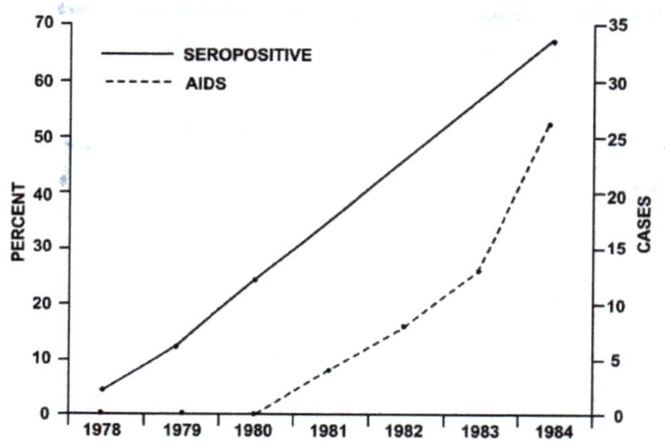

FIGURE 7.1.2 *Percent of men with human T-lymphotropic virus, type III/lymphadenopathy-associated virus antibody (seropositive) and number with acquired immunodeficiency syndrome (AIDS), by year of diagnosis, San Francisco City Clinic Cohort, 1978–1984*

Source: Jaffe HW, Darrow WW, Echenberg DF, et al. The acquired immune deficiency syndrome in a context of homosexual men. A six-year follow-up study. Ann Intern Med 1985; 103:210–4. Reprinted with permission.

By the mid-1980s, substantial concern existed about transmission of HIV through casual contact or by arthropods. Dr. Gerald Friedland and colleagues showed no evidence of transmission among close household contacts of HIV-infected patients in New York City (32). In a cover story for *LIFE* magazine, physicians from Florida had postulated that the high prevalence of AIDS in Belle Glade, a small town in southern Florida, resulted from insect transmission of HIV. Dr. Kenneth Castro and his colleagues published an extensive epidemiologic investigation in that community that did not support that hypothesis (33).

Drs. Steven McDougal and Linda Martin from CDC demonstrated that heat would inactivate HIV, providing a basis for production of clotting factor concentrate that would no longer transmit HIV infection (34). CDC laboratories also validated HIV antibody tests and provided proficiency testing materials for state public health laboratories and others. In the early HIV era, recommendations for HIV counseling and testing (35) and prevention of perinatal transmission (36) were made, and CDC provided resources and training for alternate testing and counseling sites (sites other than blood collection centers) (37). During the first 8 years of the epidemic, nearly 50 sets of recommendations and guidelines for AIDS were published in *MMWR*.

The Global Epidemic

By 1984, case reports described AIDS in Zaire (now the Democratic Republic of Congo), and a team of investigators including Dr. Joseph McCormick and Ms. Sheila Mitchell from CDC; Dr. Thomas Quinn from the National Institute of Allergy and Infectious Diseases, NIH; and Dr. Peter Piot from the Institute of Tropical Medicine in Belgium, made a joint visit to Kinshasa to verify the initial reports. Dr. Jonathan Mann was then recruited by CDC to establish a long-term project in Zaire, Project SIDA, in partnership with Dr. Bila Kapita from Mama Yemo Hospital in Kinshasa and colleagues from NIH and the Institute of Tropical Medicine. Projet SIDA would rapidly become the largest HIV/AIDS research project on the continent during the 1980s.

In 1985, CDC inaugurated and hosted in Atlanta the First International Conference on AIDS. The conference, chaired by Dr. Gary Noble of CDC, was attended by >2,000 registrants. At the conference, Dr. Mann delivered the first presentation about AIDS in Africa at a U.S. meeting and reported that the incidence of AIDS in Kinshasa was 15–30 times higher than in the United States (38).

Dr. Mann left Zaire to begin the Global Programme on AIDS at the World Health Organization. He was replaced as Project SIDA Director by Dr. Robert Ryder in 1986 and then by Dr. William Heyward in 1989. Dr. Kevin De Cock was the first Director of Projet Retro CI, CDC's second African research site, in Abidjan, C'ote D'Ivoire. Shortly thereafter, Dr. Bruce Weniger initiated CDC's HIV research site in Bangkok, Thailand.

Since the early days, CDC's response to the global HIV pandemic has been extensive. In the early 1980s, staff were detailed to, or volunteered from, many different parts of the agency. Initial CDC funding supported state and local health departments for surveillance and prevention activities, including HIV counseling and testing. In addition to these traditional CDC partners, hundreds of local and national community-based organizations were enlisted in the prevention efforts, and CDC provided support for school-based HIV education initiatives.

At CDC headquarters, the AIDS epidemic highlighted the need for behavioral and social scientists to participate in public health research.. Before 1981, only a handful of doctoral-trained behavioral and social scientists were on staff in Atlanta, but the numbers quickly grew. CDC's reputation and staff accomplishments also led to formation of the Global AIDS Program. Overall, many thousands of CDC staff have worked—and continue to work—with tens of thousands of colleagues throughout the world in the fight against AIDS. Well over 400 reports on HIV/AIDS have been published in *MMWR* since that first report in June 1981. The ongoing impact of CDC's scientific and programmatic contributions remains outstanding.

Lessons for the Future

In three decades, AIDS has emerged has a major global health problem. As the world faces the long struggle to combat the epidemic, several lessons from the early days emerge.

First, excellent surveillance of the initial AIDS cases was critical in responding to the epidemic. Surveillance was first needed to track the epidemic and direct etiologic investigations but later became critical in formulating early prevention and safety recommendations before HIV was discovered. Surveillance remains equally important now throughout the world to target resources and evaluate prevention efforts.

Second, the rapid identification of HIV as the causal agent of AIDS led to a much better understanding of transmission, natural history, and spectrum of illness. This understanding allowed for more targeted prevention efforts and paved the way for development of the first effective treatments.

Third, innovative science has in many ways exceeded the expectations of skeptics. These innovations include improvements in HIV diagnostics, such as rapid antibody testing and viral load assays; identification of zidovudine (AZT), the first antiretroviral (ARV) drug; use of ARVs to reduce perinatal transmission; effectiveness of prevention in many communities through counseling and testing, as well as behavior-based methods; and development of effective biomedical interventions, such as male circumcision, preexposure prophylaxis, and vaginal microbicides in addition to condom use and needle and syringe exchange. Finally, development of the three-drug ARV regimen (highly active antiroviral therapy [HAART]) has saved the lives of millions of persons with HIV infection in both the developed and developing worlds.

Fourth, as with most health problems where the etiology is well understood, prevention deserves primacy. Several million persons become newly infected with HIV each year, yet only approximately five to six million persons worldwide have been treated with HAART. The goal of universal HIV treatment cannot be met unless HIV incidence can be reduced. Furthermore, as long as the majority (or a substantial minority) of HIV-infected persons are unaware of their infection status, prevention and treatment efforts will be hampered.

Finally, committed persons have made—and will continue to make—the difference. Persons with HIV infection have played crucial roles in communities throughout the world by giving voice to their concerns and courageously advocating for HIV. Scientists in many disciplines who continue to discover breakthroughs for prevention and care provide hope for the future. Clinicians and caregivers and public health practitioners will pursue their work with an expanded science base.

The future of prevention and care for HIV means standing up to two societal foes, scarcity and discrimination, as much as the biologic challenge of the virus itself. Global resources for prevention and care for HIV remain severely short of the needs. Successful efforts for prevention must also include sustained and visible efforts to combat stigma and prevent discrimination.

This last lesson was emphasized by the late Jonathan Mann, who perished with his wife, HIV vaccine researcher, Mary Lou Clements-Mann, in a 1998 plane crash. Dr. Mann was the person most responsible for first calling world attention to AIDS and linking it to concerns about human rights. In one of his last public addresses, on the occasion of the 50th anniversary of the Universal Declaration of Human Rights, he stated, "Our responsibility is historic. For when the history of AIDS and the global response is written, our most precious contribution may well be that, at a time of plague, we did not flee, we did not hide, we did not separate ourselves" (*39*). The hope for the tens of millions affected by HIV currently and in the future will depend upon scientists, practitioners, and citizens working together.

References

1. CDC. *Pneumocystis* pneumonia—Los Angeles. MMWR 1981; 30:1–3.
2. Hymes, KB, Greene JB, Marcus A, et al. Kaposi's sarcoma in homosexual men: a report of eight cases. Lancet 1981; 318:598–600.
3. Walzer PD, Perl DP, Krogstad DJ, Rawson PG, Schultz MG. *Pneumocystis carinii* pneumonia in the United States: epidemiologic, diagnostic, and clinical features. Ann Intern Med 1974; 80:83–93.
4. CDC. Kaposi's sarcoma and *Pneumocystis* pneumonia among homosexual men—New York City and California. MMWR 1981; 30:305–8.
5. CDC. Revision of the case definition of acquired immunodeficiency syndrome for national reporting—United States. MMWR 1985; 34:373–5.
6. CDC. Revision of the CDC case definition for acquired immunodeficiency syndrome. MMWR 1987; 36(Suppl):82–94.
7. CDC. Impact of the expanded AIDS surveillance case definition on AIDS case reporting—United States, first quarter, 1993. MMWR 1993; 42:308–10.
8. CDC. Task Force on Kaposi's Sarcoma and Opportunistic Infections. Epidemiologic aspects of the current outbreak of Kaposi's sarcoma and opportunistic infections. N Engl J Med 1982; 306:248–52.
9. CDC. Persistent generalized lymphadenopathy among homosexual males. MMWR 1982; 31:249–51.
10. Jaffe HW, Choi K, Thomas PA, et al. National case control study of Kaposi's sarcoma and *Pneumocystis carinii* pneumonia in homosexual men: epidemiologic results. Ann Intern Med 1983; 99:145–51.
11. Rogers MF, Morens DM, Stewart JA, et al. National case-control study of Kaposi's sarcoma and *Pneumocystis carinii* pneumonia in homosexual men: Part 2. Laboratory results. Ann Intern Med 1983; 99:151–8.
12. CDC. A cluster of Kaposi's sarcoma and *Pneumocystis carinii* pneumonia among homosexual male residents of Los Angeles and Orange counties, California. MMWR 1982; 31:305–7.
13. Auerbach DM, Darrow WW, Jaffe HW, Curran JW. A cluster of cases of the acquired immune deficiency syndrome: patients linked by sexual contact. Am J Med 1984; 76:487–92.
14. CDC. *Pnemocystis carini* pneumonia among persons with hemophilia A. MMWR 1982; 31:365–7.
15. CDC. Unexplained immunodeficiency and opportunistic infections in infants—New York, New Jersey, California. MMWR 1982; 31:665–7.
16. Oleske J, Minnefor A, Cooper R, et al. Immune deficiency syndrome in children. JAMA 1983; 249:2345–9.
17. Rubenstein A, Sicklick M, Gupta A, et al. Acquired immunodeficiency with reversed T4/T8 ratios in infants born to promiscuous and drug-addicted mothers. JAMA 1983; 249:2350–6.
18. CDC. Immunodeficiency among female sexual partners of males with acquired immune deficiency syndrome (AIDS). MMWR 1983; 31:697–8.
19. Harris C, Small CB, Klein RS, et al, Immunodeficiency in female sexual partners of men with the acquired immunodeficiency syndrome. N Engl J Med 1983; 308:1181–4.
20. CDC. Possible transfusion-associated acquired immune deficiency syndrome (AIDS)—California. MMWR 1982; 31:652–4.
21. Curran JW, Lawrence DL, Jaffe HW, et al. Acquired immunodeficiency syndrome (AIDS) associated with transfusions. N Engl J Med 1984; 310:69–75.
22. CDC. Opportunistic infections and Kaposi's sarcoma among Haitians in the United States. MMWR 1982; 31:353–61.

23. Liautaud B, Laroche C, Duvivier J, et al. Le sarcoma de Kapsoi (maladie de Kaposi) est-il-frequent en Haiti? Presented at the 18th Congres des Medecins francophones de l'hemisphere Americain: Port-Au-Prince, Haita, April 1982.
24. Farmer P. AIDS and accusation: Haiti and the geography of blame, Berkeley, CA: University of California Press; 1992.
25. CDC. Acquired immune deficiency syndrome (AIDS): precautions for clinical and laboratory staffs. MMWR 1982; 31:577–80.
26. CDC. Prevention of acquired immune deficiency syndrome (AIDS): report of inter-agency recommendations. MMWR 1983; 32:101–3.
27. Barre-Sinoussi F, Chermann JC, Rey F, et al. Isolation of a T-lymphotropic retrovirus from a patient at risk for acquired immune deficiency syndrome (AIDS). Science 1983; 220:868–71.
28. Gallo RC, Salahuddin SZ, Popovic M, et al. Frequent detection and isolation of cytopathic retroviruses (HTLV-III) from patients with AIDS and at risk for AIDS. Science 1984; 224:500–3.
29. Feorino PM, Jaffe HW, Palmer E, et al. Transfusion-associated acquired immunodeficiency syndrome (AIDS): evidence for persistent infection in blood donors. N Engl J Med 1985; 312:1293–6.
30. Jaffe HW, Darrow WW, Echenberg DF, et al. AIDS, AIDS-related conditions, and exposure to HTLV-III/LAV in a cohort of homosexual men: a 6-year follow-up study. Ann Intern Med 1985; 103:210–4.
31. Morgan WM, Curran JW. Acquired immunodeficiency syndrome (AIDS): current and future trends. Public Health Rep 1986; 101:459–65.
32. Friedland GH, Saltzman BR, Rogers MF, et al. Lack of transmission of HTLV-III/LAV infection to household contacts of patients with AIDS or AIDS-related complex with oral candidiasis. N Engl J Med 1986; 314:344–50.
33. Castro KG, Lieb S, Jaffe HW, et al. Transmission of HIV in Belle Glade, Florida: lessons for other communities in the United States. Science 1988; 239:193–8.
34. McDougal JS, Martin LS, Cort SP, Mozen CM, Heidebrant CM, Evatt BL. Thermal inactivation of the acquired immunodeficiency syndrome virus, human T-lymphotropic virus–III/lymphaderopathy-associated virus, with special reference to antihemophilic factor. J Clin Invest 1985; 76:875–7.
35. CDC. Public Health Service guidelines for counseling and antibody testing to prevent HIV infection and AIDS. MMWR 1987; 36:509–15.
36. CDC. Recommendations for assisting in the prevention of perinatal transmission of human T-lymphotropic virus type III/lymphadenopathy-associated virus and acquired immunodeficiency syndrome. MMWR 1985; 34:721–6.
37. CDC. Human T-lymphotropic virus type III/lymphadenopathy associated virus antibody testing at alternate sites. MMWR 1986; 35:284–7.
38. Mann JM, Francis H, Asila PK, et al. Surveillance for acquired immunodeficiency syndrome in a central African city: Kinshasa, Zaire. JAMA 1986; 255:3255–9.
39. Mann JM. Presentation at XII International Conference on AIDS, June 28–July 3, 1998, Geneva, Switzerland.

7.2

Pneumocystis Pneumonia—Los Angeles

The First Published Account of AIDS

M.S. Gottlieb, H.M. Schanker, P.T. Fan, A. Saxon, and J.D. Weisman

Prior to the publication of this paper, in June of 1981, researchers within the halls of the CDC were already puzzling over an increase in requests for pentamidine isethionate, the drug used to treat PCP. (At the time, the CDC was the only source of pentamidine in the United States.) Around the country, cases of PCP were appearing in patients with no known cause of immune suppression, presenting a medical mystery. However, word had not spread beyond a handful of scientists.

At the same time, Dr. Michael Gottlieb and his colleagues at the University of California at Los Angeles and Cedars-Mt. Sinai Hospital were also realizing that something unusual was brewing. The appearance of several cases of PCP among otherwise healthy, young, homosexual men baffled and alarmed them. These astute clinicians notified the CDC Epidemic Intelligence Service Officer in the Los Angeles Department of Health Services. Together they crafted and published the first account of what would later be called AIDS, alerting the medical community to a new, unknown threat. At the time, they could not have known that there were likely thousands already infected with the deadly plague, which would become one of the most lethal in human history. Within a year and a half, the modes of transmission would be elucidated, but the cause of the syndrome would not be discovered until 1983.

In the period October 1980–May 1981, 5 young men, all active homosexuals, were treated for biopsy-confirmed *Pneumocystis carinii* pneumonia at 3 different hospitals in Los Angeles, California. Two of the patients died. All 5 patients had laboratory-confirmed previous or current cytomegalovirus (CMV) infection and candidal mucosal infection. Case reports of these patients follow.

Patient 1: A previously healthy 33-year-old man developed *P. carinii* pneumonia and oral mucosal candidiasis in March 1981 after a 2-month history of fever associated with elevated liver enzymes, leukopenia, and CMV viruria. The serum complement-fixation CMV titer in October 1980 was 256; in May 1981 it was 32. The patient's condition deteriorated despite courses of treatment with trimethoprimsulfamethoxazole

Gottlieb, et al, "Pneumocystis Pneumonia – Los Angeles," *MMWR*, vol. 30, no. 21, pp. 1–3, 1981.

(TMP/SMX), pentamidine, and acyclovir. He died May 3, and postmortem examination showed residual *P. carinii* and CMV pneumonia, but no evidence of neoplasia.

Patient 2: A previously healthy 30-year-old man developed *P. carinii* pneumonia in April 1981 after a 5-month history of fever each day and of elevated liver-function tests, CMV viruria, and documented seroconversion to CMV, i.e., an acute-phase titer of 16 and a convalescent-phase titer of 28 in anticomplement immunofluorescence tests. Other features of his illness included leukopenia and mucosal candidiasis. His pneumonia responded to a course of intravenous TMP/SMX, but, as of the latest reports, he continues to have a fever each day.

Patient 3: A 30-year-old man was well until January 1981 when he developed esophageal and oral candidiasis that responded to Amphotericin B treatment. He was hospitalized in February 1981 for *P. carinii* pneumonia that responded to TMP/SMX. His esophageal candidiasis recurred after the pneumonia was diagnosed, and he was again given Amphotericin B. The CMV complement-fixation titer in March 1981 was 8. Material from an esophageal biopsy was positive for CMV.

Patient 4: A 29-year-old man developed *P. carinii* pneumonia in February 1981. He had had Hodgkins disease 3 years earlier, but had been successfully treated with radiation therapy alone. He did not improve after being given intravenous TMP/SMX and corticosteroids and died in March. Postmortem examination showed no evidence of Hodgkins disease, but *P. carinii* and CMV were found in lung tissue.

Patient 5: A previously healthy 36-year-old man with clinically diagnosed CMV infection in September 1980 was seen in April 1981 because of a 4-month history of fever, dyspnea, and cough. On admission he was found to have *P. carinii* pneumonia, oral candidiasis, and CMV retinitis. A complement-fixation CMV titer in April 1981 was 128. The patient has been treated with 2 short courses of TMP/SMX that have been limited because of a sulfa-induced neutropenia. He is being treated for candidiasis with topical nystatin.

The diagnosis of *Pneumocystis* pneumonia was confirmed for all 5 patients antemortem by closed or open lung biopsy. The patients did not know each other and had no known common contacts or knowledge of sexual partners who had had similar illnesses. Two of the 5 reported having frequent homosexual contacts with various partners. All 5 reported using inhalant drugs, and 1 reported parenteral drug abuse. Three patients had profoundly depressed *in vitro* proliferative responses to mitogens and antigens. Lymphocyte studies were not performed on the other 2 patients.

Editorial Note: *Pneumocystis* pneumonia in the United States is almost exclusively limited to severely immunosuppressed patients (1). The occurrence of *pneumocystosis* in these 5 previously healthy individuals without a clinically apparent underlying immunodeficiency is unusual. The fact that these patients were all homosexuals suggests an association between some aspect of a homosexual lifestyle or disease acquired through sexual contact and *Pneumocystis* pneumonia in this population. All 5 patients described in this report had laboratory-confirmed CMV disease or virus shedding within 5 months of the diagnosis of *Pneumocystis* pneumonia. CMV infection has been shown to induce transient abnormalities of *in vitro* cellular-immune function in otherwise healthy human hosts (2,3). Although all 3 patients tested had abnormal cellular-immune function, no definitive conclusion regarding the role of CMV infection in these 5 cases can be reached because of the lack of published data on cellular-immune function in healthy homosexual males with and without CMV antibody.

In 1 report, 7 (3.6%) of 194 patients with pneumocystosis also had CMV infection; 40 (21%) of the same group had at least 1 other major concurrent infection (1). A high prevalence of CMV infections among homosexual males was recently reported: 179 (94%) had CMV viruria; rates for 101 controls of similar age who were reported to be exclusively heterosexual were 54% for seropositivity and zero for viruria (4). In another study of 64 males, 4 (6.3%) had positive tests for CMV in semen, but none had CMV recovered from urine. Two of the 4 reported recent homosexual contacts. These findings suggest not only that virus shedding may be more readily detected in seminal fluid than urine, but also that seminal fluid may be an important vehicle of CMV transmission (5).

All the above observations suggest the possibility of a cellular-immune dysfunction related to a common exposure that predisposes individuals to opportunistic infections such as pneumocystosis and candidiasis. Although the role of CMV infection in the pathogenesis of pneumocystosis remains unknown, the possibility of *P. carinii* infection must be carefully considered in a differential diagnosis for previously healthy homosexual males with dyspnea and pneumonia.

References

1. Walzer PD, Perl DP, Krogstad DJ, Rawson G, Schultz MG. *Pneumocystis carinii* pneumonia in the United States. Epidemiologic, diagnostic, and clinical features. *Ann Intern Med* 1974; 80:83–93.
2. Rinaldo CR, Jr., Black PH, Hirsh MS. Interaction of cytomegalovirus with leukocytes from patients with mononucleosis due to cytomegalovirus. *J Infect Dis* 1977; 136:667–78.
3. Rinaldo CR, Jr., Carney WP, Richter BS, Black PH, Hirsh MS. Mechanisms of immunosuppression in cytomegaloviral mononucleosis. *J Infect Dis* 1980; 141:488–95.
4. Drew WL, Mintz L, Miner RC, Sands M, Ketterer B. Prevalence of cytomegalovirus infection in homosexual men. *J Infect Dis* 1981; 143:188–92.
5. Lang DJ, Kummer JF. Cytomegalovirus in semen: observations in selected populations,. *J Infect Dis* 1975; 132:472–3.

similarities
↳ PCP
- ↑ fever + liver function
- candida inf
- CMV inf

7.3

U.S. Drops Charges Against AIDS Pioneer

Sheryl Stolberg

THE FEDERAL GOVERNMENT FRIDAY RELUCTANTLY DROPPED charges of scientific misconduct against Dr. Robert C. Gallo, the pioneering researcher who has spent the past decade fighting accusations that his role in the discovery of the AIDS virus was tainted by failure to give proper credit to French scientists.

The decision by the Office of Research Integrity reversed an earlier guilty finding. It came just three days before a hearing was to begin on Gallo's appeal and brought an official end to what may be the most closely watched ethics probe in modern medical science.

It did not lay to rest the international controversy over who discovered the AIDS virus. In the wake of the ruling, French scientists once again demanded full credit for the discovery and all royalties from the blood test it made possible—despite a 1987 accord in which France and the United States agreed to share credit and split the money.

Gallo was cleared last year of the most serious allegation, a charge that he stole the virus from the Pasteur Institute in Paris. But, in a serious blot on his career, he was found guilty of scientific misconduct for failing to acknowledge the contribution of French scientists to his work.

Government investigators made clear Friday that they are still troubled by his actions in the early to mid-1980s, saying they withdrew the charges solely as "a practical matter." A recent legal decision, they said, set "a new and extremely difficult standard" for proving scientific misconduct.

"Clearly, we weren't happy to do it," said Dr. Lyle W. Bivens, who heads the Office of Research Integrity. "We felt that we couldn't proceed with our case."

But the 56-year-old researcher, who has vehemently denied wrongdoing, declared that he was "delighted" by the ruling.

"I have been completely vindicated," Gallo said in a brief statement. "I will now be able to redouble my efforts in the fight against AIDS and cancer."

Widely regarded as a brilliant scientist, Gallo is known as much for his brusque manner as for his contributions to AIDS and cancer research. His lab at the National Cancer Institute is working on an AIDS vaccine, and on gene therapy treatments for AIDS and cancer. He has also helped develop drugs that are being tested for Kaposi's sarcoma, a cancer common to AIDS patients.

Friday's decision was not entirely a surprise. Last week, in a related case, an appeals panel overturned a judgment against Dr. Mikulas Popovic, who had carried out crucial AIDS experiments under Gallo's direction.

Like Gallo, Popovic was found guilty of scientific misconduct last year by the Office of Research Integrity, an arm of the U.S. Department of Health and Human Services. When Popovic won his appeal, it became apparent that Gallo—whose hearing was set to begin Monday morning—would win as well.

In the Popovic decision, the appeals board ruled that false statements alone were not enough to warrant a finding of scientific misconduct. Rather, the board said, the agency would have to prove that the statements were deliberately deceptive, that they had a significant effect on the research conclusions of the paper and that there was no possibility of honest error.

Bivens said it made no sense to go forward under those terms, "in the face of virtual certainty that we would lose." He added that his office intends to work toward legislation that would make such cases easier to prove.

Controversy has swirled around Gallo's research since 1984, when he published a paper in the prestigious journal *Science* that described how he had discovered the virus that causes AIDS. At the time, researchers worldwide were racing to find the cause of the mysterious new disease.

One year earlier, researchers in the laboratory of Dr. Luc Montagnier at the Pasteur Institute in Paris had published similar findings, saying they had isolated a virus taken from AIDS patients, but were uncertain whether it caused the disease. Calling the virus LAV, they sent two samples to Gallo's lab.

When Gallo's paper appeared in *Science*, critics accused him of stealing the virus from the French and taking credit for their work. Although Gallo denied the claims, later analysis showed that the virus he had isolated was nearly identical to that of the French, indicating that it may have been the same virus.

In 1985, when the AIDS blood test was licensed, the French sued the U.S. government over credit for the discovery of the virus. That suit was settled in 1987 with an agreement signed by President Ronald Reagan and French Prime Minister Jacques Chirac naming Gallo and Montagnier as co-discoverers.

France is now trying to renegotiate that agreement. In a statement Friday, lawyers for the Pasteur Institute said the U.S. government is "obligated by both conscience and its commitment to scientific integrity" to give them full credit.

Although the matter was the subject of international negotiations, the U.S. government did not launch a formal ethics probe until 1989, after the *Chicago Tribune* published an extensive article detailing the charges against Gallo.

The government took three years to investigate. Last December, the Office of Research Integrity cleared Gallo of the charge that he stole the virus from the French, but concluded that he had "falsely reported" the role that the French samples had played in his work in an intentional effort to mislead colleagues and gain credit for himself.

The agency also found that Gallo had failed to give proper credit to American scientists who developed the cell culture in which his researchers grew the AIDS virus. The report also charged that Gallo withheld the AIDS culture from other laboratories, slowing the pace of research.

Gallo appealed. "The charges against Gallo were false," said his lawyer, Joseph Onek, on Friday. "They were always false. The government, despite all this rigmarole, withdrew the case because it knew it could not prove these false charges."

Gallo is a dumb stuck up man

Section VIII

Origin of HIV

8.1

The Origin and Diversity of the HIV-1 Pandemic

Joris Hemelaar

This review examines the enormous progress that has been made in the past decade in understanding the origin of HIV, HIV genetic variability, and the impact of global HIV diversity on the pandemic. Multiple zoonotic transmissions of simian immunodeficiency virus (SIV) have resulted in different HIV lineages in humans. In addition, the high mutation and recombination rates during viral replication result in a great genetic variability of HIV within individuals, as well as within populations, upon which evolutionary selection pressures act. The global HIV pandemic is examined in the context of HIV evolution, and the global diversity of HIV subtypes and recombinants is discussed in detail. Finally, the impact of HIV diversity on pathogenesis, transmission, diagnosis, treatment, the immune response, and vaccine development is reviewed.

Global Epidemiology of HIV

HIV-1 remains a global health problem of unprecedented dimensions. Since the recognition of acquired immunodeficiency syndrome (AIDS) in 1981 and the discovery of human immunodeficiency virus (HIV) as the causative agent in 1983, 60 million people have become infected with HIV, 25 million of whom have since died [1–3]. Although the percentage of people living with HIV globally has stabilised since 2000, the overall number of people infected with HIV has steadily increased to an estimated 33.3 million in 2009 (Box 8.1a) [3].

Box 8.1a: Further sources of information

- Global epidemiology: http://www.unaids.org/en/KnowledgeCentre/HIVData/default.asp
- Los Alamos National Laboratory HIV sequence database: http://www.hiv.lanl.gov/content/sequence/HIV/mainpage.html
- Circulating recombinant forms (CRFs) composition, structure and reference strains: http://www.hiv.lanl.gov/content/sequence/HIV/CRFs/CRFs.html

Joris Hemelaar, "The Origin and Diversity of the HIV-1 Pandemic," *Trends in Molecular Medicine*, vol. 18, no. 3, pp. 182–192.

This review examines the HIV pandemic from an evolutionary perspective, starting with the zoonotic origin of HIV. High mutation and recombination rates during viral replication create a viral diversity in the host that is subject to evolutionary selection pressures by host restriction factors and the immune response. The timing and spread of the global HIV pandemic is examined in the context of HIV evolution, and the global diversity of HIV subtypes and recombinants this has generated is discussed in detail. Finally, the impact of HIV diversity on key aspects of HIV infection—such as pathogenesis, transmission, clinical management, the immune response and vaccine development—is discussed, as well as ways in which our understanding of HIV diversity can be harnessed to combat HIV.

HIV as a Zoonosis

origin

HIV originated from multiple zoonotic (see Glossary) transmissions of simian immunodeficiency virus (SIV) from nonhuman primates into humans in West and Central Africa. Cross-species transmission probably occurred in the process of hunting and butchering of primates for bushmeat and the capture, trade and keeping of monkeys as pets [4]. More than 40 different nonhuman primate species harbour SIV infections, with each species carrying a species-specific virus [5]. Independent zoonotic transmission events from nonhuman primates to humans have generated several HIV lineages: HIV type 1 (HIV-1) groups M, N, O and P and HIV type 2 (HIV-2) groups A–H. The size of the epidemic caused by each group varies considerably. HIV-1 group M is responsible for the global HIV pandemic (approximately 33 million infected individuals), group O causes a few tens of thousands of infections in West–Central Africa, group N has been found in a handful of people in Cameroon and group P was recently identified in two individuals originating from Cameroon [6–10]. It is conceivable that further HIV lineages in humans will be discovered in the future, as all HIV lineages may not yet have been identified and new cross-species transmissions may take place in the future.

Glossary

Ancestral sequence: a sequence that represents the ancestor from which a given group of more recent sequences have descended, reconstructed by computer modelling based on an evolutionary model.

Centre-of-tree sequence: a sequence, obtained via computer modelling, whereby the average evolutionary distance to each tip of a phylogeny is minimised.

Consensus sequence: a sequence in which each amino acid is the most commonly found at that position in the group of sequences studied (e.g. within a subtype).

Host restriction factors: cellular proteins expressed by the host which limit the ability of HIV/SIV to infect or replicate in cells of a particular species. HIV restriction factors include APOBEC, TRIM5α, and tetherin.

KIR (killer immunoglobulin-like receptors): activating and inhibitory receptors on natural killer (NK) cells which recognise MHC class I–peptide complexes.

Molecular clock: a statistical model that describes the relationship between time and genetic distances among sequences.

Nef (negative factor): viral protein associated with cytoplasmic membranes which induces complex changes in trafficking, signal transduction, and gene expression, including down-modulation of CD4 and MHC class I molecules from the cell surface.

Phylogenetics: the study of the evolutionary relationships between organisms based on their genetic relatedness.

Tetherin: a cellular membrane protein that inhibits release of HIV particles by tethering mature viral particles to the cell surface.

Time to the most recent common ancestor (tMRCA): estimated time to the most recent sequence from which all sequences in the examined group have directly descended, as determined by phylogenetic and molecular clock analysis, usually expressed as the year AD.

Vpu (viral protein U): integral membrane protein expressed by HIV-1 whose main functions are the targeting of CD4 for degradation by the ubiquitin–proteasome pathway and the inhibition of tetherin.

Zoonosis: an infectious disease transmitted from animals to humans, or the event of cross-species transmission.

HIV-1 groups M and N originate directly, but independently, from SIVcpz found in the chimpanzee *Pan troglodytes troglodytes* in West–Central Africa (Figure 8.1.1) [11,12]. SIVcpz itself arose through recombination between ancestors of SIVrcm from red-capped mangabeys (*Cercocebus torquatus*) and SIVgsn from greater spot-nosed monkeys (*Cercopithecus nictitans*) within chimpanzees or an intermediate host [13]. Isolated wild-living *P. t. troglodytes* chimpanzee communities in South–Eastern and South–Central Cameroon form natural reservoirs of SIV which gave rise to HIV-1 groups M and N, respectively. Whereas group N has remained confined to a small number of individuals in Cameroon (13 individuals identified so far with an estimated prevalence of 0.1% in Cameroon) [14], group M spread south via the Congo river to what is now Kinshasa in the Democratic Republic of the Congo (DRC) (formerly Leopoldville, Zaire), from where the global HIV-1 epidemic was probably initiated [...] [12].

OH review

HIV-1 group O and the newly discovered group P are related to SIVgor identified in wild-living Western lowland gorillas (Gorilla gorilla gorilla) in Cameroon (Figure 8.1.1) [8,12,15]. SIVgor itself is thought to be derived from an ancestor of a divergent SIVcpz lineage in chimpanzees [16]. It is possible that HIV-1 groups O and P were derived from independent transmissions of SIVgor strains from gorillas to humans. Although this seems the most probable scenario for group P (given its close clustering with SIVgor sequences in phylogenetic analyses), it cannot be ruled out that group O originated from chimpanzees transmitting related viruses directly to humans as well as to gorillas [8,12,15,16]. Group O infections have not spread significantly beyond Cameroon, Gabon and Equatorial Guinea and the prevalence of group O in Cameroon has remained stable and very low (approximately 1.1%) [9,17]. Group P has so far only been identified in 2 individuals originating from Yaounde, Cameroon [8,10].

Timing of Cross-Species Transmissions

The earliest direct evidence of HIV infection in humans was found retrospectively in a serum sample and a lymph node biopsy specimen stored in 1959 and 1960, respectively, in Kinshasa in the DRC

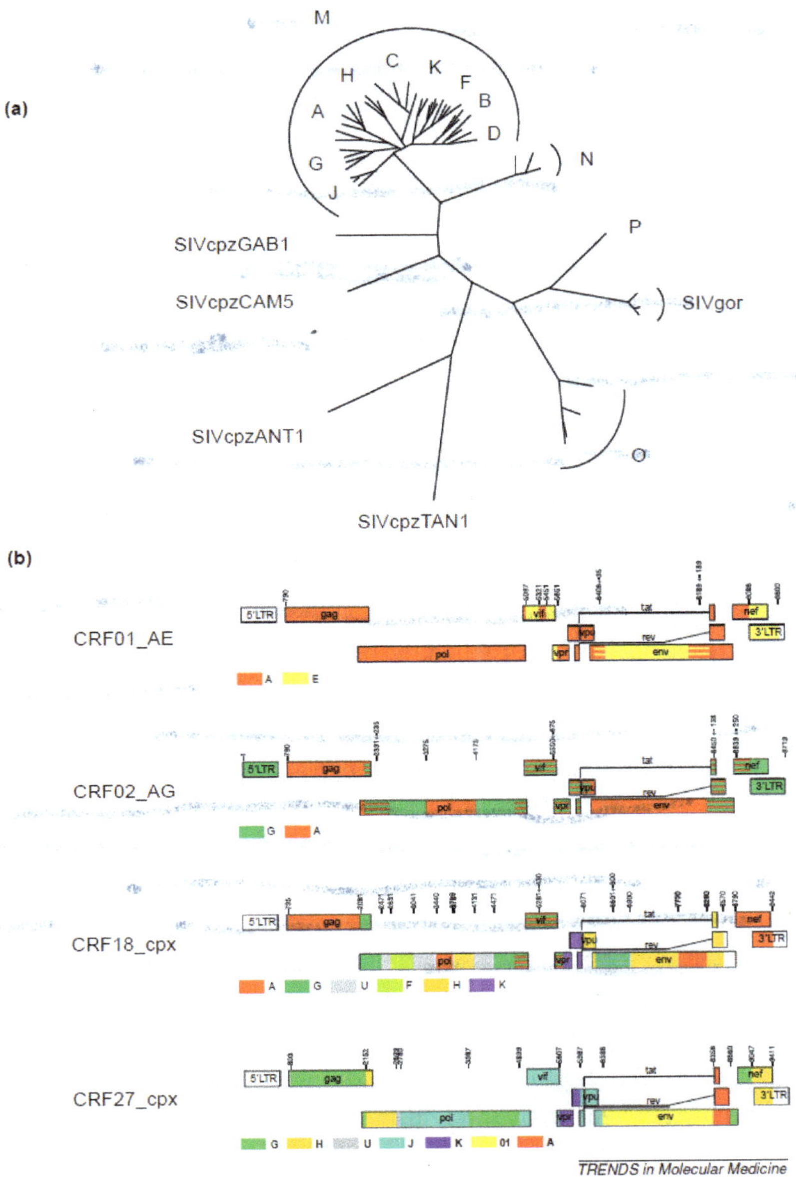

FIGURE 8.1.1 *(a) Phylogenetic tree of SIV and HIV-1. Phylogenetic tree based on polymerase sequences of reference sequences of SIV and HIV-1 [97]. Sequences were aligned using ClustalW2 [ClustalW2 program: http://www.ebi.ac.uk/Tools/msa/clustalw2/] and a rootless tree was built with the Phylip software package using the maximum likelihood method and the Drawtree program [PHYLIP software: http://evolution.gs.washington.edu/phylip.html]. HIV-1 group M subtypes A–D, F–H, J and K are indicated. Circulating recombinant forms clustering with M group subtypes have been omitted for clarity. HIV-1 groups N, O and P are also indicated. For SIV from chimpanzees two SIVcpz sequences derived from each of the Pan troglodytes subspecies troglodytes (SIVcpzCAM5 and SIVcpzGAB1) and schweinfurthii (SIVcpzANT and SIVcpzTAN1) were included. Three representative sequences for SIV derived from gorilla (Gorilla gorilla gorilla) were included (SIVgor). (b) Recombinant structures of CRFs. The subtype compositions of selected CRFs are shown [Los Alamos National Laboratory (http://www.hiv.lanl.gov/content/sequence/HIV/CRFs/CRFs.html)].*

[18,19]. As well as providing direct evidence of the age of the HIV epidemic in humans, these samples have been instrumental in the validation and extrapolations of molecular clock computer programs used to estimate the time to the most recent common ancestors (tMRCAs) and evolutionary rates of various HIV lineages [19,20].

HIV-1 group M appears to be the oldest HIV lineage in humans, with an estimated tMRCA in the first two or three decades of the 1900s (Table 8.1.1) [19,20]. The tMRCA shared between group M and SIVcpz is estimated at 1853 (1799–1904) [21]. Cross-species transfer is therefore inferred to have taken place sometime between 1853 and the early 1900s, although there is some uncertainty, given the size of the confidence intervals. The estimated date of origin of the group O radiation, circa 1920 (1890–1940), is very similar to the tMRCA of group M (Table 8.1.1) [22]. Estimation of the tMRCA of group P awaits identification of further infections, as only two different sequences are available, precluding relevant phylogenetic analysis [8,10]. Cross-species transmission of HIV-1 group N probably took place later in the 20th century as the tMRCA is estimated to be as recent as 1963 (1948–1977) and the tMRCA shared between group N and SIVcpz is 1921 (1885–1955) [21]. Although groups M and N are both derived from SIVcpz*Ptt* from chimpanzees in Cameroon, they have distinct times of origin and have spread to very different extents. Conversely, group O appears to have originated at a similar time as group M but has only infected several thousand people. Although the time of origin of group P is unknown, its prevalence appears very low [10]. It is tempting to speculate whether these differences are due to chance or whether there are identifiable molecular factors responsible for differences in cross-species transmission and subsequent adaptation and spread. A possible explanation for some of these findings comes from the extent to which different HIV groups have overcome the host restriction factor tetherin [23]. Tetherin prevents viral particle release [from] infected cells by linking viral and cellular membranes. Although Nef protein confers resistance to tetherin in chimpanzees and gorillas, Nef is unable to do so in humans due to a deletion in the cytoplasmic region of human tetherin. Instead, Vpu in HIV-1 group M is able to efficiently counteract human tetherin while retaining the ability of Vpu to downregulate CD4. Vpu of group N is able to inhibit tetherin to some extent but is no longer able to downregulate CD4. By contrast, Vpu proteins of groups O and P are unable to antagonise human tetherin (although they can still downregulate CD4) [23]. Further elucidation of the molecular differences between these HIV lineages may shed further light on their origin, transmission and pathogenesis.

HIV Genetic Diversity in Individuals

One of the most important factors in the worldwide spread of HIV is its enormous genetic variability and rapid evolution. This genetic variability of HIV results from the high mutation and recombination rates of the reverse transcriptase enzyme, which lacks a proof-reading mechanism [24], together with high rates of virus replication [25]. Insertions and deletions in the viral genome are also frequent occurrences. These mechanisms result in the rapid generation of genetically diverse viral populations within each infected individual. Viral sequences within a single individual can differ by up to 10% [26].

Recent studies on newly infected individuals have shown that a large proportion of productive infections are initiated by a single infectious unit (a single virus or infected cell), whereas the remainder are the result of multiple variants [27–31]. This dramatic reduction in viral diversity from a diverse

TABLE 8.1.1 Time to the most recent common ancestors (tMRCA) of HIV-1 groups, subtypes, and CRFs

HIV-1 group	tMRCA[a]	CI[b]	Refs
Group M	1921	1908–1933	[19]
Group M	1920/1937	1902–1949*	[98]
Group M	1931	1915–1941	[20]
Group O	1920	1890–1940	[22]
Group N	1963	1948–1977	[21]
HIV-1 group M subtype/CRF			
Subtype A1 (Africa)	1948	1865–1969	[63]
Subtype A1	1954	1939–1968	[34]
Subtype B/D	1949/1954	1935–1964*	[98]
Subtype B/D	1950	1938–1959	[20]
Subtype B/D	1954	1946–1961	[99]
Subtype D	1944/1946	1935–1955	[34]
Subtype D (East Africa)	1958/1967	1931–1984	[63]
Subtype D	1966	1961–1971	[99]
Subtype C	1952/1955	1933–1971	[34]
Subtype C	1958	1949–1960	[42]
Subtype C	1966–1969	1959–1973	[100]
Subtype C	1967	1962–1972	[101]
Subtype C (Zimbabwe)	1972	1969–1974	[102]
Subtype C (India)	1976/1979	1972–1982	[101]
Subtype C (China)	1981	1976–1985	[101]
Subtype C' (Ethiopia)	1982	1980–1983	[103]
Subtype C (Ethiopia)	1983	1980–1984	[104]
Subtype C (Brazil)	1980–1983	1966–1988	[105]
Subtype B	1959–1966	1950–1972	[34]
Subtype B (Global and Haiti)	1966	1962–1970	[99]
Subtype B	1970/1972	1963–1978*	[98]
Subtype B	1976/1977	1974–1980	[106]
Subtype B (Brazil)	1964/1967	1946–1984	[105]
Subtype B (USA)	1967	1960–1971	[20]
Subtype B (USA/Canada)	1969	1966–1972	[99]
Subtype B (Trinidad and Tobago)	1973	1970–1976	[99]
Subtype B (Albania)	1976	1954–1986	[107]
Subtype B (South Korea)	1984	1972–1989	[108]
Subtype G	1969	1959–1978	[34]
Subtype F1 (South America)	1976	1966–1982	[109]
Subtype F (Brazil)	1977/1978	1963–1988	[105]
CRF01_AE (Africa)	1965/1969	1963–1973	[110]
CRF01_AE	1975	1970–1980	[34]

cs

HIV = J diverse

HIV-1 group	tMRCA[a]	CI[b]	Refs
CRF01_AE (Thailand)	1984	1980–1986	[20]
CRF01_AE (Vietnam, South, hetero)	1980/1981	1979–1982	[110]
CRF01_AE (Vietnam, South, IDU)	1987/1990	1987–1990	[110]
CRF01_AE (Vietnam, North)	1993/1994	1992–1995	[110]
CRF02_AG	1973	1972–1975	[111]
CRF02_AG	1975/1976	1969–1981	[34]
CRF31_BC (Brazil)	1988	1982–1992	[112]
CRF08_BC (China)	1990	1988–1991	[101]
CRF07_BC (China)	1993	1991–1995	[101]
CRF33_01B (Malaysia)	1991–1993	1987–1997	[113]

[a]tMRCAs refer to the global strains unless otherwise stated.
[b]CI, 95% confidence intervals. Where there are multiple estimates of the tMRCAs (based on the analysis of multiple different genome fragments) for a given group or subtype/CRF then the outer limits of the overlapping CIs are given.
*indicates a 99% CI.

swarm in the donor to a very limited number of variants in the recipient represents a genetic bottleneck. This reduction in diversity is dependent on the transmission route, as approximately 80% of productive infections are caused by a single virus in heterosexual transmission, but only 60% in men who have sex with men (MSM) and 40% in intravenous drug users (IDU) [27–31]. The mucosal barrier is thought to be important for this genetic bottleneck as inflammatory genital infections and hormonal contraceptives are associated with increased acquisition of multiple HIV-1 variants [29,32].

Classification and Sequence Variation in HIV-1 Groups and Subtypes

During the course of the HIV epidemics in humans the sequences of the different HIV-1 groups have diversified in the population, which has prompted further classifications. Within the pandemic HIV-1 group M nine subtypes are recognised, designated by the letters A–D, F–H, J and K. Within a subtype, variation at the amino acid level is in the order of 8–17% but can be as high as 30%, whereas variation between subtypes is usually between 17% and 35% but can be up to 42%, depending on the subtypes and genome regions examined [26]. Intra-subtype diversity continues to increase over time [33] and evolution rates may differ according to subtype [34].

Group O sequence diversity is high, which has led to a classification of sequences into clades I–V, which are as genetically distant from each other as are group M subtypes, consistent with the tMRCA of group O being similar to group M. However, there is less subtype-like signal in group O compared to group M because group O has not spread much beyond its origin in West-Central Africa [19,35,36]. All group N viruses found in humans are closely related, as are the two group P sequences [7,10].

Superinfection

Dual infection is detected in 10–20% of HIV-infected individuals in regions in Africa where different variants co-circulate [37]. Dual infection can be due to simultaneous infection with two heterologous strains (co-infection) or due to sequential infection, in which a second infection with a heterologous strain occurs after seroconversion to the initial infection has taken place (superinfection). It is now clear that superinfection with a virus from the same group M subtype (intra-subtype) as well as different subtype (inter-subtype) can occur throughout the course of infection, although the relative frequency at which these happen is uncertain [38]. Moreover, dual infection may be associated with higher viral load setpoint and more rapid disease progression [39,40].

HIV-1 Recombinants: CRFs, URFs, SGRs

Analyses of multiple genome regions and in particular full-length genome sequencing have revealed that recombination between strains is a frequent occurrence. Recombination does not appear to be limited by sequence similarity as recombination has been demonstrated between strains from different groups in HIV-1 (groups M and O) as well as between and within group M subtypes [41,42]. Intra-subtype recombination was found to be very extensive within group M subtype C [42], although such data are lacking for other subtypes.

Recombinants between different HIV-1 group M subtypes are designated as either circulating recombinant forms (CRFs) if fully sequenced and found in three or more epidemiologically unlinked individuals or as unique recombinant forms (URFs) if not meeting these criteria [43]. Newly discovered CRFs are named in the order in which they are discovered and described, and their numbering therefore does not reflect their evolutionary history or the chronological order in which they were formed. CRFs bear an extension which indicates from which 'pure' subtypes the CRF is derived (Table 8.1.2). The extension 'cpx', for complex, is given if the CRF consists of contributions from three or more different subtypes. CRFs can be true mosaics being composed of a tapestry of segments derived from many different subtypes, such as CRF18_cpx and CRF27_cpx, which are composed of five or six different subtypes as well as unclassified segments (Figure 8.1.2) [44,45]. All currently described CRFs are listed in Table 8.1.2, together with information regarding their subtype composition and geographical distribution.

TABLE 8.1.2 Circulating recombinant forms (CRFs) of HIV-1[a]

CRF	Subtype composition	Geographical distribution
CRF01_AE	A, E	South-East Asia, East Asia, Central Africa
CRF02_AG	A, G	West Africa, Central Africa, MENA
CRF03_AB	A, B	Eastern Europe and Central Asia
CRF04_cpx	A, G, H, K, U	Greece, Cyprus
CRF05_DF	D, F	Central Africa, Europe
CRF06_cpx	A, G, J, K	Central Africa, West Africa, Estonia
CRF07_BC	B′, C	China
CRF08_BC	B′, C	China
CRF09_cpx	A, G, U	West Africa, Central Africa
CRF10_CD	C, D	Tanzania
CRF11_cpx	A, G, J, CRF01_AE	Central Africa

CRF	Subtype composition	Geographical distribution
CRF12_BF	B, F	South America
CRF13_cpx	A, G, J, U, CRF01_AE, CRF11_cpx	Central Africa
CRF14_BG	B, G	Spain
CRF15_01B	CRF01_AE, B	Thailand
CRF16_A2D	A2, D	Kenya, Argentina, South Korea
CRF17_BF	BF	South America
CRF18_cpx	A1, F, G, H, K, U	Cuba, Central Africa
CRF19_cpx	A1, D, G	Cuba, Central Africa
CRF20_BG	B, G	Cuba
CRF21_A2D	A2,D	Kenya
CRF22_01A1	CRF01_AE, A1	Cameroon
CRF23_BG	B, G	Cuba
CRF24_BG	B, G	Cuba
CRF25_cpx	A, G, U	Central Africa, Saudi Arabia
CRF26_AU	A, U	Democratic Republic of the Congo
CRF27_cpx	A, E, G, H, J, K, U	Democratic Republic of the Congo
CRF28_BF	B, F	Brazil
CRF29_BF	B, F	Brazil
CRF30_0206	CRF02_AG, CRF06_cpx	Niger
CRF31_BC	B, C	Brazil
CRF32_06A1	CRF06_cpx, A1	Estonia
CRF33_01B	CRF01_AE, B	Malaysia, Singapore, Indonesia
CRF34_01B	CRF01_AE, B	Thailand
CRF35_AD	A, D	Afghanistan, Iran
CRF36_cpx	A, G, CRF01_AE, CRF02_AG	Cameroon
CRF37_cpx	A, G, CRF01_AE, CRF02_AG, U	Cameroon, Mozambique
CRF38_BF1	B, F	Uruguay
CRF39_BF	B, F	Brazil
CRF40_BF	B, F	Brazil
CRF41_CD	C, D	N.K.[b]
CRF42_BF	B, F1	Luxembourg
CRF43_02G	CRF02_AG, G	Saudi Arabia
CRF44_BF	B, F	Chile
CRF45_AKU	A, K, U	Central Africa
CRF46_BF1	B, F	Brazil
CRF47_BF	B, F	Spain
CRF48_01B	CRF01_AE, B	Malaysia
CRF49_cpx	A, C, J, K, U	The Gambia
CRF51_01B	CRF01_AE, B	Singapore

[a]Adapted from Los Alamos National Laboratory (http://www.hiv.lanl.gov/content/sequence/HIV/CRFs/CRFs.html).

[b]N.K.: not known.

The attribution and classification of CRFs is not without controversy, largely due to the (limited) availability of strains at the time of the initial classification as well as the difficulty in defining recombination breakpoints. In particular, it has been questioned whether CRF01_AE and CRF02_AG are recombinants. Large parts of the CRF01_AE genome cluster with subtype A in phylogenetic analyses, whereas the envelope region is distinct and was designated as being derived from a subtype 'E'. However, a 'pure' subtype E lineage has never been found, which led some to suggest that CRF01_AE is in fact 'subtype E' [46]. [Most] probably, however, CRF01_AE is the result of a recombination event early on in the epidemic after which the putative parental 'pure' subtype E has become extinct. This is certainly conceivable given the high frequency of unique and unclassifiable sequences found in Central and West Africa (see below) [47–51]. Similarly, it was proposed that CRF02_AG was in fact a 'pure' subtype and that subtype G was actually a recombinant of fragments of subtypes A, J and CRF02_AG [52,53]. However, others have confirmed CRF02_AG as a recombinant of subtypes A and G [54]. Moreover, the estimated tMRCAs of subtypes A and G precede those of CRF01_AE and CRF-2_AG (Table 8.1.1), and the nomenclature has remained unchanged [Los Alamos National Laboratory (http://www.hiv.lanl.gov/content/sequence/HIV/CRFs/CRFs.html)].

Some CRFs (such as CRF01_AE and CRF02_AG) were formed early on in the epidemic in Central Africa and subsequently spread to other regions where they play important roles in regional epidemics as well as globally, whereas other CRFs were formed elsewhere in the world (Tables 8.1.1 and 8.1.2) [55]. Recombination is ongoing in many places in the world where different subtypes and CRFs co-circulate, so-called 'recombination hotspots', continuously giving rise to URFs. A high prevalence of URFs (and the subtypes/CRFs involved) is found in West Africa (CRF02, CRF06_cpx and CRF09_cpx) [49], Central Africa (many different subtypes and CRFs) [51], East Africa (A, C, D) [56], South America (B, F, C) [57], Cuba (B, G, CRF18_cpx, CRF19_cpx) [58], China (B, C, CRF07_BC, CRF08_BC) [59], and South and South-East Asia (B, CRF01_AE) [60].

Once URFs are transmitted onwards in the population they can give rise to new CRFs. For example, out of the multitude of different unique B/F recombinants in South America several B/F CRFs have become established (Table 8.1.2). Some CRFs have recombined further with other subtypes or CRFs giving rise to so-called second generation recombinants (SGRs) (Table 8.1.2).

With increased global availability of sequencing techniques, it has become apparent that recombinant forms are widespread and increasing as a proportion of the total number of HIV-1 infections. Recombinants are currently estimated to be responsible for at least 20% of HIV-1 infections worldwide [55].

Central Africa is the Epicentre of the Global HIV Epidemic

The different subtypes and recombinants have distinct global distribution patterns (Figure 8.1.2) [55]. All HIV-1 group M 'pure' subtypes were found early in the epidemic in Central Africa in countries such as the DRC, Cameroon and Central African Republic (CAR) (Figure 8.1.2), further evidence of the origin of the HIV epidemic in Central Africa (Box 8.1b) [33,51,61]. Furthermore, high proportions of unique, unclassifiable sequences in addition to CRFs and URFs are found here [51,61]. Indeed, the genetic diversity in the DRC is comparable to that among global strains [51]. The isolates from the DRC fall basal to the origin of each subtype in phylogenetic analyses, indicating that the DRC and global strains have a common ancestor [33]. This distinction originates from the chance dispersal of some strains from the DRC to other geographical regions where these initiated further epidemics, the so-called 'founder effect' [33]. In this respect it is interesting to note that during the explosive expansion of the global HIV pandemic, the HIV prevalence rates in Central Africa have remained stable at around 5%, suggesting an old and mature epidemic consistent with it being the epicentre of the HIV-1 group M epidemic [62].

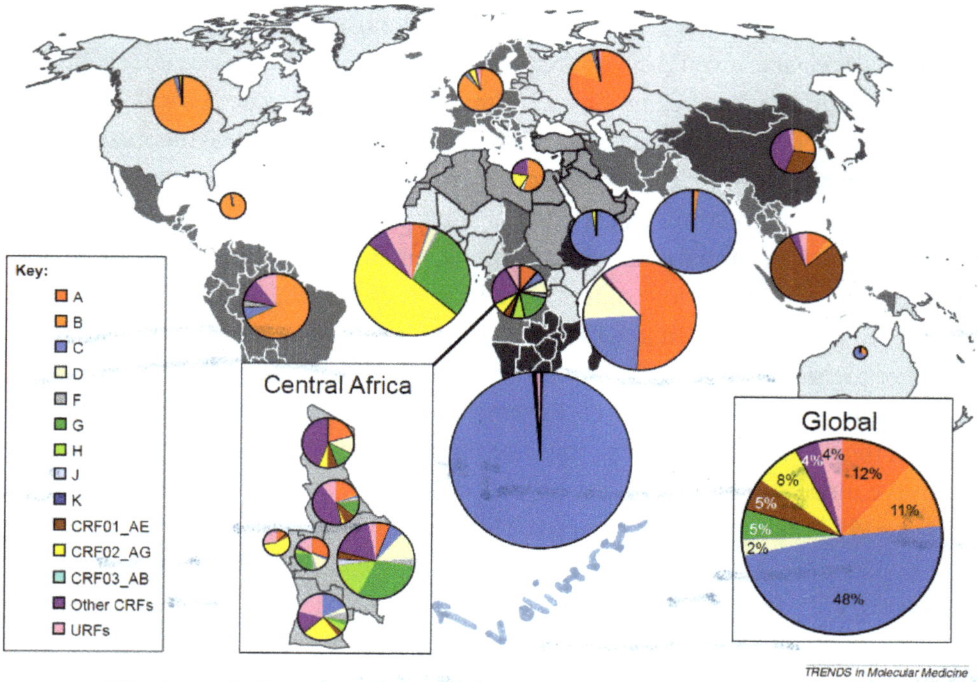

FIGURE 8.1.2 *Global distribution of HIV-1 subtypes and recombinants. In the main figure, pie charts representing the distribution of HIV-1 subtypes and recombinants from 2004 to 2007 in each region are superimposed on the regions. The relative surface areas of the pie charts correspond to the relative numbers of people living with HIV in the regions. The colours representing the different HIV-1 subtypes and recombinants are indicated in the legend on the left-hand side of the figure. The HIV-1 subtype distributions found around the world and within Central African countries are shown in the insets of the main figure, as indicated. Reproduced and adapted with permission from [55].*

Box 8.1b: Arguments for the Origin of HIV-1 in Central Africa

- Territory of chimpanzees carrying SIV strains similar to HIV-1 is in Central Africa
- Oldest known human HIV samples found in Central Africa
- All HIV groups (M, N, O, and P) are found in Central Africa
- Highest sequence diversity, and all 'pure' subtypes, are found in Central Africa
- Large proportion of unclassified unique strains in Central Africa
- High proportion and diversity of URFs and CRFs in Central Africa
- Sequences from Central Africa are basal to subtype origins in phylogenetic analyses

The explanations for the current global HIV-1 subtype distribution are probably multifactorial and include founder effects, population growth and urbanisation, cultural and sexual factors, and transport links and migration [19,63]. It is uncertain, at present, to what extent biological properties of different subtypes and recombinants play a role in their differential spread (see below).

Time of Origin of HIV-1 Group M Subtypes and Recombinants

After transmission to humans sometime around 1900, HIV-1 group M experienced a period of slow growth in the first half of the 20th century [19]. During this time, when the spread of HIV-1 group M was probably limited to Kinshasa and the surrounding area of the DRC, genetic diversification of group M in humans was already taking place. This is most clearly evidenced by the fact that the two oldest HIV-1 samples found to date, from 1959 and 1960, differed in sequence by 12% and belong to the group M subtypes D and A radiations, respectively [19]. Phylogenetic and molecular clock analysis has estimated the tMRCAs of individual group M subtypes to be between 1950 and 1970 (Table 8.1.1). As mentioned before, CRF01_AE and CRF02_AG seem to have formed shortly thereafter (Table 8.1.1). Although there is broad agreement between different studies estimating tMRCAs for different subtypes and/or CRFs, some discrepancies are evident that are probably due to differing sample sets, genome regions examined and analysis methods employed. From the middle of the past century onwards, the different 'pure' subtypes and CRF01_AE and CRF02_AG have spread across the world, each giving rise to epidemics that differ in size and geographical spread (Figure 8.1.2) [55]. The years of arrival ('founding') of some subtypes and CRFs in parts of the world outside Central Africa have been estimated as have the dates of origin of some CRFs formed outside Central Africa (Table 8.1.1).

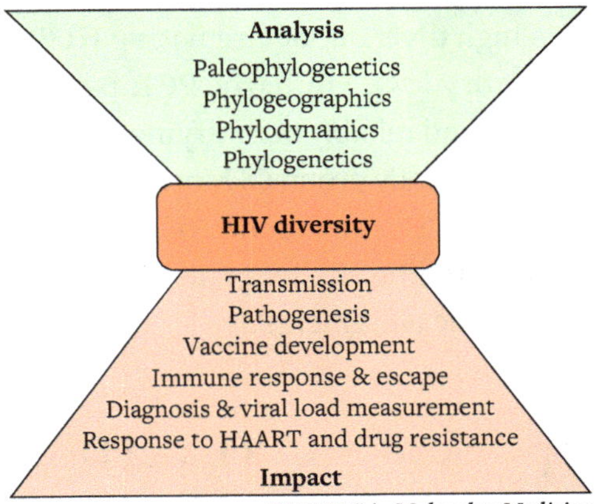

TRENDS in Molecular Medicine

FIGURE 8.1.3. *The central importance of HIV diversity. Analytic approaches which have informed our understanding of HIV diversity are listed at the top and aspects of the HIV pandemic on which HIV diversity impacts are listed at the bottom.*

The Impact of HIV Diversity

HIV diversity impacts virtually every aspect of the HIV pandemic (Figure 8.1.3). In the following sections, the effect of HIV diversity on disease progression and transmission, diagnosis and measurement of viral load, response to HAART and drug resistance, and the immune response and vaccine development will be highlighted.

Disease Progression and Transmission

The study of biological differences between HIV subtypes has been complicated by the differential distribution of HIV subtypes globally, which introduces potential confounding by host (ethnic/genetic) and environmental (co-infections, nutrition, socioeconomic) factors. Insight into the role of HIV subtypes in disease progression (as well as in transmission and viral load) has been obtained from cohort studies conducted in areas where different subtypes co-circulate, in particular East Africa. Independent studies in Uganda, Tanzania and Kenya all indicate that subtype D infection is associated with faster disease progression to death than subtype A in populations where these subtypes co-circulate [64–68]. The reduced survival was associated with lower CD4 counts in subtype D infection compared with subtype A in several studies [64,67–69]. In a Europe-an study subtype D was further noted to have a fourfold higher rate of CD4 count decline, in the absence of ARVs, compared with other subtypes in the study (A, B, C and CRF02_AG, which had similar rates of decline to one another), even when adjusted for baseline CD4 count [70]. In individuals with advanced immunosuppression, subtype D was also associated with higher rates of dementia compared with subtype A [71]. A study from Uganda found that subtype A has a higher rate of heterosexual transmission than subtype D [72]. Further studies from Uganda and Kenya found significant decreases over time in the proportion of subtype D and increases in subtype A [73,74]. These changes in the proportions of subtypes A and D are consistent with both the faster disease progression and the lower rate of heterosexual transmission of subtype D compared with subtype A.

Hiv Diagnosis and Viral Load Measurement

Although modern fourth-generation HIV-1 immunoassays are capable of detecting all known HIV-1 group M subtypes, group O and HIV-2, such advanced methodologies are often not available in resource-limited countries where most new infections occur. In field situations in Africa with a high diversity of circulating HIV strains the performance of diagnostic tests is much less satisfactory [75]. Similarly, PCR-based assays for viral load measurements have difficulty in detecting and reliably quantifying HIV-1 RNA when testing diverse genetic variants of HIV-1 from Africa, especially group O. Moreover, different assays not uncommonly yield discordant viral load results [76]. The emergence of new variants and ensuring that the assays detect them is therefore a continuing challenge, as nondetection or inefficient detection can lead to erroneously low viral load measurements.

Response to HAART and Drug Resistance

A large number of studies conducted in African and Asian countries using various different drug regimens in a variety of settings have demonstrated that different group M subtypes have similar susceptibilities to currently used antiretroviral drugs, which were originally developed based on subtype B [77]. A large global collaboration reported that each of the 55 known subtype B drug-resistance mutations were found in at least one non-B subtype. By contrast, of 67 resistance mutations found in at least one non-B subtype, only 61 were also seen in subtype B isolates, indicating that several novel mutations occur in non-B subtypes [78]. With an increasingly diverse epidemic, even in developed countries previously dominated by subtype B [55], care must be taken to examine sequences for all known resistance mutations in cases of treatment failure. For several resistance-associated mutations the mutational pathway is shorter in some non-B subtypes than in subtype B [79]. These differences in resistance pathways may impact on cross-resistance and selection of second-line regimens.

Immune Response to HIV and Escape

The immune response drives HIV evolution in individuals by positive selection of escape mutations, the occurrence of which is limited by the impact of mutations on viral fitness [80]. The effects of the $CD8^+$ cytotoxic T cell (CTL) responses mediated through human HLA molecules are observed at the population level where HIV escape epitopes are becoming established [81]. Sites of HLA-mediated escape mutations were shown to correlate with sites of inter- and intra-subtype variability, indicating a role for CTLs in driving viral evolution [82]. Similarly, KIR-associated amino acid polymorphisms, which reduce the antiviral activity of natural killer (NK) cells, are selected [83]. There is also evidence that HIV-1 envelope proteins are evolving over time to become more resistant to neutralisation by antibodies [84].

HIV Vaccines and HIV Diversity

The ideal intervention for controlling the HIV pandemic is a preventive vaccine that is safe, simple, highly effective and affordable. It is, however, recognised that HIV diversity, in individuals and in populations, is one of the major challenges in the development of a globally effective HIV vaccine. Although rapid evolution and generation of escape mutants by the infecting HIV strain is an enormous challenge for the immune system to overcome, even after priming by vaccination, a further challenge is posed by the global genetic, and therefore antigenic, variability of HIV-1.

Neutralising Antibodies

Neutralising antibodies against HIV appear only at 12 weeks after initial HIV infection and the range of epitopes targeted by these initial neutralising antibodies is very narrow allowing rapid viral escape through substitutions, insertions, deletions, and glycan shifts [85]. Broad specificity neutralising antibodies recognising conserved regions of Env are rarely generated and when they do arise it is only in chronic infection, years after seroconversion. The reasons for this are not completely understood, but include the fact that some conserved regions are hidden and only exposed during conformational changes taking place during receptor binding [80]. A vaccine will thus need to prime a very early and broadly neutralising antibody response that targets multiple conserved epitopes, to preempt escape and control viral expansion.

Although antigenic variation between strains is likely to be important for antibody mediated protection, neutralisation serotypes do not appear to correlate with HIV-1 genetic subtypes [86]. Broadly neutralising antibodies targeting new epitopes continue to be discovered and defined in HIV-infected individuals, but inducing these responses in humans through vaccination remains a daunting challenge [87].

Cytotoxic T Lymphocytes

Although antibodies are crucial for preventing chronic infection, vaccine induced cell-mediated responses can potentially lower the viral load setpoint and thereby slow disease progression and reduce the rate of transmission. HIV-specific CTLs play a role in the earliest immune control of acute

HIV infection, but the initial response is narrow and the targeted epitopes rapidly escape [88]. A vaccine would therefore need to stimulate a T cell response against multiple highly conserved epitopes.

CTL responses in HIV-1 infected people show some cross-reactivity between different subtypes, although intra-subtype responses are usually stronger and more frequent than inter-subtype reactivities [89]. However, given that amino acid variation within a subtype is in the order of 8–17% (maximum 30%) and variation between subtypes is usually between 17% and 35% (maximum 42%) [26], such cross-reactivity within and between subtypes is likely to be limited.

Central Immunogen Sequences: the Importance of Being Nearest

Broadly speaking, vaccine strains can be either primary sequences (i.e. field isolates) or artificial 'central' consensus, ancestral, or centre-of-tree sequences [...] [90]. All HIV vaccines tested in Phase III efficacy trials to date were based on primary isolate sequences [91–93]. Field isolate sequences typically differ by 5–15% at the amino acid level from other primary sequences of the same subtype (and 10–30% different from other subtypes). Consensus, ancestral and centre-of-tree sequences vary by approximately 3–8% from primary sequences of the same subtype [90], and are therefore more similar to currently circulating strains and may have enhanced potential for eliciting cross-reactive responses.

A further approach is to focus on conserved regions within the HIV genome. Apart from the fact that these regions are more likely to be recognised by cross-reactive T cells, escape from the T cell response will also be limited as mutations in conserved regions usually incur higher fitness costs [94]. Another approach is to attempt to increase the depth of coverage of variants of each epitope. This may be achieved by multiple or mosaic antigen cocktails and could enhance the ability of the T cell response to respond to escape mutations [95,96].

Future Perspective

Phylogenetic analysis of HIV sequence diversity has led to important insights into the origin, evolution and spread of HIV. The diversity of HIV has a major impact on HIV diagnosis, pathogenesis, transmission, clinical management and vaccine development. Given the central role of HIV diversity in the HIV pandemic it is imperative that global molecular epidemiology surveillance is continued and improved using rigorous sampling strategies. Further elucidation of viral polymorphisms and properties associated with transmission, viral load setpoint and disease progression may lead to new approaches to disease prevention and treatment. Because events early after infection appear to dictate the natural history of HIV, better characterisation of transmitted sequences and their evolution and escape from early immune responses should identify targets for protection against HIV. This insight can then be applied in the next generation of candidate HIV vaccines (Box 8.1a).

Conflicts of Interest

I declare that I have no conflicts of interest.

Acknowledgments

The author is a recipient of an Academic Clinical Fellowship from the National Institute of Health Research, UK. I would like to thank Dr. C.F.C. Aldrich and Dr. M-E. Blais for critical reading of the manuscript. I would like to apologise to the many colleagues whose excellent work I was unable to cite because of limitations on the number of references.

References

1. Gottlieb, M.S. *et al.* (1981) *Pneumocystis carinii* pneumonia and mucosal candidiasis in previously healthy homosexual men: evidence of a new acquired cellular immunodeficiency. *N. Engl. J. Med.* 305, 1425–1431.
2. Barre-Sinoussi, F. *et al.* (1983) Isolation of a T-lymphotropic retrovirus from a patient at risk for acquired immune deficiency syndrome (AIDS). *Science* 220, 868–871.
3. UNAIDS. Report on the Global AIDS Epidemic 2010, Geneva, 2010.
4. Hahn, B.H. *et al.* (2000) AIDS as a zoonosis: scientific and public health implications. *Science* 287, 607–614.
5. Aghokeng, A.F. *et al.* (2010) Extensive survey on the prevalence and genetic diversity of SIVs in primate bushmeat provides insights into risks for potential new cross-species transmissions. *Infect. Genet. Evol.* 10, 386–396.
6. Simon, F. *et al.* (1998) Identification of a new human immunodeficiency virus type 1 distinct from group M and group O. *Nat. Med.* 4, 1032–1037.
7. Roques, P. *et al.* (2004) Phylogenetic characteristics of three new HIV-1 N strains and implications for the origin of group N. *AIDS* 18, 1371–1381.
8. Plantier, J.C. *et al.* (2009) A new human immunodeficiency virus derived from gorillas. *Nat. Med.* 15, 871–872.
9. Ayouba, A. *et al.* (2001) HIV-1 group O infection in Cameroon, 1986 to 1998. *Emerg. Infect. Dis.* 7, 466–467.
10. Vallari, A. *et al.* (2011) Confirmation of putative HIV-1 group P in Cameroon. *J. Virol.* 85, 1403–1407.
11. Gao, F. *et al.* (1999) Origin of HIV-1 in the chimpanzee *Pan troglodytes troglodytes*. *Nature* 397, 436–441.
12. Keele, B.F. *et al.* (2006) Chimpanzee reservoirs of pandemic and nonpandemic HIV-1. *Science* 313, 523–526.
13. Bailes, E. *et al.* (2003) Hybrid origin of SIV in chimpanzees. *Science* 300, 1713.
14. Vallari, A. *et al.* (2010) Four new HIV-1 group N isolates from Cameroon: prevalence continues to be low. *AIDS Res. Hum. Retroviruses* 26, 109–115.
15. Van Heuverswyn, F. *et al.* (2006) Human immunodeficiency viruses: SIV infection in wild gorillas. *Nature* 444, 164.
16. Takehisa, J. *et al.* (2009) Origin and biology of simian immunodeficiency virus in wild-living western gorillas. *J. Virol.* 83, 1635–1648.
17. Vessiere, A. *et al.* (2010) Diagnosis and monitoring of HIV-1 group O-infected patients in Cameroun. *J. Acquir. Immune Defic. Syndr.* 53, 107–110.
18. Zhu, T. *et al.* (1998) An African HIV-1 sequence from 1959 and implications for the origin of the epidemic. *Nature* 391, 594–597.
19. Worobey, M. *et al.* (2008) Direct evidence of extensive diversity of HIV-1 in Kinshasa by 1960. *Nature* 455, 661–664.
20. Korber, B. *et al.* (2000) Timing the ancestor of the HIV-1 pandemic strains. *Science* 288, 1789–1796.

21. Wertheim, J.O. and Worobey, M. (2009) Dating the age of the SIV lineages that gave rise to HIV-1 and HIV-2. *PLoS Comput. Biol.* 5, e1000377.
22. Lemey, P. *et al.* (2004) The molecular population genetics of HIV-1 group O. *Genetics* 167, 1059–1068.
23. Kirchhoff, F. (2010) Immune evasion and counteraction of restriction factors by HIV-1 and other primate lentiviruses. *Cell Host Microbe* 8, 55–67.
24. Roberts, J.D. *et al.* (1988) The accuracy of reverse transcriptase from HIV-1. *Science* 242, 1171–1173.
25. Ho, D.D. *et al.* (1995) Rapid turnover of plasma virions and CD4 lymphocytes in HIV-1 infection. *Nature* 373, 123–126.
26. Korber, B. *et al.* (2001) Evolutionary and immunological implications of contemporary HIV-1 variation. *Br. Med. Bull.* 58, 19–42.
27. Keele, B.F. *et al.* (2008) Identification and characterization of transmitted and early founder virus envelopes in primary HIV-1 infection. *Proc. Natl. Acad. Sci. U.S.A.* 105, 7552–7557.
28. Abrahams, M.R. *et al.* (2009) Quantitating the multiplicity of infection with human immunodeficiency virus type 1 subtype C reveals a non-Poisson distribution of transmitted variants. *J. Virol.* 83, 3556–3567.
29. Haaland, R.E. *et al.* (2009) Inflammatory genital infections mitigate a severe genetic bottleneck in heterosexual transmission of subtype A and C HIV-1. *PLoS Pathog.* 5, e1000274.
30. Li, H. *et al.* (2010) High multiplicity infection by HIV-1 in men who have sex with men. *PLoS Pathog.* 6, e1000890.
31. Bar, K.J. *et al.* (2010) Wide variation in the multiplicity of HIV-1 infection among injection drug users. *J. Virol.* 84, 6241–6247.
32. Sagar, M. *et al.* (2004) Identification of modifiable factors that affect the geneticdiversity of the transmitted HIV-1 population. *AIDS* 18, 615–619.
33. Rambaut, A. *et al.* (2001) Human immunodeficiency virus. Phylogeny and the origin of HIV-1. *Nature* 410, 1047–1048.
34. Abecasis, A.B. *et al.* (2009) Quantifying differences in the tempo of human immunodeficiency virus type 1 subtype evolution. *J. Virol.* 83, 12917–12924.
35. Yamaguchi, J. *et al.* (2002) Evaluation of HIV type 1 group O isolates: identification of five phylogenetic clusters. *AIDS Res. Hum. Retroviruses* 18, 269–282.
36. Yamaguchi, J. *et al.* (2004) HIV infections in northwestern Cameroon: identification of HIV type 1 group O and dual HIV type 1 group M and group O infections. *AIDS Res. Hum. Retroviruses* 20, 944–957.
37. Powell, R.L. *et al.* (2009) High frequency of HIV-1 dual infections among HIV-positive individuals in Cameroon, West Central Africa. *J. Acquir. Immune Defic. Syndr.* 50, 84–92.
38. Piantadosi, A. *et al.* (2007) Chronic HIV-1 infection frequently fails to protect against superinfection. *PLoS Pathog.* 3, e177.
39. Grobler, J. *et al.* (2004) Incidence of HIV-1 dual infection and its association with increased viral load set point in a cohort of HIV-1 subtype C-infected female sex workers. *J. Infect. Dis.* 190, 1355–1359.
40. Gottlieb, G.S. *et al.* (2004) Dual HIV-1 infection associated with rapid disease progression. *Lancet* 363, 619–622.
41. Peeters, M. *et al.* (1999) Characterization of a highly replicative intergroup M/O human immunodeficiency virus type 1 recombinant isolated from a Cameroonian patient. *J. Virol.* 73, 7368–7375.
42. Rousseau, C.M. *et al.* (2007) Extensive intrasubtype recombination in South African human immunodeficiency virus type 1 subtype C infections. *J. Virol.* 81, 4492–4500.

43. Robertson, D.L. *et al.* (2000) HIV-1 nomenclature proposal. *Science* 288, 55–56.
44. Vidal, N. *et al.* (2008) Characterization of an old complex circulating recombinant form, CRF27_cpx, originating from the Democratic Republic of Congo (DRC) and circulating in France. *AIDS Res. Hum. Retroviruses* 24, 315–321.
45. Thomson, M.M. *et al.* (2005) Identification of a novel HIV-1 complex circulating recombinant form (CRF18_cpx) of Central African origin in Cuba. *AIDS* 19, 1155–1163.
46. Anderson, J.P. *et al.* (2000) Testing the hypothesis of a recombinant origin of human immunodeficiency virus type 1 subtype E. *J. Virol.* 74, 10752–10765.
47. Tebit, D.M. *et al.* (2006) Diversity of HIV in rural Burkina Faso. *J. Acquir. Immune Defic. Syndr.* 43, 144–152.
48. Yaotse, D.A. *et al.* (2009) Genetic characterization of HIV-1 strains in Togo reveals a high genetic complexity and genotypic drug-resistance mutations in ARV naive patients. *Infect. Genet. Evol.* 9, 646–652.
49. Delgado, E. *et al.* (2008) High prevalence of unique recombinant forms of HIV-1 in Ghana: molecular epidemiology from an antiretroviral resistance study. *J. Acquir. Immune Defic. Syndr.* 48, 599–606.
50. Brennan, C.A. *et al.* (2008) The prevalence of diverse HIV-1 strains was stable in Cameroonian blood donors from 1996 to 2004. *J. Acquir. Immune Defic. Syndr.* 49, 432–439.
51. Vidal, N. *et al.* (2000) Unprecedented degree of human immunodeficiency virus type 1 (HIV-1) group M genetic diversity in the Democratic Republic of Congo suggests that the HIV-1 pandemic originated in Central Africa. *J. Virol.* 74, 10498–10507.
52. Abecasis, A.B. *et al.* (2007) Recombination confounds the early evolutionary history of human immunodeficiency virus type 1: subtype G is a circulating recombinant form. *J. Virol.* 81, 8543–8551.
53. Lemey, P. *et al.* (2009) Identifying recombinants in human and primate immunodeficiency virus sequence alignments using quartet scanning. *BMC Bioinformatics* 10, 126.
54. Bulla, I. *et al.* (2010) HIV classification using the coalescent theory. *Bioinformatics* 26, 1409–1415.
55. Hemelaar, J. *et al.* (2011) Global trends in molecular epidemiology of HIV-1 during 2000–2007. *AIDS* 25, 679–689.
56. Nyombi, B.M. *et al.* (2008) Diversity of human immunodeficiency virus type 1 subtypes in Kagera and Kilimanjaro regions, Tanzania. *AIDS Res. Hum. Retroviruses* 24, 761–769.
57. Thomson, M.M. *et al.* (2004) Analysis of near full-length genome sequences of HIV type 1 BF intersubtype recombinant viruses from Brazil reveals their independent origins and their lack of relationship to CRF12_BF. *AIDS Res. Hum. Retroviruses* 20, 1126–1133.
58. Perez, L. *et al.* (2006) HIV type 1 molecular epidemiology in Cuba: high genetic diversity, frequent mosaicism, and recent expansion of BG intersubtype recombinant forms. *AIDS Res. Hum. Retroviruses* 22, 724–733.
59. Yang, R. *et al.* (2002) On-going generation of multiple forms of HIV-1 intersubtype recombinants in the Yunnan Province of China. *AIDS* 16, 1401–1407.
60. Tee, K.K. *et al.* (2005) Emergence of HIV-1 CRF01_AE/B unique recombinant forms in Kuala Lumpur, Malaysia. *AIDS* 19, 119–126.
61. Kalish, M.L. *et al.* (2004) Recombinant viruses and early global HIV-1 epidemic. *Emerg. Infect. Dis.* 10, 1227–1234.
62. Mulanga-Kabeya, C. *et al.* (1998) Evidence of stable HIV seroprevalences in selected populations in the Democratic Republic of the Congo. *AIDS* 12, 905–910.
63. Gray, R.R. *et al.* (2009) Spatial phylodynamics of HIV-1 epidemic emergence in east Africa. *AIDS* 23, F9–F17.

64. Kaleebu, P. *et al.* (2002) Effect of human immunodeficiency virus (HIV) type 1 envelope subtypes A and D on disease progression in a large cohort of HIV-1-positive persons in Uganda. *J. Infect. Dis.* 185, 1244–1250.
65. Kiwanuka, N. *et al.* (2008) Effect of human immunodeficiency virus type 1 (HIV-1) subtype on disease progression in persons from Rakai, Uganda, with incident HIV-1 infection. *J. Infect. Dis.* 197, 707–713.
66. Lutalo, T. *et al.* (2007) Survival of HIV-infected treatment-naive individuals with documented dates of seroconversion in Rakai, Uganda. *AIDS* 21 (Suppl. 6), S15–S19.
67. Baeten, J.M. *et al.* (2007) HIV-1 subtype D infection is associated with faster disease progression than subtype A in spite of similar plasma HIV-1 loads. *J. Infect. Dis.* 195, 1177–1180.
68. Vasan, A. *et al.* (2006) Different rates of disease progression of HIV type 1 infection in Tanzania based on infecting subtype. *Clin. Infect. Dis.* 42, 843–852.
69. Kiwanuka, N. *et al.* (2010) HIV-1 viral subtype differences in the rate of CD4+ T-cell decline among HIV seroincident antiretroviral naive persons in Rakai district, Uganda. *J. Acquir. Immune Defic. Syndr.* 54, 180–184.
70. Easterbrook, P.J. *et al.* (2010) Impact of HIV-1 viral subtype on disease progression and response to antiretroviral therapy. *J. Int. AIDS Soc.* 13, 4.
71. Sacktor, N. *et al.* (2009) HIV subtype D is associated with dementia, compared with subtype A, in immunosuppressed individuals at risk of cognitive impairment in Kampala, Uganda. *Clin. Infect. Dis.* 49, 780–786.
72. Kiwanuka, N. *et al.* (2009) HIV-1 subtypes and differences in heterosexual HIV transmission among HIV-discordant couples in Rakai, Uganda. *AIDS* 23, 2479–2484.
73. Rainwater, S. *et al.* (2005) No evidence for rapid subtype C spread within an epidemic in which multiple subtypes and intersubtype recombinants circulate. *AIDS Res. Hum. Retroviruses* 21, 1060–1065.
74. Conroy, S.A. *et al.* (2010) Changes in the distribution of HIV type 1 subtypes D and A in Rakai District, Uganda between 1994 and 2002. *AIDS Res. Hum. Retroviruses* 26, 1087–1091.
75. Aghokeng, A.F. *et al.* (2009) Inaccurate diagnosis of HIV-1 group M and O is a key challenge for ongoing universal access to antiretroviral treatment and HIV prevention in Cameroon. *PLoS ONE* 4, e7702.
76. Rouet, F. *et al.* (2010) Comparison of the generic HIV viral load assay with the Amplicor HIV-1 monitor v1.5 and Nuclisens HIV-1 EasyQ v1.2 techniques for plasma HIV-1 RNA quantitation of non-B subtypes: the Kesho Bora preparatory study. *J. Virol. Methods* 163, 253–257.
77. Kantor, R. (2006) Impact of HIV-1 pol diversity on drug resistance and its clinical implications. *Curr. Opin. Infect. Dis.* 19, 594–606.
78. Kantor, R. *et al.* (2005) Impact of HIV-1 subtype and antiretroviral therapy on protease and reverse transcriptase genotype: results of a global collaboration. *PLoS Med.* 2, e112.
79. Kosakovsky Pond, S.L. and Smith, D.M. (2009) Are all subtypes created equal? The effectiveness of antiretroviral therapy against non-subtype B HIV-1. *Clin. Infect. Dis.* 48, 1306–1309.
80. McMichael, A.J. *et al.* (2010) The immune response during acute HIV-1 infection: clues for vaccine development. *Nat. Rev. Immunol.* 10, 11–23.
81. Kawashima, Y. *et al.* (2009) Adaptation of HIV-1 to human leukocyte antigen class I. *Nature* 458, 641–645.
82. Matthews, P.C. *et al.* (2009) HLA footprints on human immunodeficiency virus type 1 are associated with interclade polymorphisms and intraclade phylogenetic clustering. *J. Virol.* 83, 4605–4615.
83. Alter, G. *et al.* (2011) HIV-1 adaptation to NK-cell-mediated immune pressure. *Nature* 476, 96–100.
84. Bunnik, E.M. *et al.* (2010) Adaptation of HIV-1 envelope gp120 to humoral immunity at a population level. *Nat. Med.* 16, 995–997.

85. Wei, X. *et al.* (2003) Antibody neutralization and escape by HIV-1. *Nature* 422, 307–312.
86. Brown, B.K. *et al.* (2008) Cross-clade neutralization patterns among HIV-1 strains from the six major clades of the pandemic evaluated and compared in two different models. *Virology* 375, 529–538.
87. Scheid, J.F. *et al.* (2011) Sequence and structural convergence of broad and potent HIV antibodies that mimic CD4 binding. *Science* 333, 1633–1637.
88. Goonetilleke, N. *et al.* (2009) The first T cell response to transmitted/founder virus contributes to the control of acute viremia in HIV-1 infection. *J. Exp. Med.* 206, 1253–1272.
89. Currier, J.R. *et al.* (2003) Detection of high frequencies of HIV-1 cross-subtype reactive CD8 T lymphocytes in the peripheral blood of HIV-1-infected Kenyans. *AIDS* 17, 2149–2157.
90. Gaschen, B. *et al.* (2002) Diversity considerations in HIV-1 vaccine selection. *Science* 296, 2354–2360.
91. Rerks-Ngarm, S. *et al.* (2009) Vaccination with ALVAC and AIDSVAX to prevent HIV-1 infection in Thailand. *N. Engl. J. Med.* 361, 2209–2220.
92. Pitisuttithum, P. *et al.* (2006) Randomized, double-blind, placebo-controlled efficacy trial of a bivalent recombinant glycoprotein 120 HIV-1 vaccine among injection drug users in Bangkok, Thailand. *J. Infect. Dis.* 194, 1661–1671.
93. Buchbinder, S.P. *et al.* (2008) Efficacy assessment of a cell-mediated immunity HIV-1 vaccine (the Step study): a double-blind, randomised, placebo-controlled, test-of-concept trial. *Lancet* 372, 1881–1893.
94. Letourneau, S. *et al.* (2007) Design and pre-clinical evaluation of a universal HIV-1 vaccine. *PLoS ONE* 2, e984.
95. Barouch, D.H. *et al.* (2010) Mosaic HIV-1 vaccines expand the breadth and depth of cellular immune responses in rhesus monkeys. *Nat. Med.* 16, 319–323.
96. Santra, S. *et al.* (2010) Mosaic vaccines elicit CD8+ T lymphocyte responses that confer enhanced immune coverage of diverse HIV strains in monkeys. *Nat. Med.* 16, 324–328.
97. Leitner, T. *et al.* (2005) HIV-1 subtype and circulating recombinant form (CRF) reference sequences, 2005. In *HIV Sequence Compendium 2005* (Leitner, T. *et al.*, eds), NM, LA-UR 06-0680, Theoretical Biology and Biophysics Group, Los Alamos National Laboratory.
98. Salemi, M. *et al.* (2001) Dating the common ancestor of SIVcpz and HIV-1 group M and the origin of HIV-1 subtypes using a new method to uncover clock-like molecular evolution. *FASEB J.* 15, 276–278.
99. Gilbert, M.T. *et al.* (2007) The emergence of HIV/AIDS in the Americas and beyond. *Proc. Natl. Acad. Sci. U.S.A.* 104, 18566–18570.
100. Travers, S.A. *et al.* (2004) Timing and reconstruction of the most recent common ancestor of the subtype C clade of human immunodeficiency virus type 1. *J. Virol.* 78, 10501–10506.
101. Tee, K.K. *et al.* (2008) Temporal and spatial dynamics of human immunodeficiency virus type 1 circulating recombinant forms 08_BC and 07_BC in Asia. *J. Virol.* 82, 9206–9215.
102. Dalai, S.C. *et al.* (2009) Evolution and molecular epidemiology of subtype C HIV-1 in Zimbabwe. *AIDS* 23, 2523–2532.
103. Abebe, A. *et al.* (2001) Timing of the introduction into Ethiopia of subcluster C′ of HIV type 1 subtype C. *AIDS Res. Hum. Retroviruses* 17, 657–661.
104. Abebe, A. *et al.* (2001) Timing of the HIV-1 subtype C epidemic in Ethiopia based on early virus strains and subsequent virus diversification. *AIDS* 15, 1555–1561.
105. Bello, G. *et al.* (2008) Origin and evolutionary history of HIV-1 subtype C in Brazil. *AIDS* 22, 1993–2000.

106. Lukashov, V.V. and Goudsmit, J. (2002) Recent evolutionary history of human immunodeficiency virus type 1 subtype B: reconstruction of epidemic onset based on sequence distances to the common ancestor. *J. Mol. Evol.* 54, 680–691.
107. Salemi, M. *et al.* (2008) High-resolution molecular epidemiology and evolutionary history of HIV-1 subtypes in Albania. *PLoS ONE* 3, e1390.
108. Kim, M.S. *et al.* (2009) Timing and evolution of the most recent common ancestor of the Korean clade HIV subtype B based on nef and vif sequences. *J. Microbiol.* 47, 85–90.
109. Aulicino, P.C. *et al.* (2007) Description of the first full-length HIV type 1 subtype F1 strain in Argentina: implications for the origin and dispersion of this subtype in South America. *AIDS Res. Hum. Retroviruses* 23, 1176–1182.
110. Liao, H. *et al.* (2009) Phylodynamic analysis of the dissemination of HIV-1 CRF01_AE in Vietnam. *Virology* 391, 51–56.
111. Faria, N.R. *et al.* (2011) Phylodynamics of the HIV-1 CRF02_AG clade in Cameroon. *Infect. Genet. Evol.* DOI: 10.1016/j.meegid.2011.04.028.
112. Passaes, C.P. *et al.* (2009) Genetic characterization of HIV-1 BC recombinants and evolutionary history of the CRF31_BC in Southern Brazil. *Infect. Genet. Evol.* 9, 474–482.
113. Tee, K.K. *et al.* (2009) Estimating the date of origin of an HIV-1 circulating recombinant form. *Virology* 387, 229–234.

8.2

Colonialism in Africa Helped Launch the HIV Epidemic a Century Ago

Craig Timberg and Daniel Halperin

WE ARE UNLIKELY TO EVER KNOW all the details of the birth of the AIDS epidemic. But a series of recent genetic discoveries have shed new light on it, starting with the moment when a connection from chimp to human changed the course of history.

We now know where the epidemic began: a small patch of dense forest in southeastern Cameroon. We know when: within a couple of decades on either side of 1900. We have a good idea of how: A hunter caught an infected chimpanzee for food, allowing the virus to pass from the chimp's blood into the hunter's body, probably through a cut during butchering.

As to the why, here is where the story gets even more fascinating, and terrible. We typically think of diseases in terms of how they threaten us personally. But they have their own stories. Diseases are born. They grow. They falter, and sometimes they die. In every case these changes happen for reasons.

For decades nobody knew the reasons behind the birth of the AIDS epidemic. But it is now clear that the epidemic's birth and crucial early growth happened during Africa's colonial era, amid massive intrusion of new people and technology into a land where ancient ways still prevailed. European powers engaged in a feverish race for wealth and glory blazed routes up muddy rivers and into dense forests that had been traveled only sporadically by humans before.

The most disruptive of these intruders were thousands of African porters. Forced into service by European colonial powers, they cut paths through the exact area that researchers have now identified as the birthplace of the AIDS epidemic. It was here, in a single moment of transmission from chimp to human, that a strain of virus called HIV-1 group M first appeared.

In the century since, it has been responsible for 99 percent of all of the world's deaths from AIDS—not just in Africa but in Moscow, Bangkok, Rio de Janeiro, San Francisco, New York, Washington. All that began when the West forced its will on an unfamiliar land, causing the essential ingredients of the AIDS epidemic to combine.

It was here, by accident but with motives by no means pure, that the world built a tinderbox and tossed in a spark.

Craig Timberg and Daniel Halperin, "Colonialism in Africa Helped Launch the HIV Epidemic a Century Ago," *Tinderbox: How the West Sparked the AIDS Epidemic and How the World Can Finally Overcome It*, pp. 2–3, 31–32, 45–46, 47–48, 50–52.

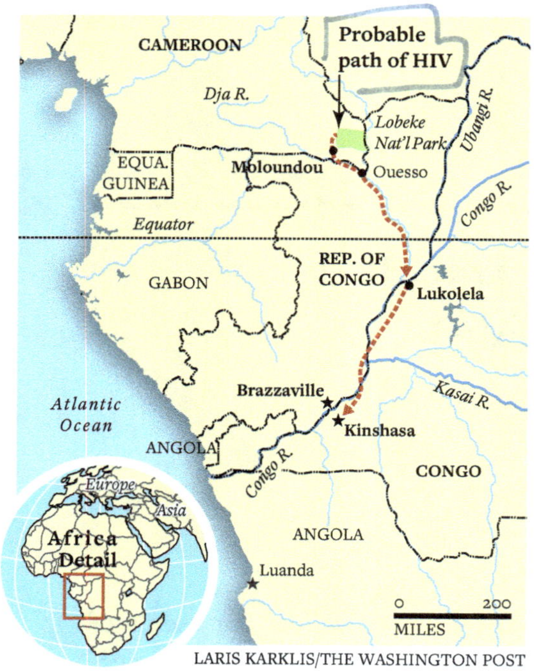

LARIS KARKLIS/THE WASHINGTON POST

The Chimps of Cameroon

Many simians, such as gorillas and monkeys, can carry a virus that resembles HIV. But scientists now know that HIV-1 group M was born from a virus circulating among a community of chimpanzees concentrated in Cameroon, a sprawling country with bustling Atlantic Ocean ports, populous highlands, and a lightly developed southern region where relatively few people live even today. This was home to the chimps.

Finding a more exact location took a remarkable degree of scientific ingenuity. An international research team led by Beatrice Hahn of the University of Alabama at Birmingham and Paul Sharp of the University of Edinburgh developed an elaborate project that involved searching for the simian virus in chimp feces collected across a vast swath of southern Cameroon.

To find a strain of the simian virus that was, on a genetic level, essentially indistinguishable from the most lethal form of HIV, the research team set up 10 stations across the region. Two of the stations were in the particularly remote southeastern corner of the nation, as far as possible from major population centers.

It was in these two stations where Hahn and Sharp's team discovered samples of the simian virus that was almost a perfect match for the HIV-1 group M that eventually killed tens of millions of humans.

This discovery, published in the journal *Science* in 2006, intensified the quest for a birth date for the virus. Again, genetic research offered the key clues.

Scientists had long known that a blood sample, preserved from 1959, showed that HIV had been circulating in Kinshasa, the capital of Congo, for several decades before the virus first drew international attention in the 1980s. In 2008, evolutionary biologist Michael Worobey sharpened that picture when he reported in the journal *Nature* the discovery of a second sample of the virus, trapped in a wax-encased lymph node biopsy from 1960.

By comparing these two historic pieces of virus and mapping out the differences in their genetic structures in his lab at the University of Arizona, Worobey determined that HIV-1 group M was much older than anyone had thought. Both samples of the virus appeared to have descended from a single ancestor at some time between 1884 and 1924. The most likely date was 1908.

Taken together, these two discoveries offered the clearest clues to the birth and early life of the epidemic.

Not far from where HIV-1 group M was born was a major river, the Sangha, flowing toward the heart of Central Africa. This section of the Sangha was not ideal for navigation because of its ribbons of sandbars and the dense vegetation along its banks.

In the especially treacherous middle section, near where Hahn and Sharp's team found the viral ancestor of HIV, few major human settlements ever developed. But there were numerous communities on the Sangha's more accessible stretches. And due south, past riverside trading towns, was the mighty Congo River itself, the superhighway of Central Africa.

Once the virus made the jump from chimp to human, a single infected person could have carried HIV down the Sangha, onto the Congo River and into Kinshasa. The Belgians had founded the city in 1881, during what historians call "The Scramble for Africa," when colonial powers carved up the continent into areas of influence. By the early 20th century Kinshasa, then called Leopoldville, was the biggest city in Central Africa, fueled by the dizzying growth of trade with the outside world.

A final, powerful bit of evidence supported the theory that Kinshasa lay at the heart of the epidemic's early movements.

Scientists studying HIV-1 group M already had found many related varieties, what scientists call subtypes, each with slightly different genetic structures and paths through the world. One, scientists discovered, had traveled east from Kinshasa toward Lake Victoria. One went south to Zambia, Botswana and South Africa. One hopped all the way across the ocean to Haiti, then to the United States and Europe.

Many others traveled not very far at all, staying in the Congo Basin. But as scientists plotted out the genetic histories of these varieties and built an extensive family tree for HIV, they all appeared to have spread from a single explosion, a big bang of the AIDS epidemic: Ground Zero was Kinshasa.

Ivory and Rubber

Powering the big bang was the burgeoning trade of colonial Africa.

Ivory may seem a touch quaint today, but in its heyday it was seen as beautiful, versatile and essential to many everyday products. It was used to make billiard balls, jewelry and cutlery. Furniture makers incorporated it into their cabinets, artists into their statues. Bagpipe makers used ivory for mounts, ferrules, buttons and mouthpieces.

When supplies of ivory gradually grew short, as colonial agents killed the once plentiful elephants by the thousands, rubber took its place as the economic lifeblood of colonialism in the Congo Basin. The first inflatable rubber tires for bicycles became popular in the 1890s. Mass production of cars soon spiked demand for rubber tires again.

The only obstacle to European companies' reaping huge profits was that collecting ivory and rubber required massive amounts of labor. Getting ivory from an elephant meant stalking the animal, killing it and cutting off its tusks. Getting rubber from vines required slashing them, collecting the oozing white sap and drying it—sometimes on the collector's own skin.

The solution to the manpower demands soon became obvious. Colonial powers created what was essentially slavery: cheap muscle at the point of a gun.

This approach was not confined to collecting ivory and rubber. These industries created tremendous new needs for infrastructure to get goods to oceangoing ships along the Atlantic coast. That meant African porters had to carry goods and supplies anyplace the steamboats couldn't reach.

Workers were needed to build railroads, trading stations, dormitories. And somebody needed to operate the steamboats, load the railroad cars, carry the tusks or gobs of rubber in from the jungle. When workers became unruly, the colonial companies deployed heavily armed soldiers to keep the cogs of these vast enterprises moving.

All these roles were filled by Africans, many imported from villages hundreds or even thousands of miles away. African life here was beyond cheap. It was disposable. Contemporary accounts by journalists and missionaries tell of colonial officials across the Congo Basin ordering mass slaughters and the torching of restive villages while creating forced settlements that resembled nothing so much as concentration camps.

The Role of African Porters

In December 1895 German colonial authorities heard reports that Cameroon's southeastern corner contained fabulously rich ivory and rubber stocks awaiting exploitation.

The Germans soon after gave authority to a colonial company to take control of the region by force. Over the next four years they extended their power all the way through southeastern Cameroon and established a trading station on the Ngoko River about 75 miles upstream from where its waters merged with the Sangha. In the wedge of land defined by these two rivers, HIV either had just been born or soon would be.

The trading station was called Moloundou, and a busy town remains there today. But at the time it was almost unimaginably remote. Few human settlements had developed among these forbidding forests. And there were only two practical ways out: by steamship down the Ngoko to the Sangha and on to the Congo River; or overland by foot to the Atlantic.

The river route was the easier of the two, and steamships transported the bulk of the ivory and rubber collected in southeastern Cameroon. But overland routes were necessary to connect Moloundou with other trading stations and inland areas rich with rubber and ivory.

For these journeys the bounty was borne by Africans who carried loads averaging 55 pounds each. At the peak of the foot traffic that would develop between inland areas and the coast, the busy way station recorded more than a thousand porters passing by on a typical day.

Trade Routes, Disease Routes

Ominously, something else followed the rubber trade through Cameroon: disease. Sleeping sickness, smallpox and skin infections were the most obvious.

Colonial authorities attempted mass inoculation campaigns for smallpox and set up quarantine zones that restricted where the porters were allowed to travel. But even so, the diseases spread.

Among them was syphilis, which arrived with the Europeans. In just a few years it reached epidemic proportions along porter routes and riverside trading posts in Cameroon and throughout the Congo Basin. It's impossible now to determine how much of this spread resulted from rapes as opposed to other kinds of encounters, but it's clear that colonial commerce created massive new networks of sexual interactions—and massive new transmissions of infections. (In later decades, transmission through the reuse of hypodermic needles in medical care probably had some role in HIV's spread as well.)

So HIV's first journey looked something like this: A hunter killed an infected chimp in the southeastern Cameroonian forest, and a simian virus entered his body through a cut during the butchering, mutating into HIV.

This probably had happened many times before, during the centuries when the region had little contact with the outside world. But now thousands of porters—both men and women—were crossing through the area regularly, creating more opportunities for the virus to travel onward to a riverside trading station such as Moloundou.

One of the first victims—whether a hunter, a porter or an ivory collector—gave HIV to a sexual partner. There may have been a small outbreak around the trading station before the virus found its way aboard a steamship headed down the Sangha River.

For this fateful journey south, HIV could have ridden in the body of these first victims, or it could have been somebody infected later: a soldier or a laborer. Or it could have been carried by a woman: a concubine, a trader.

It's also possible that the virus moved down the river in a series of steps, maybe from Moloundou to Ouesso, then onward to Bolobo on the Congo River itself.

There might even have been a series of infections at trading towns along the entire route down river. Yet even within these riverside trading posts HIV would have struggled to create anything more than a short-lived, localized outbreak.

Most of this colonial world didn't have enough potential victims for such a fragile virus to start a major epidemic. HIV is harder to transmit than many other infections. People can have sex hundreds of times without passing the virus on. To spread widely, HIV requires a population large enough to sustain an outbreak and a sexual culture in which people often have more than one partner, creating networks of interaction that propel the virus onward.

To fulfill its grim destiny, HIV needed a kind of place never before seen in Central Africa but one that now was rising in the heart of the region: a big, thriving, hectic place jammed with people and energy, where old rules were cast aside amid the tumult of new commerce.

It needed Kinshasa. It was here, hundreds of miles downriver from Cameroon, that HIV began to grow beyond a mere outbreak. It was here that AIDS grew into an epidemic.

Laying the scientific story alongside the historical one offers one final revelation. In the 1920s, as railroads became widely available, the Sangha River's value as a steamship route dwindled sharply. Global rubber prices also collapsed. The pace of human movement through the region eased.

So the improbable journey of the killer strain of HIV was feasible for only a few hectic decades, from the 1880s to the 1920s. Without "The Scramble for Africa," it's hard to see how HIV could have made it out of southeastern Cameroon to eventually kill tens of millions of people. Even a delay might have caused the killer strain of HIV to die a lonely death deep in the forest.

8.3

How Scientists Proved the Wrong Man Was Blamed for Bringing HIV to the U.S.

Deborah Netburn

A STUDY PUBLISHED ON OCT. 26 FOUND new evidence that Gaetan Dugas was not the first person in the U.S. to have HIV.

The Canadian flight attendant widely blamed for bringing HIV to the United States and triggering an epidemic that has killed nearly 700,000 people has been exonerated by science, more than 30 years after his death.

In a study published Wednesday in the journal Nature, researchers used newly available genetic evidence to show that Gaetan Dugas—who has been dubbed "Patient Zero"—could not have been the first person in the United States to have the virus that causes AIDS.

Instead, the researchers report that Dugas was one of thousands of people who were infected with the human immunodeficiency virus by the late 1970s, years before it was officially recognized by the medical community in 1981.

The genetic analysis also reveals the path taken by the most common strain of the virus after it traveled from the Caribbean to the United States. Upon arriving in New York City around 1970, it circulated and diversified for about five years before being dispersed across the country.

"There really is no question about the geographical direction of movement," said study leader Michael Worobey, an evolutionary biologist at the University of Arizona in Tucson.

The new evidence comes from two caches of serum samples taken from gay men in New York City in 1978 and 1979, and in San Francisco in 1978. (Serum is blood with the red and white blood cells removed.)

The men were participating in a study of hepatitis B, which was prevalent in the gay community at the time. They weren't tested for HIV because it wasn't known to exist back then. However, if any of them had it, there should be evidence in their blood in the form of antibodies, the proteins that our immune systems make to fight an infection.

To see if any of the men in the hepatitis B study had contracted HIV, a different group of researchers analyzed the New York City samples and found that, indeed, 6.6% of them contained HIV antibodies. Inspired by this work, Worobey and his team did a similar test for the West Coast samples and discovered HIV antibodies in 3.7% of them.

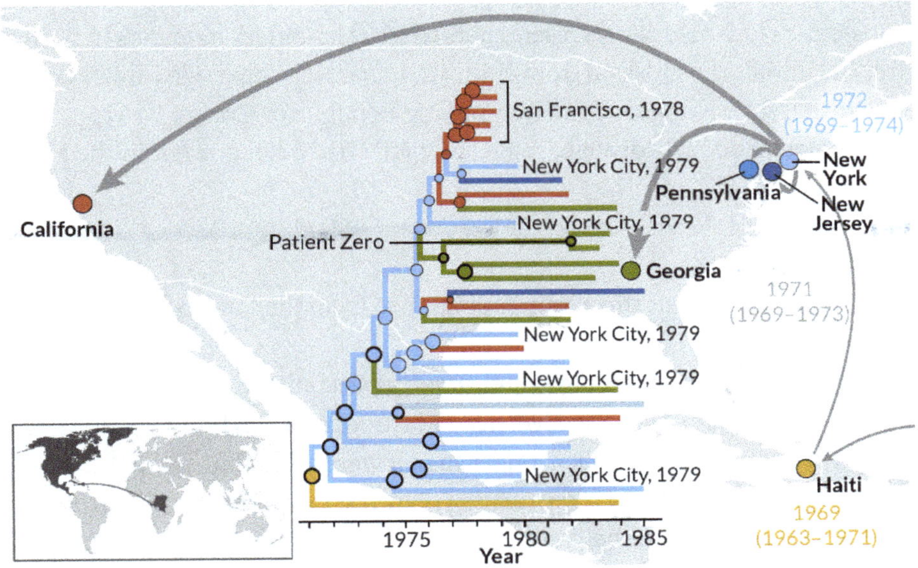

After HIV arrived in the Caribbean from Africa, it spread first to New York City and then to different locations in the United States, according to a new study. (*Worobey et al.*/Nature)

The presence of antibodies can show whether a person has contracted a certain virus, but they can't provide much detailed information about the virus itself, Worobey said. So his group's next step was to scour the serum samples for fragments of HIV RNA that may have been circulating in these men's bloodstreams.

It was a bit of a long shot. The samples were decades old, and RNA is generally too fragile to survive for long periods.

But the researchers were persistent. They selected 53 samples for attempted genetic sequencing, and they were eventually able to cobble together the full HIV genomes of eight of them—three from San Francisco and five from New York.

"It took a mixture of patience and insanity, but these old sequences are as good as a time machine," Worobey said.

Scientists track the evolution of a virus over time by tallying the number of substitutions, or mutations, in its genome.

To explain how this works, Worobey likes to conjure a cactus. (He lives in Arizona after all.)

Imagine you are staring at a saguaro with a tall central column and a couple of branches curving up like arms. If you have just a single time point—now—it's difficult to gauge the cactus' age.

However, if you could get a picture of the cactus from 10 years ago, you could calculate the growth rate for each of its branches over that time. Then you can make an educated guess about how much the cactus grows each year.

"That's what we do with HIV molecular clocks," Worobey said.

Geneticists measure how many mutations occur in the genome in a given time period. This is how they determined that HIV was first transmitted from a chimpanzee to a single human early in the 20th century in sub-Saharan Africa.

The HIV molecular clock also allows researchers to trace landmark moments in the evolution of the virus. After the initial transmission from chimp to human, the next one came when HIV began circulating in Kinshasa, the capital of the Democratic Republic of Congo. By 1960, viral samples from the city were tremendously diverse, suggesting HIV had been present in the area for a long time, Worobey said.

Around 1967, a branch of the virus known as HIV-1 group M subtype B took hold in the Caribbean and diversified in Haiti.

The new work makes clear that this strain first jumped from the Caribbean to New York City in 1970 or 1971.

By the late 1970s, when the eight serum samples were collected, the five viral genomes from New York already had a high degree of genetic diversity; the three from San Francisco did not. This indicates HIV probably was in New York much longer than it was in San Francisco.

"It appears that New York City was a key turning point," Worobey said. "New York City acts as a hub from which the virus moved to the West Coast—and eventually to Western Europe, Australia, Japan, South America and other places."

Dr. Beatrice Hahn, a professor of medicine at the University of Pennsylvania who studies the origin and evolution of immunodeficiency diseases, said she was impressed by the lengths the authors went to in order to find actual virus samples from so long ago.

Hahn, who was not involved in the research, noted that while many of the findings had been put forward before, the new study provides more convincing evidence because it was the first to isolate the complete, full-length virus genome from such early samples.

"It always helps to nail it," she said.

She added that the work does provide some new insights, including that the virus came to New York much earlier than previously recognized and that thousands of people were already infected by the time HIV was first recognized in the medical literature.

As part of this study, the authors assembled the complete HIV genome from a serum sample collected from Dugas in 1983, just one year before his death at the age of 31.

The genome was typical of HIV strains in the United States at the time, the researchers reported, and there was nothing to indicate that it had set off the epidemic here.

"In short, we found no evidence that Patient Zero was the first person infected by this lineage of HIV-1," they wrote.

So, how did this myth start?

It turns out Dugas was initially identified by the Centers for Disease Control and Prevention as case No. 057, which means he was likely the 57th patient they heard about who had been sickened by the mysterious illness.

A few years later, he participated in a study by the CDC in California that connected 40 men in 10 American cities who all had AIDS and were linked through sexual contact.

Dugas was placed near the center of this cluster, and identified as patient O for "Outside of California." But when investigators numbered the cases according to the date when each patient's symptoms started to appear, the letter O was mistaken for the number 0, and the Canadian flight attendant entered the literature with that dubious label.

In actuality, Dugas' symptoms were not reported until 1979 and 1980, considerably later than other cases in the cluster.

The medical community never released Dugas' name to the public, but journalist Randy Shilts identified him in his 1987 book "And the Band Played On" about the first five years of the American AIDS epidemic. (Shilts himself died of AIDS in 1994.)

Dugas told researchers that he averaged 250 sexual partners a year, and Shilts portrayed him as a vain and arrogant playboy who ignored doctors' orders to stop having sex to keep his infection from spreading. Media reviewers took the idea of a villainous Patient Zero and ran with it.

"Despite attempts at clarification and protest then and since, many still believe the story today," the study authors wrote.

While there are epidemiological benefits to knowing how an outbreak begins, the researchers say that doesn't mean anyone is at fault.

"Nobody should be blamed for the spread of a virus that nobody even knew about," Worobey said.

UPDATES:

5:10 p.m.: This article was updated with information about the death of Randy Shilts, the journalist who identified Gaetan Dugas as "Patient Zero."

This article was originally published at 10 a.m.

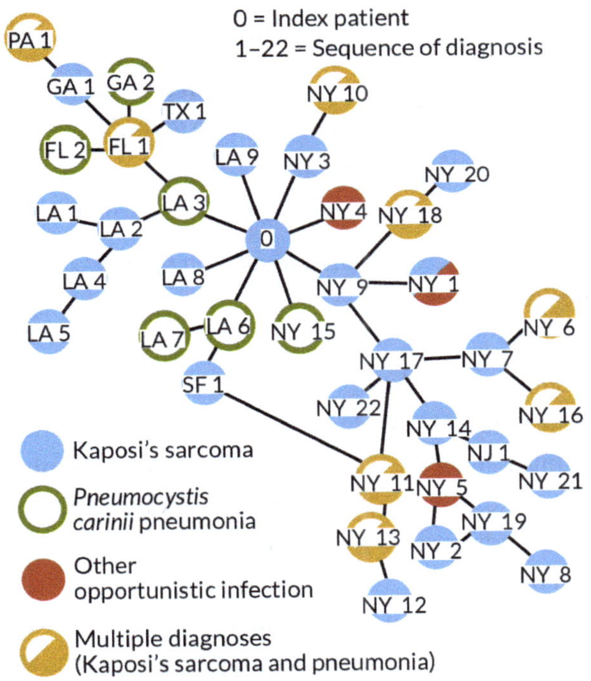

Sexual contacts among homosexual men with AIDS. Each circle represents an AIDS patient. Lines connecting the circles represent sexual exposures. Indicated city or state is place of residence of a patient at the time of diagnosis. "o" indicates Patient o.

Original Paper: Cluster of cases of the acquired immune deficiency syndrome. Patients linked by sexual contact. Auerbach DM, Darrow WW, Jaffe HW, Curran JW, Amer Journal of Medicine, 1984.

8.4

How to Prevent the Next Pandemic

An International Network for Monitoring the Flow of Viruses from Animals to Humans Might Help Scientists Head Off Global Epidemics

Nathan Wolfe

Key Concepts

- *Most human infectious diseases originated in animals.*
- *Historically, epidemiologists have focused on domestic animals as the source of these scourges. But wild animals, too, have transmitted many diseases to us, including HIV.*
- *To address the threat posed by wild animals, researchers are studying the microbes of these creatures and the people who come into frequent contact with them.*
- *Such monitoring may enable scientists to spot emerging infectious diseases early enough to prevent them from becoming pandemics.*

Sweat streamed down my back, thorny shrubs cut my arms, and we were losing them again. The wild chimpanzees my colleagues and I had been following for nearly five hours had stopped their grunting, hooting and screeching. Usually these calls helped us follow the animals through Uganda's Kibale Forest. For three large males to quiet abruptly surely meant trouble. Suddenly, as we approached a small clearing, we spotted them standing below a massive fig tree and looking up at a troop of red colobus monkeys eating and playing in the treetop.

The monkeys carried on with their morning meal, oblivious to the three apes below. After appearing for a moment to confer with one another, the chimps split up. While the leader crept toward the fig tree, his compatriots made their way up two neighboring trees in silence. Then, in an instant, the leader rushed up his tree screaming. Leaves showered down as the monkeys frantically tried to evade their attacker. But the chimp had calculated his bluster well: although he failed to capture a monkey himself, one of his partners grabbed a juvenile and made his way down to the forest floor with the young monkey in tow, ready to share his catch.

As the chimps feasted on the monkey's raw flesh and entrails, I thought about how this scene contained all the elements of a perfect storm for allowing microorganisms to jump from one species to the next, akin to space travelers leaping at warp speed from one galaxy to another. Any disease-causing agent present in that monkey now had the ideal conditions under which to enter a new type of host: the chimps were handling and consuming fresh organs; their hands were covered with blood, saliva and feces, all of which can carry pathogens; blood and other fluids splattered into their eyes and noses. Any sores or cuts on the hunters' bodies could provide a bug with direct entry into the bloodstream. Indeed, work conducted by my group and others has shown that hunting, by animals such as chimpanzees as well as by humans, does provide a bridge allowing viruses to jump from prey to predator. The pandemic form of HIV began in this way, by moving from monkeys into chimpanzees and, later, from chimpanzees into humans.

Today HIV is so pervasive that it is hard to imagine the world without it. But a global pandemic was not inevitable. If scientists had been looking for signs of new kinds of infections in Africans back in the 1960s and 1970s, they could have known about it long before it had afflicted millions of people. With a head start like that, epidemiologists might well have been able to intervene and mitigate the virus's spread. HIV is not alone in having emerged from an animal reservoir. More than half of human infectious diseases, past and present, originated in animals, including influenza, SARS, dengue and Ebola, to name a few. And today the vast interconnectedness of human populations, linked so extensively by road and air travel, allows new diseases to become pandemic more quickly, whether they come directly from wild animals, as did HIV, or indirectly, by passing from wild animals to domestic ones and then to us, as in the case of Japanese encephalitis virus and some strains of influenza. In response to these threats, my colleagues and I recently developed a bold new plan to monitor wild animals and the people who come into frequent contact with them for signs of new microorganisms or changes in the bugs' activity. We believe such eavesdropping may provide the early warning needed to stop pandemics before they start.

Stalking Viruses

Our surveillance vision grew out of research we began 10 years ago, when we initiated a study of viruses in rural villagers in the Central African country of Cameroon who hunt and butcher wild animals, as well as keep them as pets. We were trying to determine whether new strains of HIV were entering into human populations, and we suspected that these people would be at particularly high risk of infection.

To understand why we thought these Central African populations are vulnerable, consider a typical bushmeat hunter going about his day. The hunter wears only simple cotton shorts as he walks barefoot along a forest path, carrying on his back a 50-pound baboon. He has transported the animal for some miles and still has more to go before he reaches his village. As the hunter travels, the blood from his prey mingles with his own sweat and drips down his leg, flowing into open cuts along the way. Any infectious agents in the baboon's blood now have access to the hunter's circulatory system and tissues.

If the hunter had his choice, he and his fellow villagers might very well prefer pork or beef to monkey. But those forms of animal protein are rare here. And so he does what humans throughout the world have done for millennia: he hunts the local fauna, just as my friends in New Jersey do on their farm during deer season, in preparation for their annual venison dinner party. The only differences, perhaps, are that the Central African hunter relies on this food for his own survival and that of his family and that his primate quarry is more likely to transfer its viruses and other microorganisms to the hunter than is a deer, which is related to humans much more distantly.

Persuading the villagers to cooperate with us on this project was not easy. Many feared that we were going to seize their game. Only after gaining their trust could we begin collecting data. Their cooperation was essential: in addition to drawing samples of their blood for study and peppering them with questions about their health and hunting activities, we needed blood samples from their prey. We relied on them to obtain these samples by using pieces of filter paper we gave them.

Disease	Source
AIDS	Chimpanzees
Hepatitis B	Apes
Influenza A	Wild birds
Plague	Rodents
Dengue Fever	Old World primates
East African sleeping sickness	Wild and domestic ruminants
Vivax malaria	Asian macaques
West African sleeping sickness	Wild and domestic ruminants
Yellow fever	African primates
Chagas' disease	Many wild and domestic mammals

Infectious Diseases from Wild Animals. Many of the major infectious diseases of humans are believed to have come from wild animals. This fact underscores the need to monitor the microbes of wild creatures, in addition to those of lifestock. This table lists 10 such diseases and the animals from which they likely emerged.

Our analyses of the blood from the hunters and the hunted revealed several animal viruses not previously seen in humans. One agent, which we first reported in a paper published in 2004 in *Lancet*, is known as simian foamy virus (SFV), and it is a member of the same family of viruses—the so-called retroviruses—to which HIV belongs. SFV is native to most primates, including guenon monkeys, mandrills and gorillas, and each of these primate species harbors its own genetically distinctive variant of the bug. We found that all three variants had entered the hunter populations. In one particularly telling example, a 45-year-old man who reported having hunted and butchered gorillas—animals rarely pursued by subsistence hunters—had contracted gorilla SFV.

In those same Central African populations we also found a variety of retroviruses known as human T lymphotropic viruses (HTLVs), so named because of their propensity for infecting immune cells called T lymphocytes. Two of the HTLVs, HTLV-1 and HTLV-2, were already well known to affect millions of people around the world and contribute to cancer and neurological disease in some infected individuals. But HTLV-3 and HTLV-4, which we described in 2005 in the *Proceedings of the National Academy of Sciences USA*, were new to science. Given the high degree of genetic similarity between HTLV-3 and its simian counterpart, STLV-3, it appears as if this virus was picked up through hunting

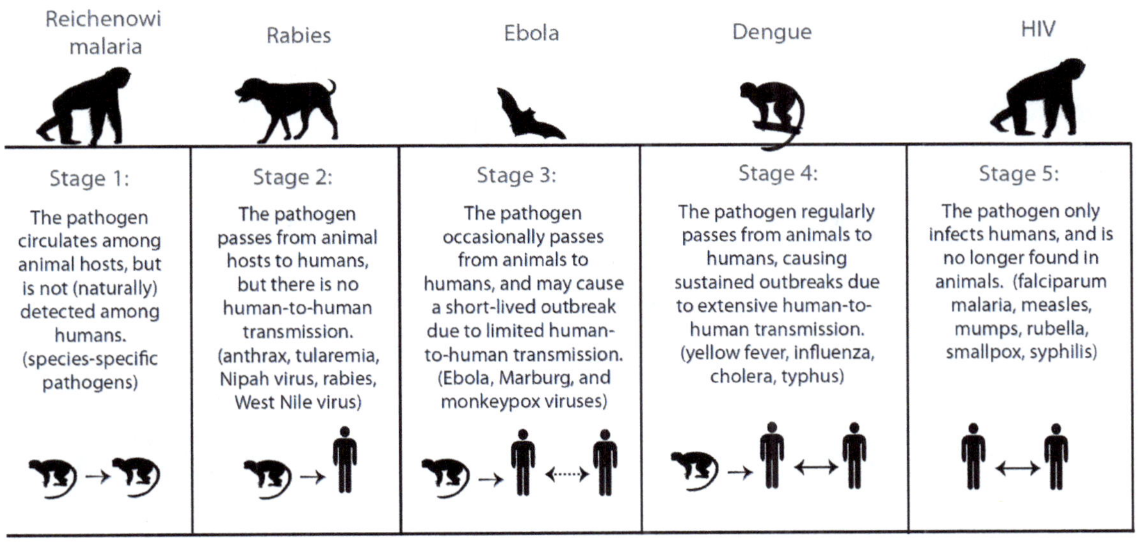

Patterns of Microbial Transmission. Animal pathogens may evolve through five stages to become exclusively human pathogens. The process is not inevitable; a microbe may remain in any stage indefinitely. The harm caused by particularly lethal agents (such as Ebola) is limited if they are still in an early stage, unable to spread easily from human to human. In contrast, a microbe which spreads readily among humans is likely to cause a pandemic.

STLV-3-infected monkeys. The origin of HTLV-4 remains unclear, but perhaps we will find its primate ancestor as we continue to explore these viruses in monkeys. We do not yet know whether SFV or the new HTLVs cause illness in people. Viruses do not necessarily make their hosts sick, and viruses that do sicken people and even spread from person to person do not always cause pandemics; often they retreat spontaneously. But the fact that SFV and HTLV are in the same family as HIV, which did spawn a global epidemic, means that epidemiologists must keep a close eye on them.

My colleagues and I have outlined five stages in the transformation of a pathogen of animals into one that specializes on humans. In stage 1, the agent lives only in animals. In stage 2, it can be transmitted to a human only from an animal. A stage 3 germ is transmitted primarily from animals to humans, but it can also spread among humans for a short time before dying out. Once the agent reaches stage 4, it can sustain longer outbreaks among humans. By the time it attains stage 5, it has become an exclusive pathogen of humans and no longer utilizes an animal host. Pathogens in stage 4 or stage 5 have the potential to cause massive human die-offs.

Forecasting the Next Pandemic

Had we been watching hunters 30 years ago, we might have been able to catch HIV early, before it reached the pandemic state. But that moment has passed. The question now is, How can we prevent the next big killers? Once my colleagues and I had determined that we could study remote populations effectively, we knew we could extend our work more broadly to listen in on viral "chatter"—the pattern of transfer of animal viruses to humans. With global surveillance, we realized, we might be able to sound the alarm about an emerging infectious disease before it boils over.

Fortunately, through partnership with Google.org and the Skoll Foundation we were able to launch the Global Viral Forecasting Initiative (GVFI), a program in which epidemiologists, public health

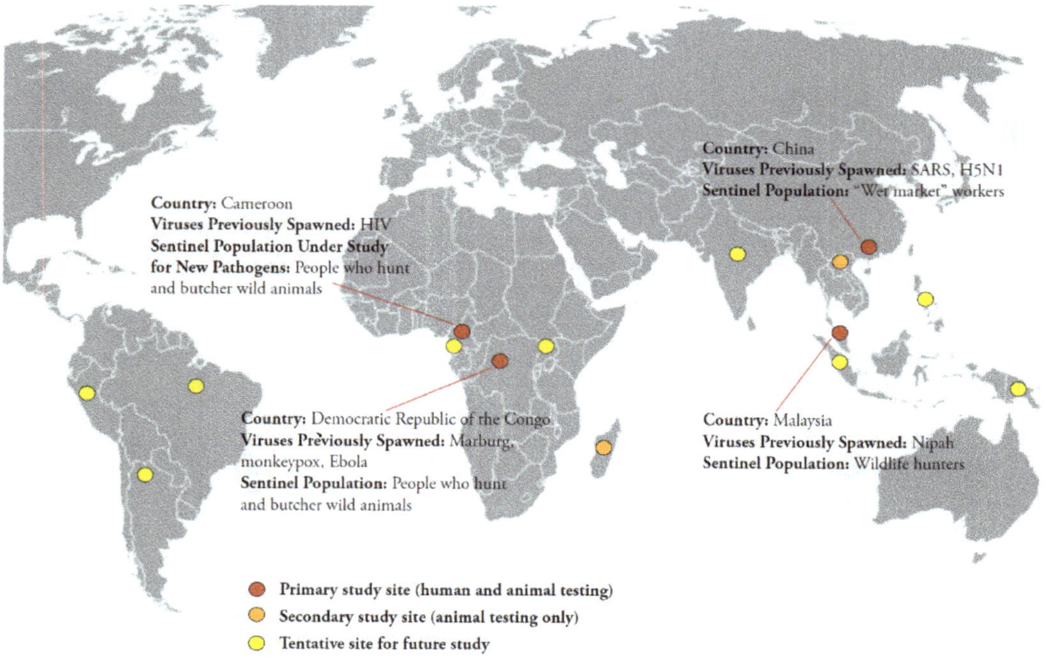

The Global Viral Forecasting Initiative (GVFI) is a surveillance program to monitor infections in wild animals and people regularly exposed to them. The aim is to detect emerging infectious diseases before they have a chance to spread into the human population. The effort currently employs 100 scientists and public health officials in several countries, particularly in tropical regions with high levels of biodiversity. Copyright © Roke (CC BY-SA 3.0) at http://commons.wikimedia.org/wiki/File:BlankMap-World-v2.png

workers and conservation biologists the world over collaborate to identify infectious agents at their point of origin and to monitor those organisms as they bubble up from animals into humans and flow outward from there. Instead of focusing narrowly on just viruses or a particular disease du jour, the GVFI works to document the full range of viruses, bacteria and parasites that are crossing over from animals into humans. Though still a fledgling effort, the GVFI now has around 100 scientists following sentinel populations or animals in Cameroon, China, the Democratic Republic of the Congo, Laos, Madagascar and Malaysia—all hotspots for emerging infectious diseases. Many of the sentinels are hunters, but we are also screening other populations at high risk of contracting diseases from wildlife, such as individuals who work in Asia's "wet markets," where live animals are sold for food.

Finding a new microorganism in a hunter is only the first step in tracking an emerging pathogen, however. We must then determine whether it causes disease, whether it is transmissible from person to person, and whether it has penetrated urban centers, where the high density of occupants could fuel its spread. The appearance in an urban center, away from the original source, would be a particularly worrisome sign of pandemic potential.

In the cases of HTLV-3 and HTLV-4, we are beginning to study high-risk populations in cities near hotspots for emerging infectious disease, regularly testing them for these viruses. Individuals with sickle cell disease who receive routine blood transfusions for their condition are one such population that could become infected early on. If we find people in these populations who are infected, we would work to initiate worldwide monitoring of blood supplies, to protect blood recipients. To that end, we are working with our long-term collaborator Bill Switzer and our colleagues at the U.S.

Centers for Disease Control and Prevention to develop new diagnostic tests to check for the presence of viruses in the blood supply. Another urgent priority would be to determine the agent's mode of transmission, which would inform tactics for blocking its spread. If an agent were sexually transmitted, for example, public health officials could launch awareness campaigns urging condom use, among other precautions.

Governments can also take measures to keep new viruses from entering the blood banks in the first place. In fact, following our discoveries concerning the relation between exposure to primates and these new viruses, the Canadian government modified its blood donation policies to exclude donors who have had contact with nonhuman primates.

In addition to our forecasting efforts, the new science of pandemic prevention includes programs such as HealthMap and ProMED, which compile daily reports on outbreaks around the world, and cutting-edge cyberwarning systems such as those piloted by Google.org to use patterns in search engine data to successfully forecast influenza. Likewise, national and international surveillance and response systems of local governments and the World Health Organization will play an important role in stopping the next plague.

For our part, we would ultimately like to expand our surveillance network to more countries around the world, including such nations as Brazil and Indonesia, which have a tremendous diversity of animal species that could transmit pathogens to humans. Fuller development of the GVFI will be expensive: building out our network so that we have adequate staff and lab facilities for testing the sentinel populations every six months and testing the animals with which these people are in contact will cost around $30 million, and keeping it running will cost another $10 million a year. But if it succeeds in averting even a single pandemic within the next 50 years, it will more than pay for itself. Even just mitigating such an event would justify the cost.

Humans work to forecast a variety of very complex natural threats. We rarely question the logic behind trying to predict hurricanes, tsunamis, earthquakes and volcanoes. Yet we really have no reason to believe that predicting pandemics is inherently harder than predicting tsunamis. Given the enormous sums of money required to stop pandemics once they have already been established, it only makes sense to spend a portion of those public health dollars on stopping them in the first place. The ounce of prevention principle has never been more apt.

Two-Way Street

Pathogens do not jump only from animals into humans—they can also travel in the other direction. Some infectious diseases that people have transmitted, and continue to transmit, to animals include:

- Tuberculosis (cattle)
- Yellow fever (South American monkeys)
- Measles (mountain gorillas)
- Poliomyelitis (chimpanzees)

Taking Action

If investigators find signs that an emerging pathogen has spread beyond humans who have direct contact with animals into the mainstream population, they will sound an alarm. Protecting the blood supply will be one important step toward preventing a pandemic. This measure will require rapid development and deployment of a diagnostic test for the germ.

The Threat From Pets

Wild animals and farm animals are not the only potential sources for the next major pandemic. Fido and Fluffy—and other pets, too—could harbor pathogens devastating to humans. This possibility arises when pets come into contact with germ-carrying wild animals. The germs can jump into pets, which can then transmit these agents to their owners.

More to Explore

1. Naturally Acquired Simian Retrovirus Infections in Central African Hunters. Nathan D. Wolfe et al. in *Lancet,* Vol. 363, No. 9413, pages 932–937; March 20, 2004.
2. Emergence of Unique Primate T-Lymphotropic Viruses among Central African Bushmeat Hunters. Nathan D. Wolfe et al. in *Proceedings of the National Academy of Sciences USA,* Vol. 102, No. 22, pages 7994–7999; May 31, 2005.
3. Bushmeat Hunting, Deforestation, and Prediction of Zoonotic Disease Emergence. Nathan D. Wolfe et al. in *Emerging Infectious Diseases,* Vol. 11, pages 1822–1827; December 2005.
4. Origins of Major Human Infectious Diseases. Nathan D. Wolfe, Claire Panosian Dunavan and Jared Diamond in *Nature,* Vol. 447, pages 279–283; May 17, 2007.
5. The Global Viral Forecasting Initiative Web site: www.gvfi.org

Section IX

Does HIV Cause AIDS?

9.1

The HIV AIDS Connection

The National Institute of Allergy and Infectious Diseases, U.S. National Institutes of Health

AIDS WAS FIRST RECOGNIZED IN 1981 and has since become a major worldwide pandemic. Abundant evidence indicates that AIDS is caused by HIV, or the human immunodeficiency virus, which was discovered in 1983. By leading to the destruction and/or functional impairment of cells of the immune system, notably $CD4^+$ T cells, HIV progressively destroys the body's ability to fight infections and certain cancers.

Why is There Overwhelming Scientific Consensus That HIV Causes AIDS?

Before HIV infection became widespread in the human population, AIDS-like syndromes occurred extremely rarely, and almost exclusively in people with known causes of immune suppression, such as chemotherapy and underlying cancers of certain types. A marked increase in unusual infections and cancers characteristic of severe immune suppression was first recognized in the early 1980s in homosexual men who had been otherwise healthy and had no recognized cause for immune suppression.

An infectious cause of AIDS was suggested by geographic clustering of cases, links among cases by sexual contact, mother-to-infant transmission, and transmission by blood transfusion. Isolation of HIV from patients with AIDS strongly suggested that this virus was the cause of AIDS. Since the early 1980s, HIV and AIDS have been repeatedly linked in time, place, and population group. The appearance of HIV in the blood supply has preceded or coincided with the occurrence of AIDS cases in every country and region where AIDS has been noted. People of all ages from many risk groups—including men who have sex with men, infants born to HIV-infected mothers, heterosexual women and men, hemophiliacs, recipients of blood and blood products, healthcare workers and others occupationally exposed to HIV-tainted blood, and male and female injection drug users—have all developed AIDS with only one common denominator: infection with HIV.

HIV destroys $CD4^+$ T cells, which are crucial to the normal function of the human immune system. In fact, depletion of $CD4^+$ T cells in HIV-infected individuals is an extremely powerful predictor of the development of AIDS. Studies of thousands of people have revealed that most who are HIV-infected

Source: http://www.niaid.nih.gov/topics/hivaids/understanding/howhivcausesaids/pages/connection.aspx.

carry the virus for years before enough damage is done to the immune system for AIDS to develop. However, with time, a near-perfect correlation has been found between infection with HIV and the subsequent development of AIDS. Recently developed sensitive tests have shown a strong correlation between the amount of HIV in the blood and the subsequent decline in $CD4^{+}$ T cell numbers and development of AIDS. Furthermore, reducing the amount of virus in the body with anti-HIV drugs can slow this immune destruction.

9.2

The Deadly Legacy of HIV Truthers

Charlie Jane Anders

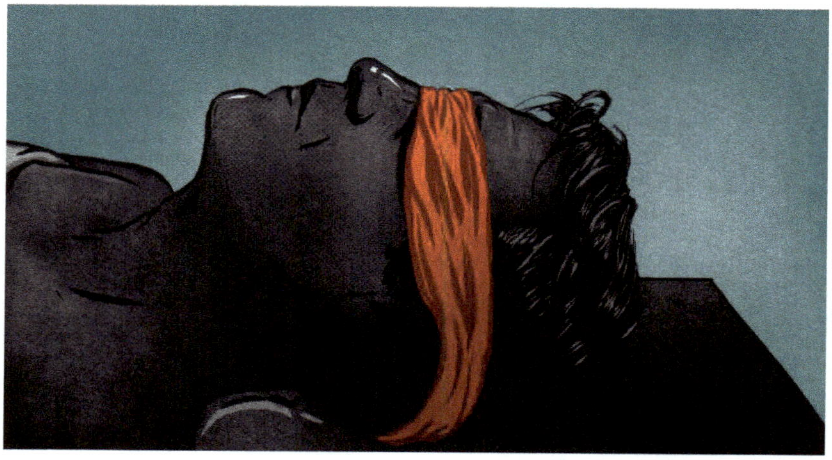

AIDS WAS A TERRIFYING MYSTERY, AND then we solved it. When researchers identified the human immunodeficiency virus as the reason why young, previously healthy people were developing rare cancers and wasting away, it was a triumph of medical science.

But even as the medical community reached a consensus that HIV caused AIDS, a counter-movement was emerging, claiming that HIV didn't exist, or that the virus existed but was harmless. The symptoms of AIDS, according to some of these people, were actually caused by HIV therapies themselves. To this day, some people continue to believe that HIV is a hoax.

The story of the HIV denialist movement demonstrates that scientific agreement is not necessarily enough. Thousands of people died because the conspiracy theory was able to outrun the facts, thriving in the climate of fear and suspicion around a grisly disease that had struck a vulnerable population. To some groups who'd been fighting on behalf of AIDS patients, it was too tidy to see a multimillion-dollar drug market emerge, to treat the same people who'd already been stigmatized and marginalized.

In the United States, the HIV denial movement led individual patients to reject medication until it was too late. In South Africa, denialists managed to win influence with the country's president, Thabo Mbeki, and his public-health policies led to an estimated 330,000 deaths that would otherwise have been preventable. Elsewhere, we may never fully know how much impact HIV denialism had—but conversations with more than a dozen HIV activists, educators, doctors, and former denialists, suggest that the denialists significantly hindered efforts at educating people about HIV and how to protect themselves.

"We Just Didn't F***ing Trust Anybody"

In the early 1980s, there was legitimate disagreement and debate over the causes of AIDS. At that point, "any theory of what was causing young people to die from these rare diseases was fair game," said University of Connecticut social psychology professor Seth Kalichman, author of the book *Denying AIDS: Conspiracy Theories, Pseudoscience, and Human Tragedy.*

But even before the virus causing AIDS was identified, the federal Centers for Disease Control put out prevention recommendations that were compatible with the idea that it was spread by a virus, said Jim Curran, who coordinated the CDC's AIDS taskforce beginning in 1981. "We did that because we thought it would be very important," Curran said—and, he said, there was already enough agreement that the condition was spreading like a virus.

And when scientists did identify HIV as the cause of AIDS, "it was obviously true from the very beginning," said Curran, who is now the Dean of the Rollins School of Public Health at Emory University. This was a new virus, which was shown to kill immune cells, or lymphocytes, in a petri dish. "Basically, everyone who has AIDS has the virus," Curran said, "and people who didn't have AIDS didn't have the virus."

But some people refused to accept the consensus. "After the virus was proven to cause AIDS, these guys came out of the woodwork," Curran said. "They had no credibility. It was so counter-intuitive."

One of the people who doubted the news was Stephen Kovacev. Kovacev remembers when he first heard that we'd found the cause of AIDS. It was 1984, and President Reagan was running for re-election. Reagan had been eager to sweep the AIDS crisis under the rug, so Kovacev immediately suspected a trick.

At this time, Kovacev had been a gay rights activist for a dozen years, having moved to New York's Christopher Street in the wake of the Stonewall riots. He'd survived protests, clashes with the police, and "brutal" treatment from a homophobic medical establishment that treated him "like a pariah" when he sought treatment for anal warts. After all of this, plus Watergate and Vietnam, said Kovacev, "how could you trust anything that came from any institution?"

So Kovacev was skeptical about a neat and tidy explanation for AIDS—and then he heard that a reputable scientist, Peter Duesberg at U.C., Berkeley, was saying he believed that HIV was a harmless virus, that had nothing to do with causing AIDS. (Duesberg still believes this.) So Kovacev and his friends didn't know what to think.

"We weren't denialists," Kovacev said of his fellow activists at the time. "We just didn't fucking trust anybody."

From early on, the HIV skeptics took two tacks, according to George Carter, director of the Foundation for Integrative AIDS Research. Either they said that HIV was harmless and had little or nothing to do with AIDS (as Duesberg argued), or they claimed that the virus actually didn't exist (or had "never been isolated"), and all we could point to were antibodies, not a virus.

drugs

There was also the pervasive claim that "drugs cause AIDS," Carter said, including heroin, amphetamines and cocaine. "Sorry, but if recreational drugs cause AIDS, there should be a helluva lot of dead straight people."

bioweapon

Meanwhile, former KGB and Stasi operatives have since admitted that there was a coordinated misinformation campaign on the part of the USSR and East Germany in the 1980s, aimed at spreading the idea that AIDS was a bioweapon created by the United States—which was successful at getting stories into the London *Sunday Express* and the CBS Evening News. In the 1990s, this gave rise to widespread beliefs that AIDS had been specifically designed to target black people, writes Nicoli Nattrass, the Director of the AIDS and Society Research Unit at the University of Cape Town in South Africa.

"All their ideas are arguable nonsense," said Carter of the denialists. This is, Carter said, "sadly proven by every HIV-positive denialist with whom I had these arguments, dying of AIDS."

Alternative Treatments

But to Kovacev, and people like him, there seemed to be some valid debate over whether the virus actually had anything to do with the disease. Soon, Kovacev was going to weekly meetings of HEAL AIDS, which met at the Gay and Lesbian Center.

HEAL AIDS was originally focused on finding alternative, non-toxic treatments for AIDS, but increasingly became focused on spreading the message that HIV was a hoax. [...] And Kovacev remembers reading New York's gay newspaper, the *New York Native*, which became dedicated to attacking the science behind HIV. (The *Native* folded in early 1997.)

A lot of the denialists rallied around Duesberg, who had real scientific credentials in spite of his viewpoints on HIV. Duesberg never seemed interested in starting a movement, but he "attracted some real fringe characters," said Kalichman. "They kind of tagged onto him."

The idea of using vitamins and health supplements as an alternatives to the early HIV drugs like AZT definitely appealed to Kovacev. In 1985, he and his partner, Kevin, had started the first "organic raw foods" store in New York. "We had friends that were healthy and went on AZT, and died," Kovacev told me in a phone conversation, adding that he asked: "What's really going on? Oh, is this Nazi Germany again? Are they trying to get rid of us?"

Kovacev's partner Kevin died of AIDS in 1990, on World AIDS Day, and his second partner died five years later. Kovacev himself had been diagnosed with AIDS, but didn't want to take any of the single-drug therapies that were available.

"By 1995, I was dying. I was pretty much going to be out of here," Kovacev said. "I had lost the will to live." He credits his "spiritual godmothers," including Amy Belle Olatunji the wife of famous drummer Baba Olatunji, with convincing him to keep living. And when the new multi-drug "cocktail" therapies came along in 1996, he decided to try them. These drugs were the first things he'd tried which actually raised his T-cell count, after years of taking health supplements—and when he saw his immune system get stronger on HIV drugs, that's when he finally believed that HIV and AIDS had to be related.

In 1997, Kovacev became the first person with full-blown AIDS to run the Boston Marathon.

The Dangerous Power of Virodene

Meanwhile, South Africa's HIV-denialist nightmare also began with a focus on alternative treatments. In 1997, then-Vice President Thabo Mbeki and other top ANC officials championed a "cure" for AIDS called Virodene—which turned out to contain an industrial solvent called dimethylformamide that causes irreversible (and often fatal) liver damage.

The creators of Virodene, University of Pretoria scientists Olga Visser and her husband Jacques Siegfried "Zigi" Visser, were invited to speak at a cabinet meeting, where Olga Visser told ANC leaders that Virodene "destroyed" AIDS. They were greeted with a standing ovation.

"With hindsight, Virodene was the start" of South African denialism, said Nathan Geffen, a long-time South African HIV activist and author of the book *Debunking Delusions*. At the time, activists just saw the Virodene incident as a "temporary aberration."

Later, after Mbeki became president in 1999, his health minister Manto Tshabalala-Msimang threw her support behind a retired Dutch nurse named Tine van der Maas who promoted a miracle AIDS cure called "Africa's Solution," whose ingredients included extract of African potato, olive green leaf and grapefruit seeds.

Tshabalala-Msimang also became known as "Dr. Beetroot" because she claimed a diet of beets, African potatoes, garlic and lemons could treat AIDS. She also supported a vitamin salesman, Matthias Rath, who claimed his supplements could reverse the progress of AIDS.

"An Epidemic Within an Epidemic"

South Africa's HIV denialism was home-grown, but it gained strength from the denialist community in the United States. When Mbeki became President, he held an AIDS conference, in which he flew in overseas "experts" like Duesberg.

"The remarkable thing about Mbeki's presidential panel was that it was really divided evenly between credible scientists and discredited denialists," Kalichman said. "And the people he seemed to listen to were the discredited denialists. And remarkably, they're all white Western European and American men. His scientists were primarily South African. They were racially diverse, and they were from his country. Some of the really most renowned AIDS scientists in the world were on that panel. And they were South African."

"Denialism has been an epidemic within an epidemic," said HIV educator Ntando Yola, who works with the Desmond Tutu HIV Foundation.

When former President Nelson Mandela tried to question Mbeki's AIDS policies at a 2002 African National Congress meeting, Mandela was publicly humiliated by top ANC officials, who were keen to show loyalty to Mbeki. They accused Mandela of breaking party discipline and undermining Mbeki, and ANC leader Ngoako Ramatlhodi described the other ANC officials as "like a pack of wild dogs, tearing their prey," and said that after this "vicious mauling," Mandela "looked twice his age, old and ashen."

After this, Mandela paid a visit to HIV-positive activist Zackie Achmat, a leader of the Treatment Action Campaign (TAC), who was challenging Mbeki's policies in court. Mandela was photographed with Achmat, wearing a shirt Achmat had given him that read "HIV-positive," in an attempt to fight the stigma around HIV.

The TAC succeeded in winning a 2002 court order that forced the government to provide anti-retroviral (ARV) drugs to prevent mother-to-child transmission of HIV. But the Mbeki government still resisted providing ARVs to the general population, so the TAC embarked on a "civil disobedience" program, including a 14,000-person protest at Parliament and protests at police stations.

"There were about 200 of us sitting inside a police station, demanding that they either arrest the Minister of Health or us," said Geffen. "We were actually occupying the whole police station." But the Cape Town police, who were sympathetic to their viewpoint, refused to arrest the activists for a long time, until the police finally relented and "symbolically charged" them, releasing them immediately. In Durban, there was one protest where the police used tear gas and beat protesters.

"Survey after survey showed there wasn't much support for these AIDS-denialist views," said Geffen. "People went along with it because it suited them politically."

After the civil disobedience campaign, the government agreed to provide ARVs to everyone with HIV—but this was followed by "years of 'malicious compliance' from the government," said Marcus Low, the TAC's head of Policy Communications and Research.

By all accounts, South Africa now has one of the best treatment programs in the world, with an estimated 3 million people receiving ARVs. South Africa's long history of "achieving freedom through civil action" was what allowed the TAC to turn the tide against denialism, said Yola: "People believed that standing up against a resistant force for what is possible will eventually yield results."

The Foo Fighters and Harpers Magazine

Around the time that Mbeki was flying denialist "experts" into South Africa, denialism was becoming a serious national movement in the United States.

In 2000, while the Foo Fighters were touring on their breakout album *There Is Nothing Left to Lose*, bass player Nate Mendel came across a book by a leading denier called Christine Maggiore, and shared it with the other band members, including former Nirvana drummer Dave Grohl. The Foo Fighters ended up playing a benefit concert for Maggiore's HIV-denialist organization, Alive and Well, at which Maggiore spoke and copies of her book were handed out. (I tried to reach Mendel to see if he still denies a link between HIV and AIDS, but he did not respond.)

Around the same time, San Francisco and Atlanta branches of ACT UP, a prominent national organization aimed at raising awareness about AIDS, turned towards debunking the "myth" of HIV. For a while there were two ACT UP organizations in San Francisco, and one became dedicated to spreading the message that "HIV does not cause AIDS and that it is the use of anti-HIV medications which make people get sick and die."

Rates of new HIV infections had been steadily going down since the early 1990s, but in 2000-2001, they started going back up again, said Jeff Sheehy, longtime AIDS activist and director of communications with the UCSF AIDS Research Institute. People were feeling more optimistic about treatment options, they were tired of using condoms, and they were feeling "fatigue from having been scared for so long."

"I think people just got burned out by the early 2000s on the notion of condoms," Carter said.

So Sheehy and other activists in San Francisco worked harder to spread the message that HIV was still a serious threat, and people needed to use condoms and get tested—and this, Sheehy said, "brought the wrath of the denialists down on us."

"I received a death threat," said Sheehy. "All of us would receive harassing phone calls in the middle of the night [and] at work. One person was being followed in the Castro, when he was walking his dog. People got calls like, 'I know where your kids go to school.'" One denialist dumped used cat litter on the head of the San Francisco AIDS Foundation at a public forum. Someone even phoned in a bomb threat to the *San Francisco Chronicle*, within a couple months after 9/11.

The message to HIV educators, Sheehy said, was "you're an enemy of the gay community, and we're going to silence you."

Finally, ACT UP San Francisco spokesman David Pasquarelli and one other activist were arrested and jailed. (The other activist said he didn't agree with Pasquarelli's views on HIV, but felt that HIV-prevention campaigns were aimed at suppressing gay sexuality.)

Kalichman said that 2001 was the peak of denialism in the United States, and it was spurred by two factors. The internet had made denialist materials easier to find, and meanwhile people could see that a world leader, Mbeki, had adopted these views.

And in much the same way that Jenny McCarthy became the face of anti-vaccine activists, Christine Maggiore was the most prominent spokesperson for HIV deniers. (And in fact, Maggiore was also famous for not vaccinating her children.) An HIV-positive woman who had been a successful businesswoman and promoted alternative medicine, Maggiore was an appealing presence, and she played well in the media, said Tara C. Smith, a professor of Public Health at Kent State who blogs about HIV at ScienceBlogs.

One of Maggiore's biggest defenders, the journalist Celia Farber, wrote a 2006 cover story for Harper's Magazine, in which she more or less accused drug companies of inventing AIDS in order to sell lethal drugs.

"Maggiore appeared in various media outlets after she refused to take medications while pregnant and breast-feeding her children," said Smith. "She was in the media again when her daughter, Eliza Jane, died of AIDS." (*Law and Order: SVU* did an episode loosely based on this case.) And then Maggiore herself died in 2008 of AIDS-related pneumonia.

The Decline of Denialism

"After losing Maggiore and her life story, I think the denialism movement has lost some momentum and prominence," said Smith. "The death of one of their most prominent faces is a tough blow."

Likewise, "AIDS denialism is dead in South Africa," said Geffen. "It pretty much died with the removal of Mbeki from power."

By the time John Strangis became an HIV denialist in 2012, the movement was already pretty marginalized. Strangis told me that he never went to any denialist conventions, because the movement no longer had enough money, or a large enough membership, to organize any.

Strangis felt attracted to the HIV denialists, because he already believed in a number of other conspiracy theories and "it was quite simple for me to assimilate this new information into my belief system." Adds Strangis, "as a person living with HIV, the possibility that HIV was a lie was quite reassuring." Soon, Strangis became one of the most active spokespeople for the movement, posting videos on YouTube and appearing on internet radio shows.

A lot of Strangis' fellow denialists, he said, believed other bizarre theories, like the idea that "the International Space Station is a hoax and doesn't exist." And, he added, "the president of Rethinking AIDS himself now believes pathogenic viruses do not exist in any shape or form."

In fact, HIV denialists often have the same characteristics as other conspiracy theorists, like climate change skeptics, Kalichman said. "There's always a rogue scientist, who has credentials but has lost credibility," he said. There's also always some powerful organization—either the government, the World Health Organization, the United Nations, or Big Pharma—that's "trying to cover up the truth." There is a basic playbook, Smith has written: Identify a sinister conspiracy; accuse the establishment of practicing a "religion" and "having 'faith' in the 'dogma' of germ theory and HIV causation"; cherry-pick the literature, and take findings out of context; move the goal posts; and so on.

I asked Smith what she meant by "moving the goal posts," and she replied: "They say HIV was never isolated. We give them excellent electron micrographs of the virus. They say 'OK, it's a virus, but it doesn't cause disease.' They say that Koch's postulates haven't been proven to conclusively show HIV causes AIDS. We give them examples of medical workers who were accidentally exposed to the virus and later developed AIDS. They say they must have undisclosed drug addictions or other causes for the immune decline. They never accept the science—they just keep changing the target of their disbelief."

"There's a subsection of the population that is inclined to doubt people speaking for the government, or professors with white hair, medical school faculty [or] people who claim to know something," said Arthur L. Reingold, professor and Head of Epidemiology at the UC Berkeley School of Public Health. "It ranges from evolution to global warming to vaccine safety to HIV and AIDS."

Strangis' wife, who's also HIV-positive, was hospitalized in 2011 for pneumocystis pneumonia, after she had stopped taking her meds in 2007. Strangis said the denialist community always claimed that the medical establishment was too quick to blame HIV, if someone became sick with an unrelated condition: "There's an old denialist saying: If you're positive, you can get hit by a bus, car, gunshot, etc., and it would still be deemed an AIDS death," Stangis said.

In June 2014, Strangis' wife became pregnant, and they decided to allow the doctors to treat her, to avoid passing HIV on to their son. "We agreed to the treatment because we did not want any problems with the authorities who would see our denial of treatment as child abuse, but also because I did not want to risk being wrong and my son having to live with the burden of HIV since birth," said Strangis—adding that they were "verbally assaulted" by their fellow denialists for choosing to accept treatment.

After their son was born, Strangis' wife became ill again and nearly died—but when she received HIV treatments in the hospital, she recovered. At that point, Strangis finally decided to leave the movement. By now, he had noticed Facebook posts showing that four other members of the movement had died of AIDS, and many others had become sick.

It's Not Over

Denialism still gets articles in reputable scientific journals, and is still influencing people, to this day.

In 2010, Kalichman did a survey of 266 men and 77 women living with HIV/AIDS, and found that one out of five of them agreed with statements like "there is no proof that HIV causes AIDS" or "HIV treatments do more harm than good." The more frequently someone used the internet, the readier they were to believe that there was no proof that HIV causes AIDS.

"We have to remember that there's still a lot of harm that comes from AIDS denialism," said Kalichman.

And in South Africa, the government is still dragging its feet on providing Pre-Exposure Prophylaxis (PrEP) to HIV-negative people, based partly on bad science about HIV transmission, said Brian Kanyemba, a key populations community engagement officer with the Desmond Tutu HIV Foundation in Cape Town.

Nor are "miracle cures" for HIV a thing of the past. Kanyemba told me that his sister was born with HIV, and she had been doing well on ARVs. Then she went to a Pentecostal church, where they gave her "special water" to drink and told her that she was cured of HIV. She stopped taking her medications, and died last summer. Since then, Kanyemba has been campaigning for the South African Health Ministry to crack down on churches, and their supposed cures for the virus.

And we'll never know exactly how much damage HIV denialism did outside of South Africa, where the impact has been well-documented. Some experts, like Reingold, say it was just a "blip" in the United States. Others say denialism was one factor among many that hindered HIV education: "It tends to reinforce the denial of risk," says Curran. But all we have are anecdotes.

For example, Sheehy knew a hairdresser in St. Mark's Place in New York who insisted that HIV didn't cause AIDS—and thus, safer sex was unnecessary. Sheehy and the hairstylist got into an argument while he was getting his hair cut: "He's a really nice kid and a sweetheart, but it was kind of an unpleasant conversation." Sheehy vowed never to go back to that hairdresser again, and later he heard that the kid had tested positive for HIV.

Art by Jim Cooke. Additional research/transcription by Levi Gadye. Thanks also to Liz Highleyman and Rich Juzwiak for the advice.

2002 TAC activist brought ART case to court force Mbeki to give ART to HIV+

9.3

World Aids Day

Russia Stands on Brink of Unprecedented HIV Crisis as Thousands of Victims Deny It Even Exists

As the international community marks World Aids Day on 1 December, Oliver Carroll investigates the growing community of Russians who refuse to accept scientific facts about their disease

Oliver Carroll

YOU CAN OFTEN CHART THE STORY of an HIV denialist live on social media. From dismissing the scientific truth about the virus to the development of Aids symptoms and ultimately to death, the progression is as predictable as it is heartbreaking.

"They said that if I don't give my son the therapy, he'd die over the New Year holidays. Of course, I didn't give him anything," wrote Sofia Kuzmina on 20 March 2013. Seven months pass, and she writes again. "Now he isn't smiling, he isn't sitting in his buggy. They killed my son. He's like a phoenix. Damned you Aids!" The boy died just before his fourth birthday.

This year, Russia recorded the third highest number of new HIV cases anywhere in the world. But trust in doctors remains low, and a joined-up public health policy lacking. Within the cracks, a cult of pseudoscience has taken root. Thousands, perhaps tens of thousands of Russians now deny the basic facts about HIV. In the last three years alone, there have been at least 70 deaths attributable to HIV denialism, many of them young children.

Two weeks ago, authorities were finally moved to action. A regional court in Perm, western Siberia, took up the case of a woman who had ignored the protestations of doctors, and over three years withheld treatment from her dying eight-year-old son. The mother was sentenced to 18 months home arrest, the first ever punishment of its kind.

Meanwhile, a trial is ongoing in neighbouring Tyumen, over the death of a two-year-old girl denied treatment by HIV-sceptic parents.

For Kirill Vorobyev, a doctor specialising in infectious diseases, it is a case of too little and—quite evidently—too late. Why, he asks, did social services do nothing in the case of a 10-year-old girl who died in August in St Petersburg? Activists, after all, had repeatedly raised the alarm several times during the child's excruciating final months. For whatever reason, those in charge chose not to take her away from her foster father, a local priest.

"And what is 18 month home arrest in any case?" says Vorobyev. "That is a very lenient sentence for murder."

Since 2014, Vorobyov has managed a social media group on Vkontakte, Russia's Facebook, designed to counteract bogus online information about HIV. His group monitors Russia's denial communities for clues about people, especially children, who might be at risk. When possible, they alert the authorities and try to pull people away. Sometimes they are successful, but more often than not they are not.

HIV denialism can be a closed group, says Vorobyov, and the ties that bind leaders to new victims are strong: "Sometimes, there's nothing you can do."

"Denialism is usually a coping mechanism for people in crisis," says former HIV denialist Julia Vereshchagina. Vereshchagina found out her positive diagnosis in 2007, after being tested without her consent during a routine appendicitis operation. She found out the news after doctors paid a visit to her parents' house. They incorrectly told her mother that she had not just HIV, but full-blown Aids.

"That's when my denialism began—I understand the way I was told had a colossal effect on how I accepted things later," she says.

A positive diagnosis handled badly is often the main trigger for HIV denialism, agrees Kirill Barsky, programme director of Steps, an HIV patient group in Moscow. Vereschagina's case is an extreme example of how not to inform patients, but it isn't unique. Typically, Russians will discover their fate from an A4 envelope, he says. They won't even have to open it; the diagnosis will already be written on the doctor's white face.

Proper psychological support is unusual. If they are lucky, patients will be told about antiretroviral therapy, and about the possibility of extending their life expectancy to near-normal levels. Or they might not. Just as likely, they will come away with the impression they have contracted the modern-day plague, with no more than a couple of years of life left.

So desperate patients turn to alcohol, drugs, and then they turn to the internet. Here they make a discovery that HIV doesn't have to exist. That HIV doesn't cause Aids. That it's the toxic medicine and anal sex that cause Aids. Change the lifestyle, bathe yourself in hot springs, give yourself a silver enema, and everything will be just fine. Perhaps you'd like to buy this miracle cure for cancer too? These are, after all, very fertile grounds for all kinds of swindlers.

Russia's army of HIV conspiracists include prominent TV personalities like Alexander Gordon, but perhaps its most influential is a woman called Olga Kovekh. A former military doctor, Kovekh was, at least until recently, a regular "expert" on federal TV. She has dished out advice about the widest spectrum of medical conditions—doubting the existence of pneumonia, the benefit of vaccinations, and even suggesting TB could be cured with the proper administration of ham sandwiches. But it was on HIV where her wisdom was most pernicious. Her shadowy role advising the parents of young HIV denial victims has been so well documented that a local publication took to calling her "Dr. Death."

The Independent tried on several occasions to speak with Kovekh, but unsuccessfully. In a series of aggressive messages, it was told by an anonymous administrator on the doctor's Vkontakte group—likely by Kovekh herself—to "mind its own f***ing business".

"It's like a sect: you're either with them, and that's OK, or you doubt things—and that means you're not praying properly," says ex-denialist Vereschagina. "If you're not getting better, it means you aren't following the recommendations, or you're depressed. I remember one denialist asked me if I had contracted HIV from stress."

For the quietly spoken head of the Federal Aids Centre, Vadim Pokrovsky, dealing with "demagoguery" is part of the job. It has accompanied his life's work at every step, he says—right from the moment he began looking for HIV-positive patients in what was then the Soviet Union.

"People used to dismiss the disease as a disease of capitalism, saying that Russia couldn't possibly have it because there was no prostitution here," he says. "Incidentally, that was also untrue."

It took a little while, but Pokrovsky and his team eventually documented the first HIV case in 1985, involving a migrant from South Africa, and the first case involving a Russian two years later. "Only when the top officials came and saw them did they believe such people existed," he says.

In the mid-1980s, not all of the scientific arguments had been settled. It wasn't yet proven that HIV caused Aids, whether this happened in all patients, or whether HIV was a co-morbid condition.

Famously, the American scientist Peter Duesberg wrote a paper in the *Cancer Research* journal claiming the "Aids virus is not sufficient to cause Aids and there is no evidence ... that it is necessary for Aids." Duesberg's arguments are the basis of the ideas of Russia's HIV denialists today. But they have been debunked conclusively, and Duesberg has been disowned by the scientific community.

"Three decades after the discovery of the virus, it all looks frankly absurd," says Pokrovsky.

When it appeared in 1996, so-called combination antiretroviral therapy transformed HIV outcomes. It is now not only effective at reducing viral loads to undetectable levels, but is also well-tolerated in patients. The UN has called for it to be at the centre of a push to curb the epidemic worldwide. It calls its model 90-90-90: if you catch 90 percent of infections, treat 90 percent of them immediately, and achieve undetectable viral loads in 90 percent of the treated cases, you'll be in a good place.

Russia might be a world leader in testing, with 25 million tests administered last year. But on the treatment front, it is sorely lacking. Owing to shortages and the problems with the financing of drugs, perhaps only 30 percent of affected Russians are treated.

"In effect, there are several hundred thousand people waiting in line for the drugs," says Vinay Saldanha, UNAids Regional Director for Eastern Europe and Central Asia. "Those are several hundred people who could be transmitting the virus."

Treatment has already made inroads into the epidemic in traditional hotspots such as Africa, says Saldanha. But Russia remains far from a breakthrough. What is worse, the epidemic looks to be moving to a new phase, making a definitive transition from vulnerable groups to the main population. Already half of new cases in Russia are now from heterosexual contact.

"That is enough to raise concerns that the country is heading the same route as Africa, where heterosexual sexual contact is now the main transmission," says Pokrovsky. "HIV is most definitely a problem for all Russians."

After a long time in relative denial, there are signs the Russian government is beginning to treat the problem with the seriousness it deserves. Last year, a new state strategy was drawn up, one that would commit Russia to a 75 percent reduction in new cases by 2020, and to achieving proper treatment rates of 60 percent in the same timeframe.

Buried in the second half of the strategy is also a promise to criminalise HIV denialism by the end of 2018.

"It's is a positive turn, no doubt, but so far it is also only words and promises," says Pokrovsky. "Until they deliver on it, and on money, the problem isn't going to go away."

9.4

Christine Maggiore, Vocal Skeptic of AIDS Research, Dies at 52

Woman and Her Husband Sued Los Angeles County for Finding that Daughter Died of Aids-Related Pneumonia

Anna Gorman and Alexandra Zavis

UNTIL THE END, CHRISTINE MAGGIORE REMAINED defiant.

On national television and in a blistering book, she denounced research showing that HIV causes AIDS. She refused to take medications to treat her own virus. She gave birth to two children and breast-fed them, denying any risk to their health. And when her 3-year-old child, Eliza Jane, died of what the coroner determined to be AIDS-related pneumonia, she protested the findings and sued the county.

On Saturday, Maggiore died at her Van Nuys home, leaving a husband, a son and many unanswered questions. She was 52.

According to officials at the Los Angeles County coroner's office, she had been treated for pneumonia in the last six months. Because she had recently been under a doctor's care, no autopsy will be performed unless requested by the family, they said. Her husband, Robin Scovill, could not be reached for comment.

Jay Gordon, a pediatrician whom the family consulted when Eliza Jane was sick, said Monday that Maggiore's death was an "unmitigated tragedy."

"In the event that she died of AIDS-related complications, there are medications to prevent this," said Gordon, who disagrees with Maggiore's views and believes HIV causes AIDS. "There are medications that enable people who are HIV-positive to lead healthy, normal, long lives."

Diagnosed with HIV in 1992, Maggiore plunged into AIDS volunteer work—at AIDS Project Los Angeles, L.A. Shanti and Women at Risk. Her background commanded attention. A well-spoken, middle-class woman, she was soon being asked to speak about the risks of HIV at local schools and health fairs. "At the time," Maggiore told *The Times* in 2005, "I felt like I was doing a good thing."

All that changed in 1994, she said, when she spoke to UC Berkeley biology professor Peter Duesberg, whose well-publicized views on AIDS—including assertions that its symptoms can be caused by recreational drug use and malnutrition—place him well outside the scientific mainstream.

Intrigued, Maggiore began scouring the literature about the underlying science of HIV. She came to believe that flu shots, pregnancy and common viral infections could lead to a positive test result. She later detailed those claims in her book, *What if Everything You Thought You Knew About AIDS Was Wrong?*

Maggiore started Alive & Well AIDS Alternatives, a nonprofit that challenges "common assumptions" about AIDS. She also had a regular podcast about the topic.

Her supporters expressed shock Monday over her death but were highly skeptical that it was caused by AIDS. And they said it would not stop them from questioning mainstream thinking.

"Why did she remain basically healthy from 1992 until just before her death?" asked David Crowe, who served with Maggiore for a number of years on the board of the nonprofit Rethinking AIDS. "I think it's certain that people who promote the establishment view of AIDS will declare that she died of AIDS and will attempt to use this to bring people back in line. But you can only learn so much from an unfortunate death."

Brian Carter, who facilitated local peer groups with Maggiore, said the movement would remain strong.

"Christine was only part of this. There is an outstanding number of prominent rethinkers, independent thinkers, doctors, scientists, lawyers who question AIDS causation."

Though they run counter to the scientific consensus about AIDS, such beliefs can have a major effect. In South Africa, where about 5.7 million people live with HIV, the government refused until 2005 to fund antiretroviral treatment, citing questions about the effectiveness of the drugs that inhibit the replication of HIV.

Federal health officials and other experts say the link between HIV and AIDS has been shown in hundreds of studies and the prescription of antiretroviral drugs has helped reduce the pandemic to a chronic but manageable disease in the United States. Researchers from the Harvard School of Public Health calculated earlier this year that the South African government's delay in introducing treatment between 2000 and 2005 cost more than 330,000 lives in that country.

Craig Thompson, executive director of AIDS Project Los Angeles, said Maggiore was an effective and powerful advocate, in part because she was a woman living with HIV. But he said her message discouraging testing and treatment was dangerous.

"It's just really sad that she never could understand and never could trust the medical community, unlike the rest of the world," Thompson said.

Maggiore's friends said she underwent a holistic "cleanse" last month that left her feeling ill.

"She was telling me that she wasn't feeling great," Carter said, adding that he questioned whether the pneumonia was related to AIDS.

As an advocate, Maggiore counseled HIV-positive pregnant women on how to avoid pressure to use the drug AZT as a method to reduce the chances of transmission to their babies. She considered the drug toxic.

Maggiore gave birth to her son, Charlie, and his younger sister, Eliza Jane, at home and breast-fed both, although research indicates that it increases the risk of transmission. Eliza Jane Scovill died in 2005 from what the coroner ruled was AIDS-related pneumonia. Maggiore and Scovill, however, hired a pathologist who concluded that the girl died of an allergic reaction to the antibiotic amoxicillin.

After Eliza Jane's death, Los Angeles police investigated whether Maggiore and Scovill were negligent in not testing the girl for HIV. In 2006, the Los Angeles County district attorney's office decided not to file criminal charges against Maggiore, saying that it would have been difficult to prove criminal negligence because Maggiore had sought medical advice. Friends said that Maggiore never fully recovered after the death of her daughter and that she had trouble even sleeping and eating. Her preteen son, Charlie, has tested HIV negative.

Last year, Maggiore and Scovill sued Los Angeles County and others on behalf of their daughter's estate, charging that the autopsy report lacked proper medical and scientific evidence for the declared cause of death. The case is pending.

Section X

Immunology

10.1

The Immune System

The National Institutes of Health

THE IMMUNE SYSTEM IS A NETWORK of **cells, tissues,** and **organs** that work together to defend the body against attacks by "foreign" invaders. These are primarily **microbes**—tiny **organisms** such as **bacteria, parasites,** and **fungi** that can cause infections. **Viruses** also cause infections, but are too primitive to be classified as living organisms. The human body provides an ideal environment for many microbes. It is the immune system's job to keep them out or, failing that, to seek out and destroy them.

The immune system is amazingly complex. It can recognize and remember millions of different enemies, and it can produce secretions (release of fluids) and cells to match up with and wipe out nearly all of them.

The secret to its success is an elaborate and dynamic communications network. Millions and millions of cells, organized into sets and subsets, gather like clouds of bees swarming around a hive and pass information back and forth in response to an infection. Once immune cells receive the alarm, they become activated and begin to produce powerful chemicals. These substances allow the cells to regulate their own growth and behavior, enlist other immune cells, and direct the new recruits to trouble spots.

Self and Nonself

The key to a healthy immune system is its remarkable ability to distinguish between the body's own cells, recognized as "self," and foreign cells, or "nonself." The body's immune defenses normally coexist peacefully with cells that carry distinctive "self" marker **molecules.** But when immune defenders encounter foreign cells or organisms carrying markers that say "nonself," they quickly launch an attack.

Anything that can trigger this **immune response** is called an **antigen.** An antigen can be a microbe such as a virus, or a part of a microbe such as a molecule.

The Structure of the Immune System

The organs of the immune system are positioned throughout the body. They are called **lymphoid organs** because they are home to **lymphocytes,** small white blood cells that are the key players in the

National Institutes of Health, "The Immune System."

immune system. Bone marrow, the soft tissue in the hollow center of bones, is the ultimate source of all blood cells, including lymphocytes. The thymus is a lymphoid organ that lies behind the breastbone. Lymphocytes known as **T lymphocytes** or **T cells** ("T" stands for "thymus") mature in the thymus and then migrate to other tissues. **B lymphocytes,** also known as **B cells,** become activated and mature into **plasma cells,** which make and release **antibodies.**

Lymphocytes can travel throughout the body using the **blood vessels.** The cells can also travel through a system of **lymphatic vessels** that closely parallels the body's **veins** and **arteries.** Cells and fluids are exchanged between blood and lymphatic vessels, enabling the lymphatic system to monitor the body for invading microbes. The lymphatic vessels carry **lymph,** a clear fluid that bathes the body's tissues.

Small, bean-shaped **lymph nodes** are laced along the lymphatic vessels, with clusters in the neck, armpits, abdomen, and groin. Each lymph node contains specialized compartments where immune cells congregate, and where they can encounter antigens.

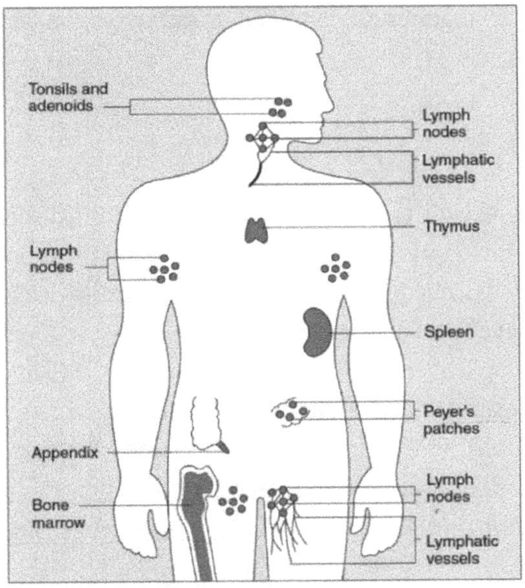

The organs of the immune system are positioned throughout the body.

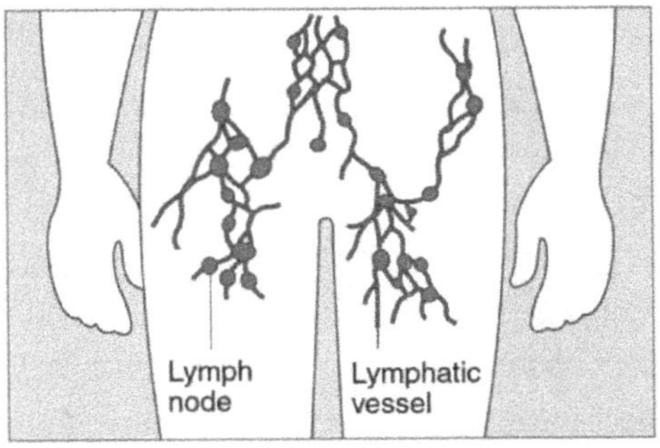

Immune cells and foreign particles enter the lymph nodes via incoming lymphatic vessels or the lymph nodes' tiny blood vessels.

Immune cells, microbes, and foreign antigens enter the lymph nodes via incoming lymphatic vessels or the lymph nodes' tiny blood vessels. All lymphocytes exit lymph nodes through outgoing lymphatic vessels. Once in the bloodstream, lymphocytes are transported to tissues throughout the body. They patrol everywhere for foreign antigens, then gradually drift back into the lymphatic system to begin the cycle all over again.

The **spleen** is a flattened organ at the upper left of the abdomen. Like the lymph nodes, the spleen contains specialized compartments where immune cells gather and work. The spleen serves as a meeting ground where immune defenses confront antigens.

Other clumps of lymphoid tissue are found in many parts of the body, especially in the linings of the digestive tract, airways, and lungs—territories that serve as gateways to the body. These tissues include the **tonsils, adenoids,** and **appendix.**

Immune Cells and Their Products

The immune system stockpiles a huge arsenal of cells, not only lymphocytes but also cell-devouring **phagocytes** and their relatives. Some immune cells take on all intruders, whereas others are trained on highly specific targets. To work effectively, most immune cells need the cooperation of their comrades. Sometimes immune cells communicate by direct physical contact, and sometimes they communicate releasing chemical messengers.

The immune system stores just a few of each kind of the different cells needed to recognize millions of possible enemies. When an antigen first appears, the few immune cells that can respond to it multiply into a full-scale army of cells. After their job is done, the immune cells fade away, leaving sentries behind to watch for future attacks.

All immune cells begin as immature **stem cells** in the bone marrow. They respond to different **cytokines** and other chemical signals to grow into specific immune cell types, such as T cells, B cells, or phagocytes. Because stem cells have not yet committed to a particular future, their use presents an interesting possibility for treating some immune system disorders. Researchers currently are investigating if a person's own stem cells can be used to regenerate damaged immune responses in immune deficiency disorders, such as **HIV** infection.

B Cells

B cells and T cells are the main types of lymphocytes. B cells work chiefly by secreting substances called antibodies into the body's fluids. Antibodies ambush foreign antigens circulating in the bloodstream. They are powerless, however, to penetrate cells. The job of attacking target cells—either cells that have been infected by viruses or cells that have been distorted by cancer—is left to T cells or other immune cells (described below).

Each B cell is programmed to make one specific antibody. For example, one B cell will make an antibody that blocks a virus that causes the common cold, while another produces an antibody that attacks a bacterium that causes pneumonia. When a B cell encounters the kind of antigen that triggers it to become active, it gives rise to many large cells known as plasma cells, which produce antibodies.

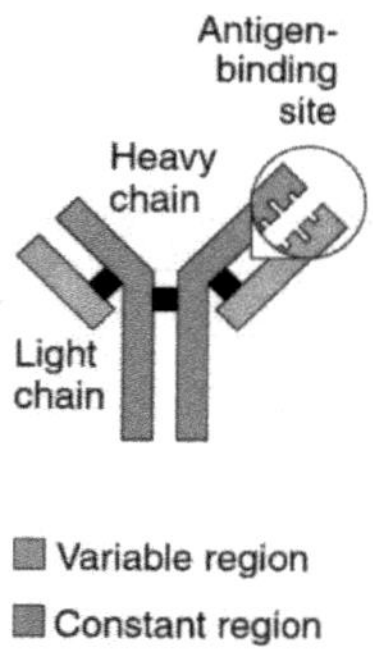

An antibody is made up of two heavy chains and two light chains. The variable region, which differs from one antibody to the next, allows an antibody to recognize its matching antigen.

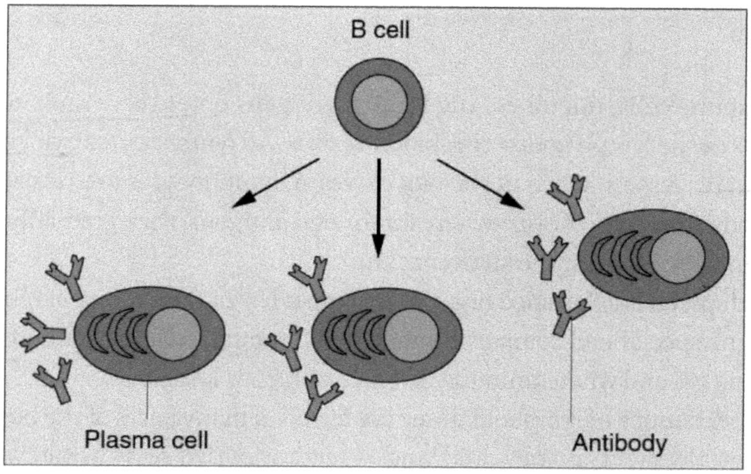

B cells mature into plasma cells that produce antibodies.

- **Immunoglobulin** G, or IgG, is a kind of antibody that works efficiently to coat microbes, speeding their uptake by other cells in the immune system.
- IgM is very effective at killing bacteria.
- IgA concentrates in body fluids—tears, saliva, and the secretions of the respiratory and digestive tracts—guarding the entrances to the body.
- IgE, whose natural job probably is to protect against parasitic infections, is responsible for the symptoms of allergy.
- IgD remains attached to B cells and plays a key role in initiating early B cell responses.

T Cells

Unlike B cells, T cells do not recognize free-floating antigens. Rather, their surfaces contain specialized antibody-like receptors (**T cell receptors**) that see fragments of antigens on the surfaces of infected cells. T cells contribute to immune defenses in two major ways: some direct and regulate immune responses, whereas others directly attack infected cells.

1. **Helper T cells,** or **Th cells,** coordinate immune responses by communicating with other cells. Some stimulate nearby B cells to produce antibodies, others call in microbe-gobbling cells called phagocytes, and still others activate other T cells.
2. **Cytotoxic T lymphocytes** (**CTLs**)—also called killer T cells—perform a different function. These cells directly attack other cells carrying foreign molecules on their surfaces. CTLs are especially useful for attacking viruses because viruses often hide from other parts of the immune system while they grow inside infected cells. CTLs recognize small fragments of these viruses peeking out from the cell membrane and launch an attack to kill the infected cell.

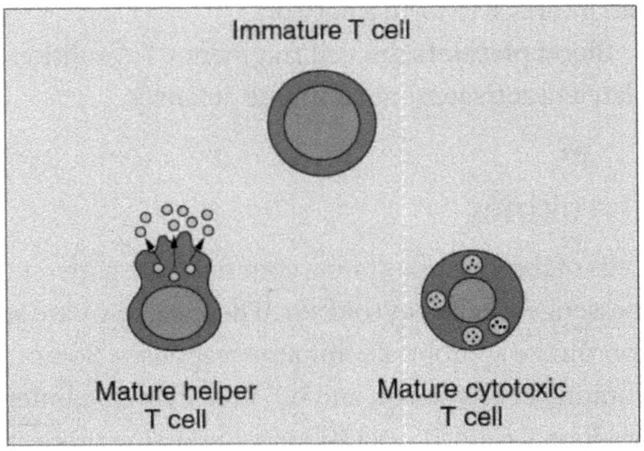

Some T cells are helper cells; others are killer cells.

T cells only recognize an antigen if it is carried on the surface of a cell by one of the body's own **major histocompatibility complex,** or **MHC,** molecules. MHC molecules are proteins recognized by T cells when they distinguish between self and nonself. A self-MHC molecule provides a recognizable scaffolding to present a foreign antigen to the T cell. In humans, MHC antigens are called **human leukocyte antigens,** or **HLA.**

T cell receptors are complex protein molecules that peek through the surface membranes of T cells. The exterior part of a T cell receptor recognizes short pieces of foreign antigens that are bound to self-MHC molecules on other cells of the body. It is because of their T cell receptors that T cells can recognize disease-causing microorganisms and rally other immune cells to attack the invaders, or kill the invaders themselves.

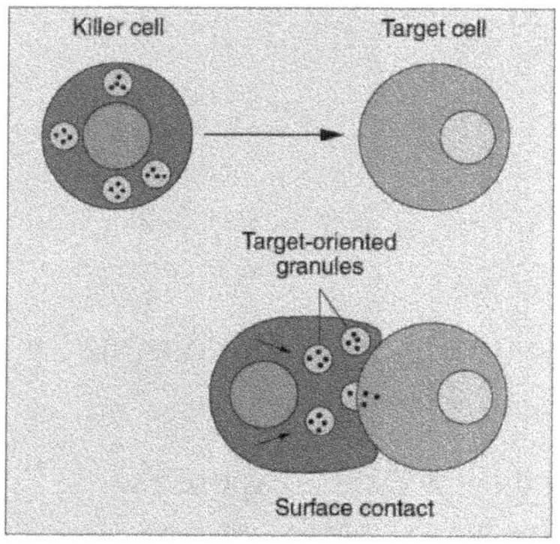

Killer cell makes contact with target cell, trains its weapons on the target, then strikes.

Natural killer (NK) cells are another kind of lethal white blood cell, or lymphocyte. Like CTLs, NK cells are armed with **granules** filled with potent chemicals. But CTLs look for antigen fragments bound to self-MHC molecules, whereas NK cells recognize cells lacking self-MHC molecules. Thus, NK cells have the potential to attack many types of foreign cells. Both kinds of killer cells slay on contact. The deadly assassins bind to their targets, aim their weapons, and then deliver a lethal burst of chemicals.

Phagocytes and Their Relatives

Phagocytes are large white blood cells that can swallow and digest microbes and other foreign particles. **Monocytes** are phagocytes that circulate in the blood. When monocytes migrate into tissues, they develop into **macrophages.** Specialized types of macrophages can be found in many organs, including the lungs, kidneys, brain, and liver.

Macrophages play many roles. As scavengers, they rid the body of worn-out cells and other debris. They display bits of foreign antigen in a way that draws the attention of matching lymphocytes and, in that respect, resemble **dendritic cells**. And they churn out an amazing variety of powerful chemical signals which are vital to the immune response.

Dendritic cells are found in the parts of lymphoid organs where T cells also exist. Like macrophages, dendritic cells in lymphoid tissues display antigens to T cells and help stimulate T cells during an immune response. They are called dendritic cells because they have branchlike extensions that can interlace to form a network.

Blood **platelets** are cell fragments. In addition to promoting blood clotting and wound repair, platelets activate some immune defenses.

Cytokines

Cells of the immune system communicate with one another by releasing and responding to chemical messengers called **cytokines.** These proteins are secreted by immune cells and act on other cells to coordinate appropriate immune responses. Some cytokines are chemical switches that turn certain immune cell types on and off. One cytokine, interleukin 2 (IL-2), triggers the immune system to produce T cells. IL-2's immunity-boosting properties have traditionally made it a promising treatment for several illnesses. Clinical studies are underway to test its benefits in diseases such as cancer, hepatitis C, and HIV infection and AIDS.

One group of cytokines chemically attracts specific cell types. These so-called **chemokines** are released by cells at a site of injury or infection and call other immune cells to the region to help repair the damage or fight off the invader. Chemokines often play a key role in inflammation and are a promising target for new drugs to help regulate immune responses.

Overview

Innate Immunity

The all-purpose "first-responder" arm of the immune system is called the **innate** immune system. In short order, the innate immune system responds with a surge of chemical signals that together cause fever, induce **phagocytosis** by macrophages, trigger the **inflammatory responses** that help control local infections, and play a range of crucial roles in defending the body against invading microbes.

Adaptive Immunity

In a delayed response, genetically identical groups of lymphocytes, called **clones,** that are already programmed to recognize specific antigens, respond to each invader individually. Such responses are called **adaptive** immunity.

Mounting an Immune Response

Infections are the most common cause of human disease. They range from the common cold to debilitating conditions like chronic hepatitis to life-threatening diseases such as AIDS. Disease-causing microbes (**pathogens**) attempting to get into the body must first move past the body's external armor, usually the skin or cells lining the body's internal passageways.

The skin provides an imposing barrier to invading microbes. It is generally penetrable only through cuts or tiny abrasions. The digestive and respiratory tracts—both portals of entry for a number of microbes—also have their own levels of protection. Microbes entering the nose often cause the nasal surfaces to secrete more protective mucus, and attempts to enter the nose or lungs can trigger a sneeze or cough reflex to force microbial invaders out of the respiratory passageways. The stomach contains a strong acid that destroys many pathogens that are swallowed with food.

If microbes survive the body's front-line defenses, they still have to find a way through the walls of the digestive, respiratory, or urogenital passageways to the underlying cells. These passageways are lined with tightly packed **epithelial cells** covered in a layer of mucus, effectively blocking the transport of many pathogens into deeper cell layers.

Mucosal surfaces also secrete a special class of antibody called IgA, which in many cases is the first type of antibody to encounter an invading microbe. Underneath the epithelial layer a variety of immune cells, including macrophages, B cells, and T cells, lie in wait for any microbe that might bypass the barriers at the surface.

Next, invaders must escape a series of general defenses of the innate immune system, which are ready to attack without regard for specific antigen markers. These include patrolling phagocytes and NK cells.

Microbes cross the general barriers then confront specific weapons of the adaptive immune system tailored just for them. These specific weapons, which include both antibodies and T cells, are equipped with singular receptor structures that allow them to recognize and interact with their designated targets.

Bacteria and Viruses

The most common disease-causing microbes are bacteria, viruses, and parasites. Each uses a different tactic to infect a person, and, therefore, each is thwarted by different components of the immune system.

Most bacteria live in the spaces between cells and are readily attacked by antibodies. When antibodies attach to a bacterium, they send signals to phagocytic cells to destroy the bound microbes. Some bacteria are eaten directly by phagocytes, which signal to certain T cells to join the attack.

All viruses, plus a few types of bacteria and parasites, must enter cells of the body to survive, requiring a different kind of immune defense. Infected cells use their MHC molecules to put pieces of the invading microbes on their surfaces, flagging down CTLs to destroy the infected cells. Antibodies also can assist in the immune response by attaching to and clearing viruses before they have a chance to enter cells.

Immunity: Natural and Acquired

Long ago, physicians realized that people who had recovered from the plague would never get it again—they had acquired immunity. This is because some of the activated T and B cells had become memory cells. Memory cells ensure that the next time a person meets up with the same antigen, the immune system is already set to demolish it.

Immunity can be strong or weak, short-lived or long-lasting, depending on the type of antigen it encounters, the amount of antigen, and the route by which the antigen enters the body. Immunity can also be influenced by inherited genes. When faced with the same antigen, some individuals will respond forcefully, others feebly, and some not at all.

An immune response can be sparked not only by infection but also by immunization with vaccines. Some vaccines contain microorganisms—or parts of microorganisms— that have been treated so they can provoke an immune response but not full-blown disease.

[...]

Infants are born with weak immune responses but are protected for the first few months of life by antibodies they receive from their mothers before birth. Babies who are nursed can also receive some antibodies from breast milk that help to protect their digestive tracts.

Vaccines

For many years, healthcare providers have used vaccination to help the body's immune system prepare for future attacks. Vaccines consist of killed or modified microbes, components of microbes, or microbial DNA that trick the body into thinking an infection has occurred.

A vaccinated person's immune system attacks the harmless vaccine and prepares for invasions against the kind of microbe the vaccine contained. In this way, the person becomes immunized against the microbe. Vaccination remains one of the best ways to prevent infectious diseases, and vaccines have an excellent safety record. Previously devastating diseases such as smallpox, polio, and whooping cough have been greatly controlled or eliminated through worldwide vaccination programs.

Immune Deficiency Disorders

When the immune system is missing one or more of its parts, the result is an **immune deficiency disorder**. These disorders can be inherited, acquired through infection, or produced as a side effect by drugs such as those used to treat people with cancer or those who have received transplants.

Temporary immune deficiencies can develop in the wake of common virus infections, including influenza, infectious mononucleosis, and measles. Immune responses can also be depressed by blood transfusions, surgery, malnutrition, smoking, and stress.

Some children are born with poorly functioning immune systems. Some have flaws in the B cell system and cannot produce antibodies. Others, whose thymus is either missing or small and abnormal, lack T cells. Very rarely, infants are born lacking all of the major immune defenses. This condition is known as severe combined immune deficiency disease or SCID.

AIDS is an immune deficiency disorder caused by a virus (HIV) that infects immune cells. HIV can destroy or disable vital T cells, paving the way for a variety of immunologic shortcomings. The virus also can hide out for long periods in immune cells. As the immune defenses falter, a person develops AIDS and falls prey to unusual, often life-threatening infections and rare cancers.

Immunology and Transplants

Each year thousands of lives in the United States are prolonged by transplanted organs including the kidneys, heart, lung, liver, and pancreas. For a transplant to "take," however, the body's natural tendency to rid itself of foreign tissue must be overridden.

One way to avoid the rejection of transplanted tissue is **tissue typing,** which ensures that markers of self on the donor's tissue are as similar as possible to those of the recipient. Every cell in the body has a double set of six major tissue antigens, and each of the antigens exists, in different individuals, in as many as 20 varieties. The chance of two people having identical transplant antigens is about one in 100,000.

A second way to avoid transplant rejection is to lull the recipient's immune system into a less active state. This can be done with powerful immunosuppressive drugs such as cyclosporine A, or by using laboratory-manufactured antibodies that attack mature T cells.

Bone Marrow Transplants

When the immune response is severely depressed—in infants born with immune disorders or in people with cancer, for example—one possible remedy is a transfer of healthy bone marrow. Once introduced into the circulation, transplanted bone marrow cells can develop into functioning B and T cells.

In bone marrow transplants, a close match is extremely important. Not only is there a danger that the body will reject the transplanted bone marrow cells, but mature T cells from the bone marrow transplant may counterattack and destroy the recipient's tissues. To prevent this situation, known as **graft-versus-host disease**, scientists use drugs or antibodies to "cleanse" the donor marrow of potentially dangerous mature T cells.

Glossary

adenoids—see tonsils.

allergen—any substance that causes an allergy.

antibody—a molecule (also called an immunoglobulin) produced by a mature B cell (plasma cell) in response to an antigen. When an antibody attaches to an antigen, it helps the body destroy or inactivate the antigen.

antigen—a substance or molecule that is recognized by the immune system. The antigen can be from foreign material such as bacteria or viruses.

antiserum—a serum rich in antibodies against a particular microbe.

appendix—lymphoid organ in the intestine.

artery—a blood vessel that carries blood from the heart to other parts of the body.

B cell or **B lymphocyte**—a small white blood cell crucial to the immune defenses. B cells come from bone marrow and develop into blood cells called plasma cells, which are the source of antibodies.

bacteria—microscopic organisms composed of a single cell. Some cause disease.

blood vessel—an artery, vein, or capillary that carries blood to and from the heart and body tissues.

cell—the smallest unit of life; the basic living unit that makes up tissues.

chemokine—a small protein molecule that activates immune cells, stimulates their migration, and helps direct immune cell traffic throughout the body.

clone—a group of genetically identical cells or organisms descended from a single common ancestor; or, to reproduce identical copies.

cytokines—powerful chemical substances secreted by cells that enable the body's cells to communicate with one another.

cytotoxic T lymphocyte (**CTL**)—a subtype of T cells that carries the CD8 marker and can destroy body cells infected by viruses or transformed by cancer.

dendritic cell—an immune cell with highly branched extensions that occurs in lymphoid tissues, engulfs microbes, and stimulates T cells by displaying the foreign antigens of the microbes on their surfaces.

enzyme—a protein produced by living cells that promotes the chemical processes of life without itself being altered.

epithelial cells—cells that make up the epithelium, the covering for internal and external body surfaces.

fungus—a member of a class of relatively primitive vegetable organisms. Fungi include mushrooms, yeasts, rusts, molds, and smuts.

gene—a unit of genetic material (DNA) inherited from a parent that controls specific characteristics. Genes carry coded directions a cell uses to make specific proteins that perform specific functions.

genome—a full set of genes in a person or any other living thing.

graft rejection—an immune response against transplanted tissue.

graft-versus-host disease—a life-threatening reaction in which transplanted cells attack the tissues of the recipient.

granule—a membrane-bound organelle (specialized part) within cells where proteins are stored before secretion.

growth factors—chemicals secreted by cells that stimulate proliferation of or changes in the physical properties of other cells.

helper T cells (Th cells)—a subset of T cells that carry the CD4 surface marker and are essential for turning on antibody production, activating cytotoxic T cells, and initiating many other immune functions.

hepatitis—the name of several viruses that cause liver diseases. These viruses include hepatitis A, hepatitis B, and hepatitis C.

histocompatibility testing—a test conducted before transplant operations to find a donor whose MHC molecules are similar to the recipient's; helps reduce the strength of transplant rejection.

human leukocyte antigen (HLA)—a protein on the surfaces of human cells that identifies the cells as "self" and, like MHC antigens, performs essential roles in immune responses. HLAs are used in laboratory tests to determine whether one person's tissues are compatible with another person's, and could be used in a transplant. HLAs are the human equivalent of MHC antigens; they are coded for by MHC genes.

immune response—reaction of the immune system to foreign substances. Although normal immune responses are designed to protect the body from pathogens, immune dysregulation can damage normal cells and tissues, as in the case of autoimmune diseases.

immunoglobulin—one of a family of large protein molecules, also known as antibodies, produced by mature B cells (plasma cells).

immunosuppressive—capable of reducing immune responses.

inflammation—an immune system reaction to "foreign" invaders such as microbes or allergens. Signs include redness, swelling, pain, or heat.

inflammatory response—redness, warmth, and swelling produced in response to infection; the result of increased blood flow and an influx of immune cells and their secretions.

innate—an immune system function that is inborn and provides an all-purpose defense against invasion by microbes.

interferon—a protein produced by cells that stimulates antivirus immune responses or alters the physical properties of immune cells.

lymph—a transparent, slightly yellow fluid that carries lymphocytes, bathes the body tissues, and drains into the lymphatic vessels.

lymph node—a small bean-shaped organ of the immune system, distributed widely throughout the body and linked by lymphatic vessels. Lymph nodes are garrisons of B and T cells, dendritic cells, macrophages, and other kinds of immune cells.

lymphatic vessels—a bodywide network of channels, similar to the blood vessels, which transports lymph to the immune organs and into the bloodstream.

lymphocyte—a small white blood cell produced in the lymphoid organs and essential to immune defenses. B cells, T cells, and NK T cells are lymphocytes.

lymphoid organ—an organ of the immune system where lymphocytes develop and congregate. These organs include the bone marrow, thymus, lymph nodes, spleen, and various other clusters of lymphoid tissue. Blood vessels and lymphatic vessels are also lymphoid organs.

macrophage—a large and versatile immune cell that devours invading pathogens and other intruders. Macrophages stimulate other immune cells by presenting them with small pieces of the invaders.

major histocompatibility complex (**MHC**)—a group of genes that controls several aspects of the immune response. MHC genes code for "self" markers on all body cells.

memory cells—a subset of T cells and B cells that have been exposed to antigens and can then respond more readily when the immune system encounters those same antigens again.

microbe or **microorganism**—a microscopic living organism. Examples include bacteria, protozoa, and some fungi and parasites. Viruses are also called microbes.

molecule—the smallest amount of a specific chemical substance. Large molecules such as proteins, fats, carbohydrates, and nucleic acids are the building blocks of a cell, and a gene determines how each molecule is produced.

monocyte—a large phagocytic white blood cell which, when entering tissue, develops into a macrophage.

natural killer (**NK**) **cell**—a large granule-containing lymphocyte that recognizes and kills cells lacking self antigens. These cells' target recognition molecules are different from T cells.

NK T cell—a T cell that has some characteristics of NK cells. It produces large amounts of cytokines when stimulated, and is activated by fatty substances (lipids) bound to non-MHC molecules called CD1d.

organ—a part of the body that has a specific function, such as the lungs.

parasite—a plant or animal that lives, grows, and feeds on or within another living organism.

passive immunity—immunity resulting from the transfer of antibodies or antiserum produced by another person.

pathogen—a disease-causing organism or virus.

phagocyte—a large white blood cell that contributes to immune defenses by ingesting microbes or other cells and foreign particles.

phagocytosis—process by which one cell engulfs another cell or large particle.

plasma cell—a large antibody-producing cell that develops from B cells.

platelet—a cellular fragment critical for blood clotting and sealing off wounds.

serum—the clear liquid that separates from the blood when it is allowed to clot. This fluid contains the antibodies that were present in the whole blood.

spleen—a lymphoid organ in the abdominal cavity that is an important center for immune system activities.

stem cell—an immature cell from which other cells derive. Bone marrow is rich in the kind of stem cells that become specialized blood cells.

T cell or **T lymphocyte**—a small white blood cell that recognizes antigen fragments bound to cell surfaces by specialized antibody-like receptors. "T" stands for the thymus gland, where T cells develop and acquire their receptors.

T cell receptor—complex protein molecule on the surfaces of T cells that recognizes bits of foreign antigen bound to self-MHC molecules.

tissue typing—see histocompatibility testing.

tissue—a group of similar cells joined to perform the same function.

tonsils and **adenoids**—prominent oval masses of lymphoid tissues on either side of the throat.

vaccine—a preparation that stimulates an immune response that can prevent an infection or create resistance to an infection. Vaccines do not cause disease.

vein—a blood vessel that carries blood to the heart from the body tissues.

virus—a particle composed of a piece of genetic material—RNA or DNA—surrounded by a protein coat. Viruses can reproduce only in living cells.

10.2

Overview of Adaptive Immunity

Cindy Gustafson-Brown

Antigen Presentation

There are two circumstances in which host cells present antigens on their surfaces.

1. Professional antigen presenting cells (APCs), including dendritic cells, macrophages, and B cells, engulf free-floating microorganisms or foreign molecules and digest them. In this case, the APC is on the attack, and the microbe is on defense. If all goes well, the APC is NOT infected. The foreign proteins are chopped up into small segments known as **peptides**. These peptides (exogenous antigens) are presented on the surface, together with MHC molecules.

   Antigens presented with **MHC Class II** are recognized by the T cell receptors of naïve **CD4 T cells**. In addition to the T cell receptor, these lymphocytes have another surface molecule known as CD4. It projects from the surface of the CD4 T cell and also binds to the MHC Class II. The interaction leads to activation of the CD4 T cell.

   Dendritic cells may also present antigens together with **MHC Class I** on the cell surface. In this case, the peptide is recognized by the T cell receptors of naïve **CD8 T cells.** In addition to the T cell receptor, these lymphocytes have another surface molecule known as CD8. It projects from the surface of the CD8 T cell and binds to the MHC Class I as well. The interaction leads to activation of the CD8 T cell.

2. A microbe infects a host cell. In this case, the microbe is on the attack, and the host cell is on the defense. The microbe begins replicating inside the host cell. The host cell communicates with the immune system by presenting pieces of all the proteins produced within (endogenous antigens, including foreign proteins) on its surface together with **MHC Class I.** In this context, foreign antigens presented with MHC Class I are recognized by the T cell receptors of activated **CD8 T cells,** also known as cytotoxic T lymphocytes (CTLs). CD8 also binds to the MHC Class I. The interaction leads the CTL to kill the infected cell.

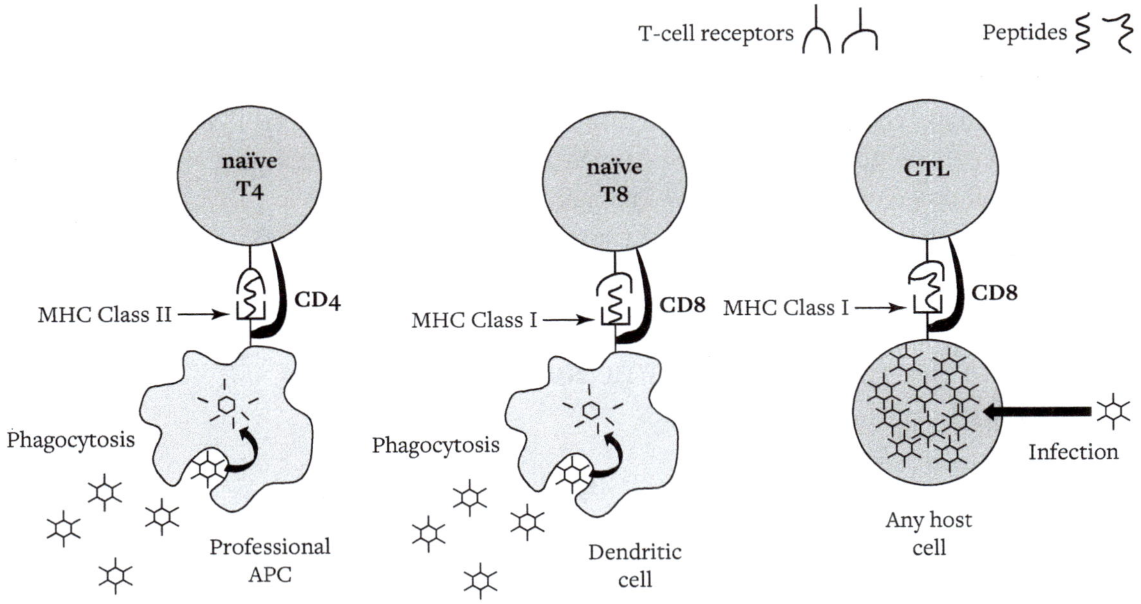

Antigen Presentation

Activation of Lymphocytes

Activation of CD4 T Cells (Helper T Cells)

1. The virus is engulfed and digested by the antigen presenting cell (APC), which may be a macrophage, dendritic cell, or B cell. This cell is NOT infected.
2. Pieces of the virus (antigen) are presented on the surface of the APC together with MHC Class II molecules.
3. A naïve CD4 T lymphocyte binds to the presented antigen via its T cell receptor(s).
4. Binding activates the CD4 T cell. It proliferates. Some of the progeny become effector CD4 T cells and begin secreting cytokines. Other progeny become long-lived memory CD4 T cells (not shown).

Activation of CD8 T Cells (Cytotoxic T Cells)

1. The virus is engulfed and digested by a dendritic cell. This cell is NOT infected.
2. Pieces of the virus (antigen) are presented on the surface of the dendritic cell together with MHC Class I molecules.
3. A naïve CD8 T lymphocyte binds to the presented antigen via its T cell receptor(s).
4. The binding of the antigen, together with cytokines from activated CD4 T cells, activates the CD8 T cell. It proliferates. Some of the progeny become cytotoxic T lymphocytes (CTLs) which subsequently kill infected host cells. Each CTL may kill many infected host cells over its lifetime. (HIV-infected host cells include CD4 T cells and macrophages.) Other progeny become long-lived memory CD8 T cells (not shown).

Activation of B Cells

1. The B lymphocyte binds to the extracellular virus (antigen) via its surface antibodies.
2. The binding of the antigen, together with cytokines from activated CD4 T cells, activates the B cell. It proliferates. Some of the progeny become plasma cells and begin secreting antibodies. Other progeny become long-lived memory B cells (not shown).
3. Antibodies in the blood and lymph (extracellular fluid) bind to a free-floating virus.
4. Macrophages engulf and digest the antibody-bound viruses.

Overview of the Adaptive Immune Response

Abbreviations

APC	antigen presenting cell
B	B lymphocyte
CTL	cytotoxic T lymphocyte (activated CD8 T cell)
MHC	major histocompatibility complex
MΦ	macrophage
TCR	T-cell receptor

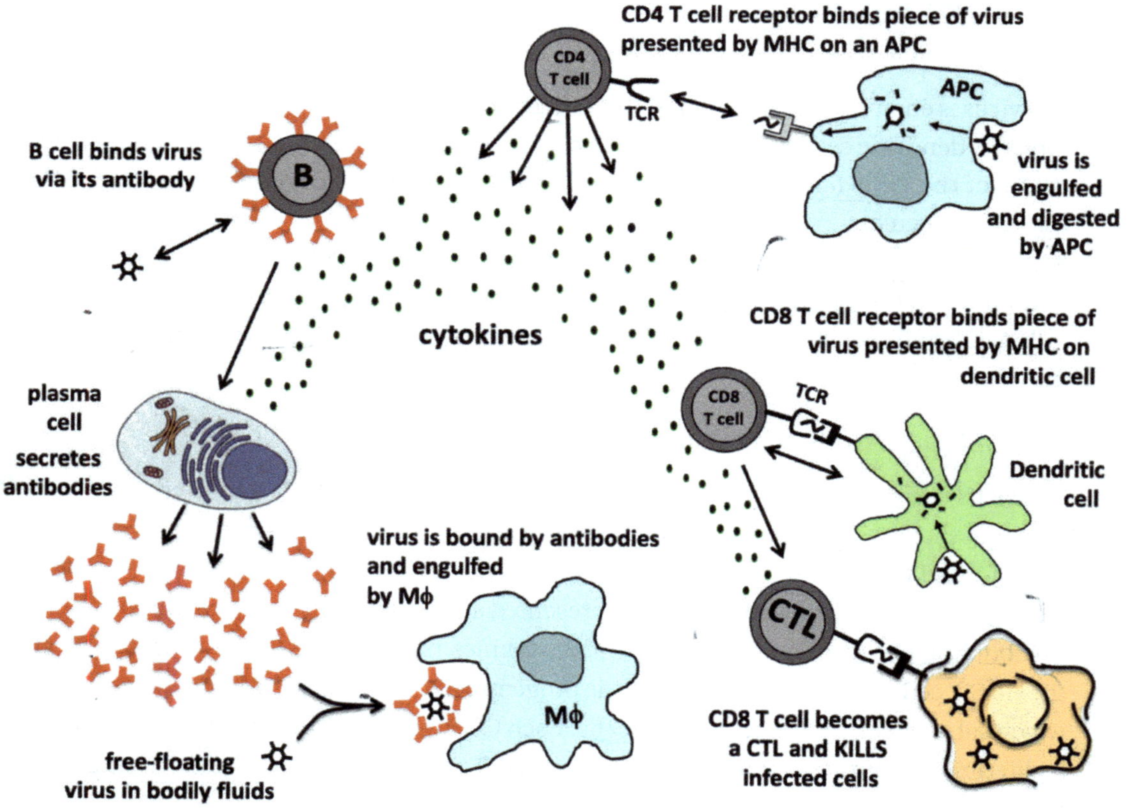

Section XI

Biology of HIV

11.1

A Primer on DNA, RNA, and Proteins

Cindy Gustafson-Brown

DNA (DEOXYRIBONUCLEIC ACID) IS AN INFORMATION-CONTAINING molecule found in the **nucleus** of a cell. It provides instructions to the cell in the form of blueprints for the construction of proteins. It is known as the **genetic material** because it is inherited, carrying biological information from one generation to the next.

In the nucleus of a single human cell are two sets of 23 pieces of DNA known as **chromosomes**. The entire set of chromosomes in a single cell is known as the **genome**. The DNA molecules which comprise the human genome are exceedingly long, totaling about six feet in length! DNA is made of subunits known as **nucleotides** linked together like beads on a string. Such molecules, composed of repeating subunits, are known as **polymers**. The longest human chromosome is nearly 250 million nucleotides in length, while the total length of one set of our 23 chromosomes is three billion nucleotides. For comparison, the single chromosome of the bacterium *E. coli* is 5 million nucleotides long.

There are four nucleotides, abbreviated A, G, T, and C. They are connected in various sequences, making up the **genetic code**. A DNA molecule is made of two such strands, which are aligned with one another based on the fact that certain nucleotides are attracted to each other. An A in one strand will bind to a T in the other. Likewise, a G in one strand will bind to a C in the other. We refer to these pairs of nucleotides as **complementary**. As a consequence of their specific pairing, the sequence in one strand will determine the sequence in the other (complementary) strand. The two strands twist around one another to form the iconic DNA double helix.

Within the genetic code are segments of information known as **genes**, just as a chapter is a cohesive section of information within the thousands of consecutive letters which comprise a book. Human cells harbor about 25,000 genes, and each gene contains a particular sequence of nucleotides, dictating how a corresponding protein will be constructed.

Proteins are also polymers—long molecules made of repeating subunits. However, proteins differ from DNA in two important ways. First, they are not nearly as long, typically hundreds or a few thousand subunits long. Second, the subunits are not nucleotides, but instead are **amino acids**. These are held together by linkages known as **peptide bonds**; therefore, proteins are often referred to as **polypeptides**. There are 20 different amino acids, whose order will determine the three dimensional shape of the resulting protein. The shape is *vital* to the function of the protein, as it will determine how the protein will behave.

Proteins, known as the "workhorses of the cell," serve in a variety of capacities. Some are structural, just as beams and girders support and give shape to a building. Structural proteins also may anchor a cell to its neighbors. Other proteins function as highways and vehicles, providing an intracellular transportation system. Some, including **hormones**, are sent out of the cell on expeditions, carrying signals near and far. Others sit on the cell surface and receive such signals, relaying information to a network of internal signaling proteins. There are also proteins on the surface which function as identification tags, so cells may recognize one another. Within the cell's plasma membrane are proteins which provide portals through which cargo is moved in and out of the cell. Finally, a large proportion of proteins are **enzymes**. These catalyze all the thousands of biochemical reactions which occur in a cell every day. Collectively these comprise the "cellular machinery."

A gene functions as a blueprint for a protein because the nucleotide sequence of the gene is used to determine the amino acid sequence of the corresponding (encoded) protein. However, physically the blueprint remains permanently in the cell nucleus, while proteins are constructed outside the nucleus in the region known as the **cytoplasm**. How does the cell get the information from the blueprint in the nucleus out to the construction site in the cytoplasm? It does what any contractor does: It makes a copy of the blueprint. That copy is in the form of a related molecule—RNA (ribonucleic acid).

Like DNA, RNA is a polymer which carries information encoded in the sequence of nucleotides. Both DNA and RNA are called **nucleic acids**; however, RNA differs from DNA in important ways. First, it is a single strand, not double like DNA. Second, instead of the nucleotide T, it carries a substitute, abbreviated U. Finally, each molecule of RNA is only the length of a single gene. When the cell needs to synthesize a particular protein, it activates, or expresses, the corresponding gene within the DNA. The sequence of nucleotides within the gene is copied, creating a matching sequence of nucleotides in a new molecule of RNA. The copying of information from DNA into RNA is known as **transcription**. In common parlance, transcription refers to the copying of information from one form (verbal) to another (written) in the same language. In the same way, molecular transcription is the copying of information from one form (DNA) to another (RNA) in the same language (nucleotides).

The new RNA travels out of the nucleus into the cytoplasm, carrying the information. For this reason, it is known as **messenger RNA** (mRNA). When the RNA reaches the cytoplasm, the blueprint can be "read" to create a protein in a process known as **translation**. In translation, information in one language (a sequence of nucleotides) is interpreted into another language (a sequence of amino acids). The genetic code is read in "words," known as **triplet codons**, consisting of three nucleotides. Each group of three nucleotides corresponds to one particular amino acid. As the RNA sequence is decoded, codon by codon, a new protein is assembled, amino acid by amino acid. In this way, the directions contained within the gene in the nucleus are faithfully followed to produce a protein with a very particular amino acid sequence in the cytoplasm.

The Central Dogma of Biology

DNA —transcription→ **RNA** —translation→ **Protein**

The flow of information from DNA to RNA to protein is key to understanding genetics and molecular biology. This concept is known as the **central dogma of biology**.

11.2

The Biology of HIV

Cindy Gustafson-Brown

Introduction to Virology

As the most abundant organisms on Earth, viruses are incredibly diverse. They have evolved to exploit every possible host, infecting bacteria, archaea, protozoa, algae, fungi, plants, and animals. The term **virus** is derived from the Latin word for poison. Although we commonly think of viruses as **pathogens** (disease-causing microorganisms), in fact, most viruses do not cause disease.

Are viruses alive? They straddle the boundary between the living and non-living world. They are infectious, spreading from host to host, sometimes causing disease. They evolve over time. However, they have been described as living a "borrowed life" (van Regenmortel & Mahy, 2004, p. 8) because they do not share the characteristics which we typically associate with "living" organisms.

- Viruses are the only organisms which are not made of cells. Instead, they resemble molecular machines, inert assemblages of chemicals apart from a cellular host.
- Viruses do not grow or divide like cells do. They cannot reproduce independently from cells. Instead, their parts are manufactured and assembled inside a cell much like cars on an assembly line. Their life cycle involves disintegration upon entering a cell and subsequent reconstitution from newly minted parts.
- They cannot "live" apart from a cellular host. They have no intrinsic source of energy. They cannot synthesize biological building blocks or macromolecules. They must cannibalize a host cell to acquire these resources and complete their life cycle.
- They are much smaller than cells. HIV is an average size virus at about 0.1 microns (μ). It would take 250,000 HIV particles to span one inch. A bacterial cell is about 20 times larger, and a human white blood cell is 100 times larger. Although cells are visible with a light microscope, viruses are not. They must be viewed with an electron microscope, which provides greater resolution of the tiniest specimens.

Due to their size and lifestyle, viruses are described as **submicroscopic, obligate intracellular parasites**.

Viral Structure

Viruses come in many shapes and sizes. They may look like rigid rods, flexible filaments, geodesic domes, amorphous blobs, or lunar landers. An intact virus is often referred to as a **virus particle.** If the virus particle is infectious, it is called a **virion.** Not all virus particles are virions; in fact in some cases, an infection may produce more defective particles than infectious ones.

All viruses are composed of similar components:

a) Genetic material	This is the viral **genome**. It is nucleic acid, either DNA or RNA. It may be single stranded or double stranded. It is often complexed with viral proteins.
b) Protein capsid	This is the protective coat surrounding the nucleic acid. It is a symmetrical shell made of many copies of one or a few proteins. The simple, geometric design of many viral capsids facilitates their spontaneous self-assembly. The capsid protects the genetic material from damage in the environment: chemicals, enzymes, mechanical forces, or UV light.
c) Lipid envelope	A lipid (fatty) envelope may surround the capsid. It is a phospholipid bilayer studded with membrane proteins. The virus steals the envelope from a cellular membrane. This is **optional**; not all viruses have an envelope. Those without one are known as **naked** viruses.

Some viruses have more elaborate structures, but this is the minimal composition of a virus.

Viral Life Cycle

All viral life cycles share some common features. They reproduce by entering and hijacking a cell, commandeering its internal machinery and transforming it into a virus factory.

a) Adsorption	The virus binds to the surface of the target cell. This attachment is a specific interaction mediated by viral proteins which bind to proteins or carbohydrates (sugars) on the surface of the cell, known as **viral receptors**.
b) Penetration	The virus penetrates the cell surface, entering the cytoplasm.
c) Uncoating	The virus capsid releases its nucleic acid into the cell. This step *may* be concomitant with penetration.
d) Viral gene expression and synthesis of viral proteins	Regulatory proteins are synthesized during the early phase and structural proteins during the late phase of the life cycle.
e) Replication of the viral genome	
f) Assembly of **progeny** viruses	Offspring, the next generation.
g) Release of progeny viruses	Thousands of new viruses may be released. Sometimes assembly and release are one continuous process.

In the first step, the receptor to which a virus prefers to bind determines its **tropism**—its preference for infecting certain cell types or tissues. This also explains why some viruses are host-specific, meaning they only infect one species. Usually this is because the virus binds a particular viral receptor found only on the cells of that species. Other viruses are more promiscuous; they may be transmitted among members of several species, due to their ability to bind receptors found in them all.

At the end of the cycle, viral infections may or may not result in the death of the host cell. If the release of progeny viruses involves the **lysis** (bursting) of the cell, it is termed a **lytic** infection. However, many enveloped viruses are able to release their progeny from host cells without rupturing the cell's outer membrane (**plasma membrane**). In some of these cases, internal damage caused by the infection itself will eventually kill the cell. But in other cases the cell may survive for a time, all the while producing and releasing viruses.

Some viruses persist inside infected cells for long periods of time—months or years. Such a virus may alternate between active and dormant states. When **active**, the viral genes are expressed, and progeny are released, often without killing the host cell. Alternatively, persistent viruses may remain dormant, their genes silent, in a condition known as **latency**. Certain stimuli may cause latent viruses to "wake up" and return to an active state in a process known as **reactivation.**

Human Immunodeficiency Virus

HIV is a type of virus known as a **retrovirus**. All retroviruses are RNA viruses (but not all RNA viruses are retroviruses). The genetic material inside the capsid is single-stranded RNA. Retroviruses are the only viruses that are **diploid**, meaning there are two copies of the genomic RNA strand. Once a retrovirus enters a cell, the RNA is copied into DNA by a unique enzyme known as **reverse transcriptase**. The term "retro" virus reflects a reversal of the central dogma of biology (DNA → RNA).

HIV Genome

The HIV genome is single-stranded RNA, 9,749 nucleotides in length, which is tiny compared to a human, or even bacterial, genome. It has the same "sense," or sequence as the viral messenger RNA (mRNA). In fact, it resembles a normal cellular mRNA in the special features at its ends. The "upstream" end, where translation of the nucleotide sequence begins, is known as the 5 prime (5′) end and has a structure known as a "5 prime cap." The "downstream" end is known as the 3 prime (3′) end. It concludes with a string of "A" nucleotides, known as a poly-A tail.

Also at both ends of the genome is a repeated sequence (R) of 150–200 nucleotides. Additionally, there are sequences at either end known as the U5 and U3 sequences, for "unique 5′ sequence" and "unique 3′ sequence," respectively.

Map of the HIV Genome

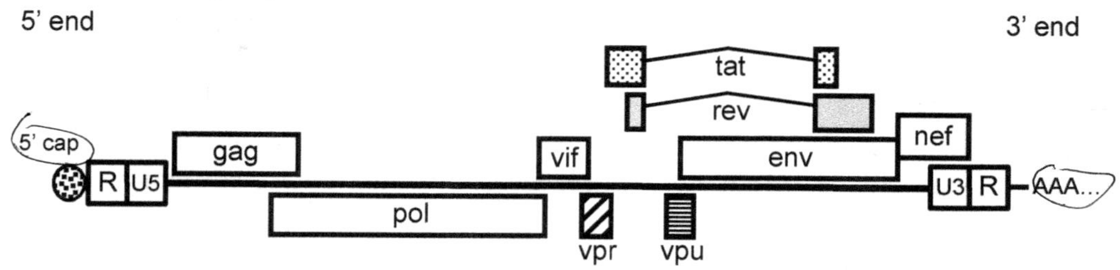

The genome harbors nine genes. Three are common to all retroviruses:

- ***gag***
  group specific **a**nti**g**en
  encoding matrix (MA, p17), capsid (CA, p24), and nucleocapsid (NC, p7) proteins
- ***pol***
  polymerase
  encoding the viral enzymes
  protease (PR), reverse transcriptase (RT), and integrase (IN)
- ***env***
  envelope
  encoding the envelope proteins, gp41 and gp120

Note that each of these genes encodes more than one protein product.

Maps of *gag, pol, and env* genes

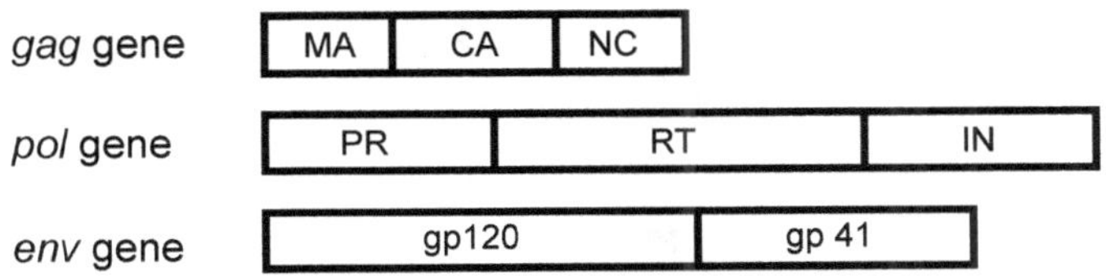

> *Tip concerning naming of proteins: HIV proteins are designated by p (protein) or gp (glycoprotein), followed by their molecular weight in kilodaltons.*

In addition, HIV has six other unique genes encoding regulatory proteins:

- ***tat***—**t**rans**a**ctivator of **t**ranscription
- ***rev***—**r**egulator of **e**xpression of **v**irion proteins
- ***vif***—**v**iral **i**nfectivity **f**actor
- ***vpr***—**v**irion **p**rotein **R**
- ***vpu***—**v**irion **p**rotein **u**nique to HIV-1
- ***nef***—**n**egative **ef**fector

Structure of HIV

HIV contains two single-stranded copies of the RNA genome. The RNA is bound to many copies of the **nucleocapsid** protein (p7), which protects and stabilizes the nucleic acid. Also attached to the genome are the viral enzymes **reverse transcriptase** and **integrase**. The surrounding, conical-shaped capsid is composed of about 1500 copies of **capsid** protein (p24). The capsid and its contents are known as the viral **core**. Other accessory proteins are packaged inside the virus as well, including **protease**.

The core, in turn, is enclosed in a spherical, lipid **envelope**, undergirded by a layer of **matrix** protein (p17). Protruding from the envelope are the viral **spikes**. Each spike is a trimer, containing three copies of the transmembrane protein **gp41** and three copies of the surface protein **gp120**. gp41 anchors gp120 to the membrane. Both are glycoproteins, meaning they are proteins that are highly glycosylated, or covered in sugar. In fact, half of the mass of gp120 is made up of sugar chains, which form a protective cloak masking the surface of the virus, effectively hiding it from attack by antibodies.

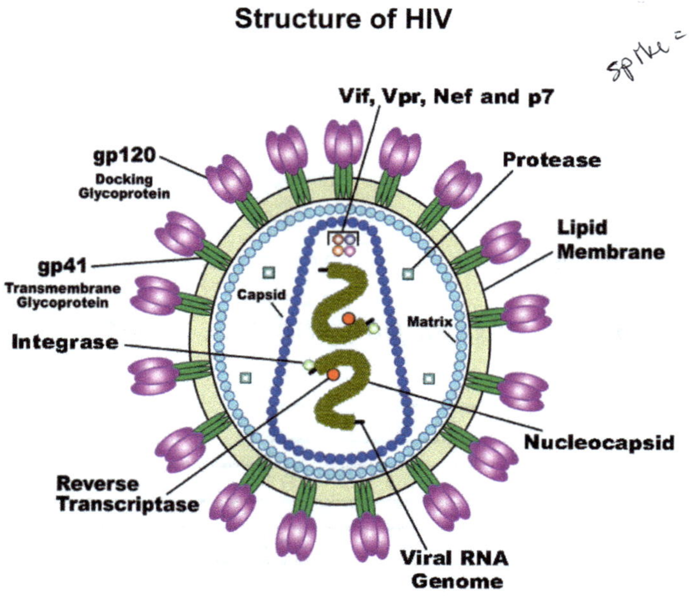

(U.S. National Institutes of Health)

Life Cycle of HIV

It takes approximately two days for HIV to complete its life cycle. The series of steps is similar to that described for all viruses with some modifications.

Adsorption—The gp120 protein on HIV is responsible for binding to target cells. It first binds to the viral receptor, the cell surface protein CD4. This protein is found on two types of white blood cells, which are primary targets for HIV, macrophages, and (helper) CD4 T cells. (Note that when HIV binds to T cells, the viral receptor is CD4, *not* the T cell receptor.) Upon binding to CD4, gp120 undergoes a structural change and then must bind a second viral receptor, or **coreceptor**, on the cell. Two chemokine receptors[1] are commonly co-opted by HIV for use as coreceptors, and particular strains of HIV have a preference for one or the other. When HIV is sexually transmitted to a new host, it is usually an **R5 strain**. Such strains have a preference for the coreceptor CCR5 found

1 Note the different uses of the term "receptor." A **viral receptor** is any protein on the surface of a cell which is bound by a virus, regardless of its usual function. A **chemokine receptor** is a surface protein on white blood cells which normally binds to chemokines (signaling molecules) and relays the signal to the interior of the cell. A **T cell receptor** is an antigen-binding protein on the surface of T cells.

on macrophages and memory CD4 T cells. Over time the virus will mutate, eventually evolving into a more lethal **X4 strain**, with a preference for the coreceptor CXCR4 found on naïve CD4 T cells. X4 strains lead to the rapid decline of the immune system.

Years ago it was observed that some people were repeatedly exposed to HIV without becoming infected. Studies of such cases led to the discovery that some of these subjects harbor a mutation in the gene encoding the CCR5 protein. Those with one mutant and one normal version of the gene (heterozygous) have a reduced amount of CCR5 on their cells and have a decreased risk of HIV infection. If they become infected, they progress more slowly to AIDS. Those with two mutant versions of the CCR5 gene (homozygous mutant) have no CCR5 protein on their cells and are almost never infected with HIV sexually. One percent of Caucasians are homozygous for this mutation and 18% are heterozygous.

Penetration and uncoating—Penetration of HIV into a target cell is dependent upon membrane **fusion**. Once gp120 has bound to CD4 and a coreceptor, it peels back to reveal gp41 beneath it. Subsequently gp41 springs out like a harpoon toward the host cell, embedding its distal end in the plasma membrane. Now the gp41 protein bridges the virus and the cell with one end traversing the viral envelope and the other penetrating the cell membrane. This unstable configuration collapses, as the protein folds in half, pulling the two membranes into close proximity. When they touch the lipids flow into one another and the membranes fuse. The involvement of several viral spikes leads to the formation of a **fusion pore** through which the viral core passes into the cytoplasm of the cell. The capsid is shed, releasing the genomic RNA and associated proteins. The viral envelope, together with the spikes, remains behind—now a contiguous part of the plasma membrane.

Recently, scientists have observed evidence that prior to fusion, HIV may be taken into the cell by a process known as **endocytosis.** During endocytosis, the plasma membrane invaginates, forming a pocket on the cell surface. As it moves farther inward, a membrane-enclosed compartment (vesicle) buds into the cytoplasm like a bubble within a bubble. External particles, including viruses bound to the membrane, may be carried within the vesicle into the cell. If HIV enters by endocytosis, fusion occurs between the viral envelope and the vesicle membrane, releasing the capsid into the cytoplasm (Miyauchi et al., 2009, pp. 433–444).

Synthesis and integration of viral DNA—Reverse transcriptase (RT), a large and multifaceted enzyme, makes a DNA copy (**cDNA**) of the RNA genome. This requires that the one protein carry out three different enzymatic activities:

- RNA-dependent DNA polymerase
  RT copies a single RNA strand into a complementary DNA strand, resulting in an RNA/DNA hybrid.
- RNase H enzyme
  RT degrades the RNA strand from the RNA/DNA hybrid.
- DNA-dependent DNA polymerase
  RT copies the single DNA strand into a complementary DNA strand, resulting in a double-stranded DNA.

When RT produces the cDNA it copies some extra material from one end of the genome onto the other and vice versa. This creates a longer region which is repeated at each end, known as the **long terminal repeat**, or **LTR**.

Once the cDNA copy is complete, it is bound by cellular and viral proteins (including integrase), forming the circular, **pre-integration complex** (**PIC**). The PIC migrates through a nuclear pore into the cell nucleus.

Inside the nucleus, the accompanying enzyme integrase mediates the integration of the viral DNA into a host-cell chromosome in three steps.

- It cuts one host chromosome at a *random* location.
- It inserts the viral DNA.
- It seals one of the two strands at each end of the inserted DNA.

Cellular DNA repair mechanisms will spontaneously splice the remaining strand at each end, so the viral DNA is fully incorporated into the chromosome. Once integrated, the viral DNA is known as a **provirus.** In recently infected individuals, up to 1% of the CD4 T cells harbor a provirus.

Comparison of HIV genomic RNA and HIV provirus

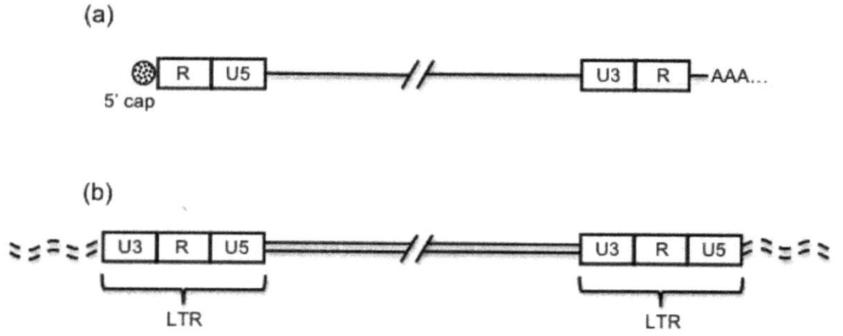

(a) HIV genomic RNA, (b) HIV provirus integrated into a host chromosome

Where in the host genome can the provirus be integrated? In each cell, only a subset of genes is actively expressed at one time. Those which are not transcriptionally active, are tightly folded and therefore inaccessible. As a consequence the HIV provirus can only be inserted into an active (unfolded) chromosomal region. But among these regions, the location is random.

The integration of viral DNA into the genome of an infected cell is *irreversible*. Once established, the provirus is permanent, will be replicated along with the cellular DNA, and is passed down to all future generations of that cell.

On rare occasions the integration of the provirus may damage a critical cellular gene, resulting in cell death. Another infrequent but possible outcome is that the provirus may integrate adjacent to a gene normally involved in cell division. If the viral DNA causes the aberrant regulation of its neighbor, then the cell might be driven to proliferate excessively and become cancerous. (Most HIV-associated cancers do not arise in this way.)

Summary of the HIV-1 replication cycle

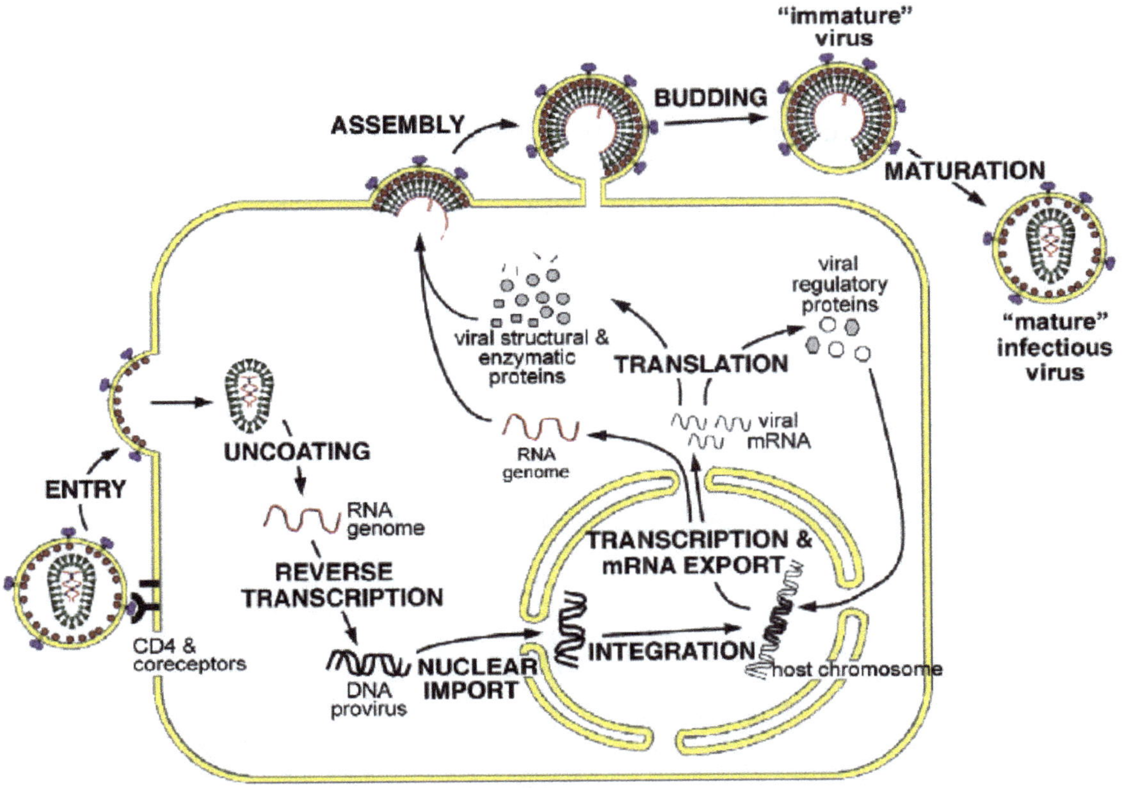

Ganser-Pornillos, et al, 2008 Current Opinion in Structural Biology, 18:203–217

Expression of HIV Genes—Not all the HIV genes are expressed at once. There are phases during which early genes and then late genes are activated. The first genes to be expressed are regulatory, controlling the unfolding sequence of events. Only later do the genes encoding enzymes and structural proteins become active.

During viral gene expression, nearly the entire length of the HIV provirus is transcribed into one long piece of RNA. This RNA may undergo a splicing process which trims it into smaller pieces. In fact, alternative splicing events result in over 25 variations of viral RNA. When these RNAs leave the nucleus, they are used in the cytoplasm for the translation of different viral proteins. In addition, full-length HIV RNA, arriving in the cytoplasm, may either be translated to produce Gag and Pol proteins or packaged in its entirety into a newly forming capsid. In other words, full-length viral RNA may be used as mRNA (translated) or as genomic RNA (packaged).

Because some HIV genes encode more than one protein, translation of some viral mRNAs results in extra long strings of amino acids spanning the length of two or three different proteins. Initially, these consecutive proteins are linked together and are known as **polyproteins**. For example, expression of *gag* results in a matrix-capsid-nucleocapsid polyprotein, which is needed in large amounts when the production of viral progeny kicks into high gear. The *pol* gene is not expressed as abundantly as *gag*; new viruses require only a few copies of the enzymes but hundreds of the structural proteins. When the occasional Pol proteins are synthesized, they always tag along with Gag, resulting in an even larger MA-CA-NC-PR-RT-IN polyprotein!

Assembly and release of progeny viruses—At this point, the cell has produced two of the three components necessary to build a new virus: the genetic material and the proteins. Transcription provides the new genomes. Translation of the mRNA generates the proteins (enzymes and structural proteins). These make their way to the cell surface where the assembly of progeny commences just beneath the plasma membrane.

Gag polyprotein and virus assembly

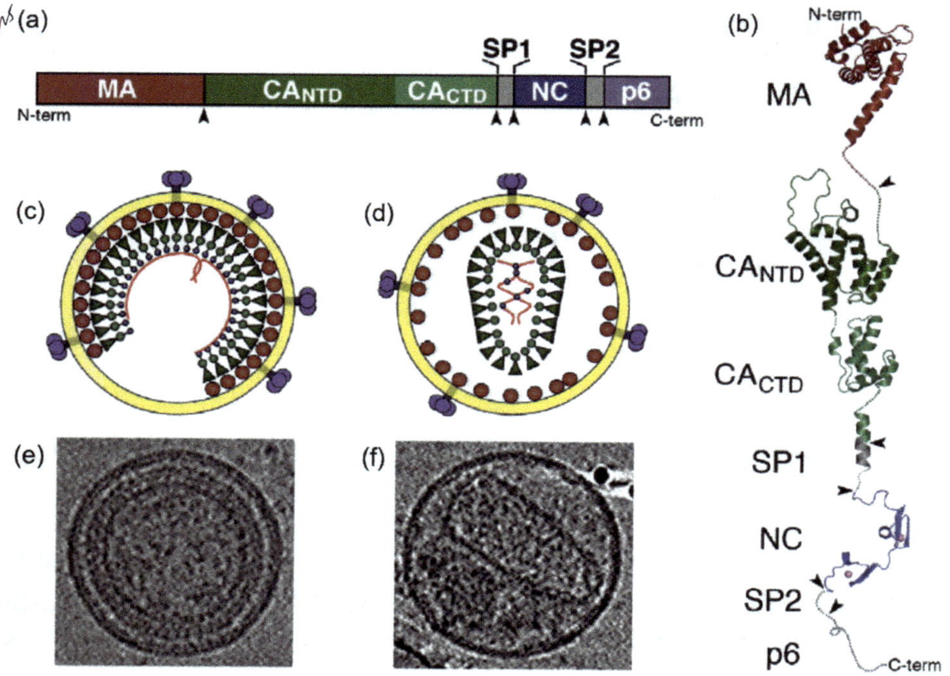

(a) HIV-1 Gag polyprotein domain structure, showing the locations of MA, CA_{NTD}, CA_{CTD}, SP1, NC, SP2, and p6. (b) Structural model of the extended Gag polypeptide, derived from high-resolution structures and models of isolated domains. Unstructured and linker regions are represented by dashed lines. PR cleavage sites are indicated by the arrowheads in (a) and (b). Schematic models of the immature (c) and mature (d) HIV-1 virions. Central slices through tomograms of immature (e) and mature (f) HIV-1 particles derived by electron cryotomography. The spherical virions are approximately 130 nm in diameter. Abbreviations: MA = matrix, CA = capsid, NTD = N terminal domain, CTD = C terminal domain, NC = nucleocapsid, SP1 = spacer peptide 1, SP2 = spacer peptide 2. *Ganser-Pornillos, et al, 2008 Current Opinion in Structural Biology, 18:203–217*

Steps in the HIV replication cycle

1. Adsorption
   a. binding of gp120 to CD4
   b. binding of gp120 to CCR5 or CXCR4

2. Penetration
   a. possible endocytosis
   b. membrane fusion (mediated by gp41)

3. Uncoating

   Capsid opens, spilling out RNA and enzymes

4. Reverse transcription and integration

   a. viral ssRNA → viral dsDNA (reverse transcriptase)

   (reverses the Central Dogma)

   b. viral DNA and integrase **migrate** into nucleus

   c. viral DNA is **integrated** into a host chromosome

5. Expression of HIV genes

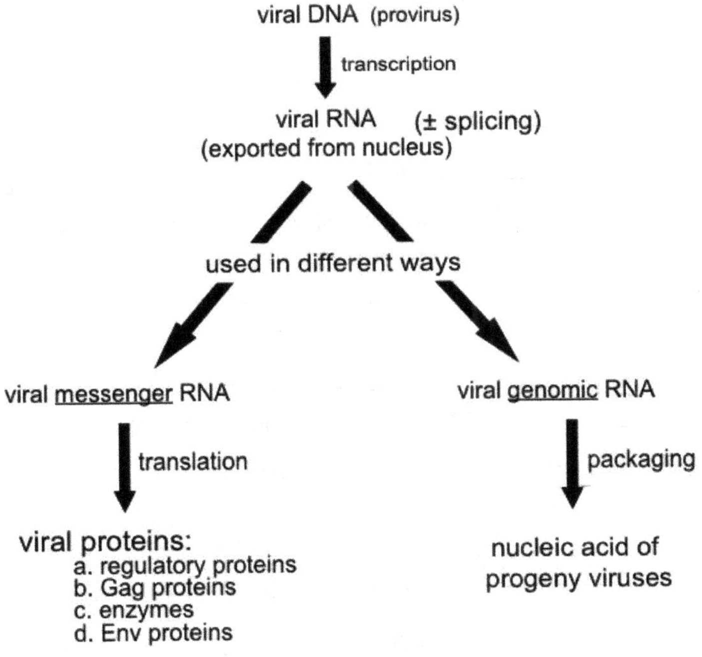

6. Assembly and release

   at the cell surface

7. Maturation

   HIV protease cleaves polyproteins

How do viruses get the final component—the lipid envelope? They swipe it from the plasma membrane. Remember that a viral envelope is not only lipid; it also contains proteins. HIV encodes two proteins that are integral to the envelope: gp41 and gp120. These are initially synthesized as a single polypeptide, which is cleaved by a cellular enzyme. (Enzymes that cut proteins are known as **proteases**.) Immediately following synthesis and cleavage, gp41 and gp120 are trafficked to the plasma membrane where they congregate in patches and attract the other viral components to join them.

Once all the parts are in place at the plasma membrane, they associate with each other in a way that draws the viral assembly into a spherical structure, pulling the membrane around it like saran wrap. Once the new virus has formed completely, the thin tube of membrane still connecting it to the cell pinches off, releasing the nascent HIV. This is known as **budding**.

Maturation—When the progeny are initially released from the cell, they are immature and not infectious. This is because their Gag and Pol proteins are still attached to each other. Maturation requires that these proteins be released, but how? The virus carries an enzyme that functions like molecular scissors—the HIV **protease**. Even while it is still part of a polyprotein itself, the protease can commence its work cutting apart the Gag and Pol components. The cleavage may begin as the virus is in the process of budding, and once it is complete, the initially spherical capsid is remodeled, taking on the conical shape characteristic of a mature virion. The progeny are ready to infect the next cell and start the cycle again!

Functions of HIV Accessory Proteins

- **Tat** up-regulates transcription of HIV genes.
- **Rev** regulates the splicing and nuclear export of HIV transcripts. The export of variably spliced HIV mRNAs from the nucleus to be translated into the cytoplasm determines whether early (Tat, Rev, Nef) or late (Vif, Vpr, Vpu, Gag, Pol, Env) gene products are synthesized. High levels of Rev promote the synthesis of late gene products.
- **Nef** causes internalization and destruction of CD4 from the surface of the infected cell. Nef also inhibits expression of MHC class I on the surface of the infected cell.
- **Vpu** causes the destruction of CD4 as it is synthesized in the host cell. Vpu also enhances the release of progeny virions from infected cells by down-regulating a protein called BST-2, or tetherin, from the cell surface. BST-2 is a cellular defense protein which tethers the emerging virions to the cell surface, preventing them from escaping to infect neighboring cells.
- **Vif** degrades another cellular defense protein, APOBEC3G, which would otherwise enter progeny viruses during budding and irreparably mutate their genomes.
- **Vpr** promotes nuclear import of the HIV pre-integration complex from the cytoplasm. It also promotes transcription of HIV genes. Furthermore, Vpr regulates cell cycle progression and apoptosis.

The Rapid Mutation Rate of HIV

Reverse transcriptase is an error-prone enzyme, which cannot proofread its handiwork like the cellular DNA polymerase that normally copies our chromosomes. It is so sloppy in fact that it incorporates one or more errors into every new HIV strand. These errors in DNA sequence are known as mutations. As a consequence, each generation of HIV progeny is mutant compared to its parent. The rapid pace of mutation exceeds that of any other known organism and quickly produces a large collection of genetic variants, known as **quasispecies**, within the body of a single host. Strikingly, the genetic diversity of HIV produced in a single human patient is greater than the total global diversity of influenza virus during any flu season.

How do the mutations alter the virus form and function? Each protein is encoded by a gene and, therefore, may change shape if the gene mutates. When the nucleotide sequence of the gene changes, this may alter the sequence of amino acids in the encoded protein. In some cases, the mutation will cause the protein to fold up differently, taking on a new shape. If the mutation affects a structural protein, it may modify the form of the virus. A mutation in an enzyme or regulatory protein may alter the activity of the protein or completely disable it, rendering the protein nonfunctional.

As reverse transcriptase synthesizes the viral DNA, it introduces mutations randomly at locations throughout the sequence. Any HIV gene may be affected with three possible outcomes. A silent mutation is a change in the nucleotide sequence which has no effect at all on the encoded protein. On the other hand, many of the errors do change the amino acid sequence of the protein. In most cases this is detrimental, rendering the progeny defective. However, HIV is incredibly prolific, generating several billion progeny each day in an infected patient, so even if most of them are defective, there are plenty of functional virions remaining. Because of the enormous numbers of progeny, the mutation rate is a net benefit; some of the random mistakes provide the virus a significant advantage in adapting to the obstacles it will face. Mutant strains become specialized for the infection of certain cell types or adapted to thrive in particular compartments of the body (e.g., lymph nodes or the brain). (Remember that tropism is the preference of a virus to infect specific cells or tissues.) Mutations affect the replication rate and transmissibility of populations of viruses in the body and the ways in which viruses kill cells—increasingly virulent and infectious strains often arise after several years. The ramifications for the human host are severe. The virus may be able to evade immune attack, the protective effect of vaccines, and the risk of antiviral medications.

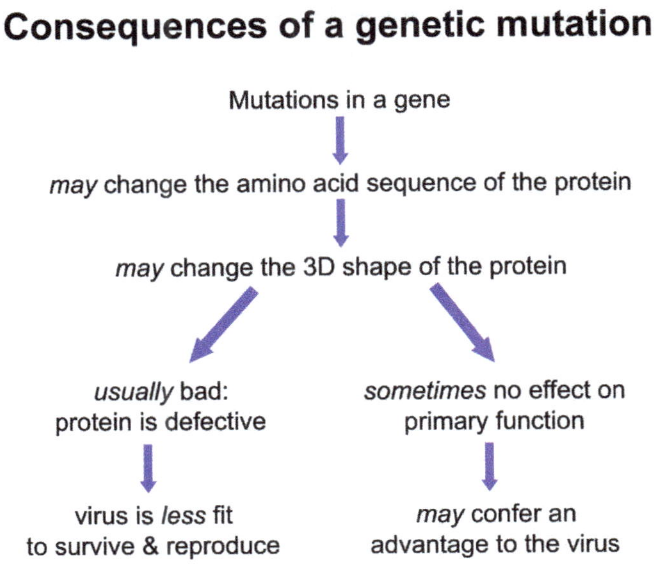

The HIV gp120 *protein* is the primary target of the **humoral immune response**, but the gp120 *gene* repeatedly mutates, resulting in a surface protein which disguises itself over and over. As each new version of gp120

takes its place on the envelope of viral progeny, it becomes unrecognizable to pre-existing antibodies, and the immune system must start over, as if it has met a new invader. This creates an enormous challenge for the immune system, which eventually is not able to keep up an effective response. Similar problems face the **cellular immune response**, which recognizes several different HIV proteins. These also mutate, although not as rapidly as gp120.

Moreover, it complicates the production of an effective **vaccine**. Immunizations provide the immune system a "sneak preview" of a pathogen based on the shapes of its proteins. As the virus evolves new strains arise that "look" different to the immune system compared to the virus contained in the vaccine. Consequently, the vaccine will not be protective against strains that have significantly mutated.

Another threat which the virus may face is **antiretroviral medications.** These drugs attack the virus at several points in its life cycle, usually binding to a viral protein and disabling its normal function. Random mutations may occur in the genes encoding the viral proteins, changing their amino acid sequence and, therefore, their shape. As a result, the target is no longer recognized or bound by the drug. When this occurs, the virus becomes **resistant** to the drug.

Reference

Miyauchi, K., Kim, Y., Latinovic, O., Morozov, V., & Melikyan, G. (2009). HIV enters cells via endocytosis and dynamin-dependent fusion with endosomes. *Cell, 137*, 433–444.

van Regenmortel, M., & Mahy, B. (2004). Emerging issues in virus taxonomy. *Emerg Infect Dis.* 10(1): 8–13.

Credit

Fig. 11.2c: Source: U.S. National Institutes of Health.

Fig. 11.2e: Barbie K. Ganser-Pornillos, Mark Yeager, and Wesley Sundquist, "Summary of the HIV-1 Replication cycle," *Current Opinion in Structural Biology*, vol. 18, no. 2. Copyright © 2008 by Elsevier B.V. Reprinted with permission.

Fig. 11.2f: Barbie K. Ganser-Pornillos, Mark Yeager, and Wesley Sundquist, "Gag polyprotein and virus assembly," *Current Opinion in Structural Biology*, vol. 18, no. 2. Copyright © 2008 by Elsevier B.V. Reprinted with permission.

Section XII

Testing

12.1

HIV Testing in the United States

Kaiser Family Foundation

Key Facts

- HIV testing is integral to HIV prevention, treatment, and care. Knowledge of one's HIV status is important for preventing the spread of disease, yet 15% of people with HIV do not know they are infected. Studies show that those who learn they are HIV positive modify their behavior to reduce the risk of HIV[1,2,3]
- Overall about half (46%) of nonelderly adults in the United States (U.S.) have ever been tested for HIV, including 8% in the last year. The Centers for Disease Control and Prevention (CDC) recommends routine HIV screening in health-care settings for all adults, aged 13–64, and repeat screening for those at higher risk.
- Early knowledge of HIV status is critical for linkage to medical care and treatment that can reduce morbidity and mortality and improve quality of life.[4] Treatment guidelines recommend starting antiretroviral treatment as soon as one is diagnosed with HIV.[5] Individuals with HIV who have an undetectable viral load, typically as a result of effective antiretroviral therapy, cannot sexually transmit HIV to others.[6]
- Most people with health insurance—both public and private—have access to HIV testing, often at no cost. And, for those without insurance, HIV testing can often be obtained at little or no cost in community settings.

KEY DATES in the History of HIV Testing[7]

1981: First AIDS case reported

1984: Human immunodeficiency Virus (HIV) identified

1985: First test for HIV licensed (ELISA)

1987: First Western Blot blood test kit

1992: First rapid test

1994: First oral fluid test

1996: First home and urine tests

2002: First rapid test using finger prick

2003: Rapid finger prick test granted CLIA (Clinical Laboratory Improvement Amendments) waiver

2004: First rapid oral fluid test (also granted CLIA waiver)

2006: CDC recommends routine HIV screening in U.S. health care settings[8]

2007: CDC launches Expanded HIV Testing Initiative in U.S.

2007: WHO/UNAIDS global guidelines recommend routine HIV screening in health care settings[9]

2010: First test approved that detects both antigen and antibodies[10]

2012: First rapid oral fluid home test[11]

2013: USPSTF gives routine HIV screening an "A" rating[12]

2013: First rapid test approved that detects both antigen and antibodies, and distinguishes between acute and established HIV-1 infection[13]

2015: Centers for Medicare and Medicaid Services announces Medicare coverage of annual HIV screening for all beneficiaries 15–65, and for those older and younger beneficiaries at "increased risk" for HIV[14]

2019: USPSTF reaffirms its "A" rating for HIV screening

Testing Statistics

- Among the more than 1.1 million people with HIV in the U.S., an estimated 15% do not know they are infected and this share accounts for nearly 40% of new transmissions.[15, 16] Studies show that those who learn they are HIV positive modify their behavior to reduce the risk of HIV transmission.[17]
- Through earlier detection, raising awareness of HIV status, and linkage to care and treatment, testing could play an important role in addressing the U.S. epidemic.
- According to the CDC's Behavioral Risk Factor Surveillance System (BRFSS) about half (46%) of U.S. adults, aged 18–64, reported ever having been tested for HIV, including 8% who reported being tested in the last year (see Figure 12.1.1).

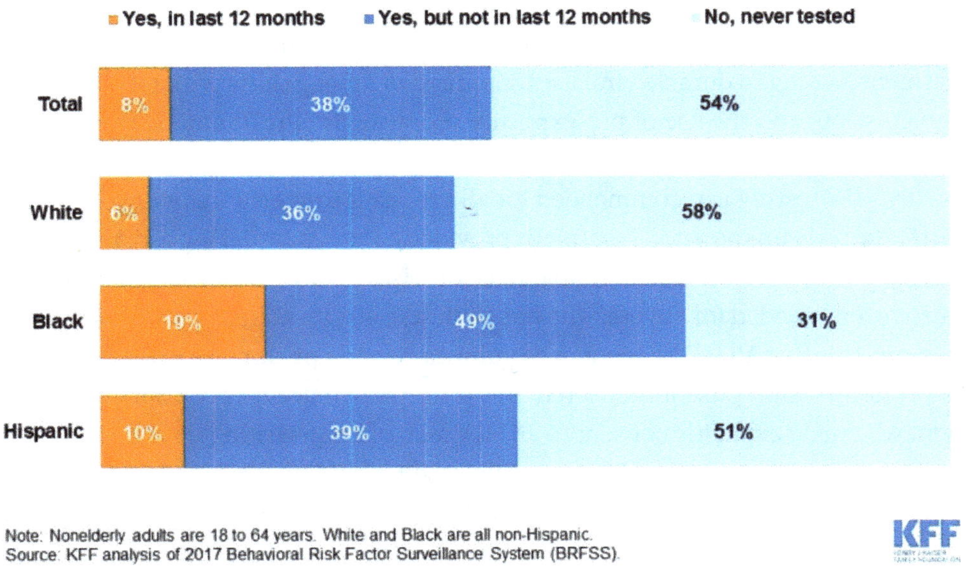

FIGURE 12.1.1 Percent of Nonelderly Adults who Reported Being Tested for HIV, by Race/Ethnicity, 2017.

- HIV testing varies by state, age, race/ethnicity, and other factors.[18,19,20,21,22] For example, Blacks and Latinos are more likely to report recent testing and having ever been tested for HIV than whites (e.g. 68% and 49% vs 46%, respectively have ever been tested).[23] (See Figure 12.1.1)
- According to a 2014 survey of gay and bisexual men in the U.S., relatively few report being tested as regularly as is often advised. Seven in 10 say they have been tested at some point in their lives, 1 in 5 say they were tested within past six months, and 3 in 10 say they've never been tested for HIV, a share that rises to 44 percent among those under age 35.[24]
- Findings from a recent CDC analysis of a decade of testing data suggests that some people at risk for HIV are not getting tested as frequently as recommended.[25]

Testing Recommendations and Requirements

The U.S. Centers for Disease Control and Prevention (CDC) recommends **routine HIV screening in health-care settings** for all adults, aged 13–64, and repeat screening at least annually for those at higher risk.[26,27] Per the CDC individuals who may benefit from at least annual screening include:[28]

- sexually active gay or bisexual men (some of whom may benefit from more frequent testing, such as every 3 to 6 months)
- individuals who have had sex with an HIV-positive partner
- individuals who have had more than one partner since their last HIV test
- those who have shared needles or works to inject drugs
- people who have exchanged sex for drugs or money
- individuals who have another sexually transmitted disease, hepatitis, or tuberculosis
- those who have had sex with someone who has participated in any of the above activities or with someone with an unknown sexual history

Certain factors are known to reduce the risk of HIV transmission including condom use, antiretroviral treatment leading to durable viral load suppression among those with HIV, which prevents further transmission, and the use of pre-exposure prophylaxis (PrEP) among those at increased risk for HIV.[29]

Additionally, HIV testing is recommended for all pregnant women and for any newborn whose mother's HIV status is unknown.[30] Treatment provided to pregnant HIV-positive women and to their infants for 4–6 weeks after delivery can reduce the risk of transmitting HIV to 1% or less.[31] HIV testing is also recommended for anyone who has been sexually assaulted.

CDC recommends that all HIV screening be **voluntary**, and **opt-out** (patient is notified that the test will be performed and consent is inferred unless the patient declines) vs. **opt-in** (test is offered to the patient who must explicitly consent to an HIV test, often in writing).[32]

HIV testing is **mandatory** in the U.S. in certain cases, including for: blood and organ donors;[33] military applicants and active duty personnel;[34] federal and state prison inmates under certain circumstances;[35,36] and newborns in some states.[37] As of January 2010, HIV testing is no longer mandatory for those wishing to [immigrate] to the United States or for refugees.[38]

Insurance Coverage of HIV Testing

Most insurers now broadly cover HIV testing, many without cost-sharing, in part due to a decision made by the United States Preventive Services Task Force (USPSTF), an independent panel that assess the net benefit of preventive services and assigns a subsequent letter grade (A–D). Under the ACA, any "A" or "B" graded preventive services must be provided by most insurers without cost-sharing; in addition, traditional Medicaid programs, while not required to provide USPSTF top graded services are incentivized to do so. In 2013, the USPSTF gave HIV screening an "A" rating for all adolescents and adults, ages 15 to 65.[39] It also gave an "A" grade to HIV screening for pregnant women. Both of these recommendations were reaffirmed in 2019.[40] The current insurance coverage landscape of HIV testing is as follows:

- **Private Insurance:** Most private plans cover HIV testing without cost-sharing. All plans created after the ACA was signed in 2010 must cover.[41, 42]
- **Medicaid:** All Medicaid programs cover "medically necessary" HIV testing and most cover routine HIV screening.
    - Traditional Medicaid Programs: While all Medicaid programs must cover "medically necessary" HIV testing,[43] coverage of "routine" HIV screening is an optional benefit in traditional (non-expansion) Medicaid programs. Still, most states (42 states and DC) do cover routine HIV screening; only eight cover just "medically necessary" testing (AL, FL, GA, ME, MS, NE, SD, and VA).[44] Among the 43 states that cover routine HIV screening, 15 (CA, CO, DE, HI, KY, LA, MT, NH, NJ, NV, NY, OH, OR, WA and WI) cover all USPTSF "A" and "B" graded services and have sought an additional 1% increase in their federal matching rate (FMAP) for these services under Sec. 4106 of the ACA.[45]
    - Medicaid Expansion Programs: In addition to covering medically necessary testing, Medicaid programs expanded under the ACA are required to cover preventive services rated "A" or "B" by the USPSTF, including HIV screening, without cost-sharing. To date 37 states and DC have expanded their Medicaid programs.[46]
- **Medicare:** In April 2015, following the 2013 USPSTF recommendation and a subsequent National Coverage Determination, CMS expanded Medicare coverage to include annual HIV testing for beneficiaries ages 15–65 regardless of risk, and those outside this age range at increased risk without cost-sharing.[47] Additionally, Medicare will cover up to three tests for pregnant beneficiaries.[48]
- **Uninsured:** For those without insurance coverage (or wishing not to use their insurance), HIV testing can be obtained at little or no cost in some community based settings (e.g., stand-alone HIV testing sites, community health centers, mobile testing clinics).

Testing Sites and Policies

HIV testing is offered at CDC-funded testing sites (accounting for more than 3 million tests) and in other public and private settings, including free-standing HIV counseling and testing centers, health departments, hospitals, private doctor offices, STD clinics, and mobile testing units.[49] The overall positivity rate at CDC funded test sites was 0.9% in 2017, including testing among those newly and previously diagnosed. The positivity rate for new diagnoses was 0.4% but was substantially higher for certain sub-populations (e.g. 3.2% for black men who have sex with men).[50] Among CDC-funded testing sites, non-health care facilities have a higher rate of clients testing HIV-positive than do health care and correctional facilities.[51]

All states/territories have moved to **HIV name reporting** (in addition to reporting AIDS cases) where a person's name is reported to the state if they test HIV positive. The state then reports the number of unique positive HIV tests to CDC (no names or other personally identifying information are reported to CDC; only clinical and basic demographic information are forwarded). This is considered **confidential** HIV testing. There is also **anonymous** HIV testing offered at some testing sites where identifying information is not collected.

Testing Techniques

HIV tests aim to detect the virus by looking for evidence of the body's immune response (antibodies), proteins on the surface of the virus (antigens), or genetic material from the virus (RNA). Detectable antibodies usually develop within 3–8 weeks after infection, but may take longer; the period after initial infection with HIV before detectable antibodies develop is the "window period."[52] In 2010, the FDA approved the first HIV diagnostic test that detects both antibodies and antigen, a component of the virus that triggers the production of antibodies.[53] In 2013, the FDA approved the first rapid antigen-antibody test, the first test also to distinguish between acute and established HIV-1 infection.[54] Tests for antigen allow for earlier detection of HIV because they can detect the virus before the body has mounted a response, although there will still be a window period of approximately two weeks after initial infection during which no test can detect the virus. RNA, or nucleic acid tests, which detect the virus itself in the blood, are also available, but not routinely used for screening. The test may be used in cases where there has been a high-risk exposure to HIV and as a follow-up test to a positive antibody test.[55]

The current HIV diagnostics in the U.S. differ based on type of specimen tested (whole blood, serum, or plasma; oral fluid; urine); how the specimen is collected (blood draw/venipuncture; finger prick; oral swab; via urination); where the test is done (laboratory; point-of-care site; at home); and how quickly results are available (conventional or rapid).[56,57] The main types of tests are:

- **Conventional Blood Test:** Blood sample drawn by health care provider; tested at lab. Results: less than an hour to several days.
- **Conventional Oral Fluid Test:** Oral fluid sample collected by health care provider, who swabs inside of mouth; tested at lab. Results: a few days to two weeks.
- **Rapid Tests:**[58] Whole blood finger prick or venipuncture; plasma; oral fluid sample collected depending on complexity of rapid test and individual administering test. Results: approximately 10 minutes. If test is negative, no further testing is needed. If positive, test must be confirmed with a more specific test through conventional method. Some rapid tests have been granted CLIA waivers which allow them to be used outside traditional laboratories.

- **Home Tests:** There are two approved home tests, one of which is performed with a finger prick finger with a lancet, placing drops of blood on treated card, and mailed to lab for testing. An identification number on the card is used when phoning for results; counseling and referral available by phone. Results: in approximately three days. The other is a rapid oral fluid test for home use. Results: approximately 20 minutes. Both home tests may be purchased from drug stores and online.[59]
- **Urine Test:** Urine sample collected by health care provider; tested at lab. Results: a few days to two weeks.

After an HIV Test

Following an HIV test, individuals who test positive can expect a confirmatory test and linkage to HIV care and treatment. It is considered a best practice to initiate antiretroviral treatment as soon as possible after diagnosis.[60] Doing so facilitates the best possible clinical outcomes for the HIV positive individual and is also a prevention opportunity, as once that individual has an undetectable viral load they cannot transmit HIV to others.[61] Individuals who test HIV negative but who are at high risk for the infection, may be referred to additional prevention services such as PrEP which can reduce the risk of HIV acquisition through sex by more than 90%.[62]

Endnotes

1. Li, Z., et al. CDC, *Vital Signs*: HIV Transmission Along the Continuum of Care—United States, 2016 *Weekly*/March 22, 2019/68(11);267–272.
2. CDC, *MMWR* 55(RR14); September 2006.
3. CDC, *MMWR* 52(15); April 2003.
4. CDC, *MMWR* 55(RR14); September 2006; CDC, *MMWR* 52(15); April 2003.
5. U.S. Department of Health and Human Services, *Guidelines for the Use of Antiretroviral Agents in Adults and Adolescents with HIV;* (https://aidsinfo.nih.gov/guidelines/html/1/adult-and-adolescent-arv/0) updated October 2018.
6. CDC, HIV Basics: Prevention (https://www.cdc.gov/hiv/basics/prevention.html); updated January 2019.
7. KFF, Global HIV/AIDS Timeline (http://kff.org/hivaids/timeline/global-hivaids-timeline/).
8. CDC, *MMWR* 55(RR14); September 2006.
9. WHO/UNAIDS Press Release, "WHO and UNAIDS issue new guidance on HIV testing and counselling in health facilities (http://www.who.int/mediacentre/news/releases/2007/pr24/en/);" May 2007.
10. FDA Consumer Information, "Fourth Generation HIV Diagnostic Test Approved, permitting earlier detection of infection;" June 2010.
11. FDA Approval Letter, July 3, 2012 Approval Letter, OraQuick In-Home HIV Test (http://www.fda.gov/BiologicsBloodVaccines/BloodBloodProducts/ApprovedProducts/PremarketApprovalsPMAs/ucm310592.htm).
12. U.S. Preventive Services Task Force, "Human Immunodeficiency Virus (HIV): Screening; (http://www.uspreventiveservicestaskforce.org/Page/Topic/recommendation-summary/human-immunodeficiency-virus-hiv-infection-screening)" April 2013.
13. FDA Consumer Information, "First rapid diagnostic test to detect both HIV-1 antigen and HIV-1/2 antibodies approved."

14. Centers for Medicare & Medicaid Services, "Decision Memo for Screening for the Human Immunodeficiency Virus (HIV) Infection (CAG-00409R) (http://www.cms.gov/medicare-coverage-database/details/nca-decision-memo.aspx?NCAId=276);" April 2015.
15. CDC. Li, Z. et al. *Vital Signs*: HIV Transmission Along the Continuum of Care—United States, 2016 68(11); 267–272
16. CDC. Li, Z. et al. *Vital Signs*: HIV Transmission Along the Continuum of Care—United States, 2016 68(11); 267–272
17. CDC, *MMWR* (https://www.cdc.gov/mmwr/preview/mmwrhtml/rr5514a1.htm) 55(RR14); September 2006.
18. KFF analysis of 2017 Behavioral Risk Factor Surveillance System (BRFSS).
19. CDC, Behavior Risk Factor Surveillance System. (https://www.cdc.gov/brfss/index.html)
20. CDC, National Health Interview Surveys (http://www.cdc.gov/nchs/nhis.htm).
21. CDC, *MMWR* (http://www.cdc.gov/healthyyouth/data/yrbs/pdf/2015/ss6506_updated.pdf) 65(6); June 2016.
22. CDC, *MMWR* (https://www.cdc.gov/mmwr/volumes/67/wr/mm6724a2.htm?s_cid=mm6724a2_e) 67(24); June 2018.
23. KFF analysis of 2017 Behavioral Risk Factor Surveillance System (BRFSS).
24. KFF, *HIV/AIDS In The Lives Of Gay And Bisexual Men In The United States* (http://kff.org/hivaids/report/hivaids-in-the-lives-of-gay-and-bisexual-men-in-the-united-states/); September 2014.
25. CDC, *MMWR* (https://www.cdc.gov/mmwr/volumes/67/wr/mm6724a2.htm?s_cid=mm6724a2_e) 67(24); June 2018.
26. CDC, *MMWR* 55(RR14); September 2006.
27. CDC, *MMWR* (https://www.cdc.gov/mmwr/volumes/66/wr/mm6631a3.htm) 66(31); August 2017.
28. CDC. HIV Testing 101 (https://www.cdc.gov/hiv/pdf/library/factsheets/hiv-testing-101-infosheet.pdf). February 2018.
29. CDC, HIV Basics: Prevention (https://www.cdc.gov/hiv/basics/prevention.html); updated February 27, 2018.
30. CDC, *MMWR* (https://www.cdc.gov/mmwr/preview/mmwrhtml/rr5514a1.htm) 55(RR14); September 2006.
31. CDC, HIV Among Pregnant Women, Infants, and Children (https://www.cdc.gov/hiv/group/gender/pregnantwomen/index.html); 2018.
32. CDC, *MMWR* (https://www.cdc.gov/mmwr/preview/mmwrhtml/rr5514a1.htm) 55(RR14); September 2006.
33. FDA, "Keeping Blood Transfusions Safe: FDA's Multi-layered Protections for Donated Blood," Publication No. FS 02-1; February 2002.
34. U.S. Department of Defense, Instruction Number 6485.01; October 2006.
35. U.S. Federal Bureau of Prisons, *Legal Resource Guide to the Federal Bureau of Prisons*; November 2008.
36. U.S. Department of Justice, Bureau of Justice Statistics, *HIV in Prisons, 2007–2008*; December 2009.
37. KFF/NASTAD, *The National HIV Prevention Inventory*; July 2009.
38. CDC, "Final Rule Removing HIV Infection from U.S. Immigration Screening (http://www.cdc.gov/immigrantrefugeehealth/laws-regs/hiv-ban-removal/final-rule.html)."
39. U.S. Preventive Services Task Force, "Human Immunodeficiency Virus (HIV): Screening; (http://www.uspreventiveservicestaskforce.org/Page/Topic/recommendation-summary/human-immunodeficiency-virus-hiv-infection-screening)" April 2013.

40. U.S. Preventive Services Task Force, "*Human Immunodeficiency Virus (HIV) Infection: Screening* (http://www.uspreventiveservicestaskforce.org/Page/Topic/recommendation-summary/human-immunodeficiency-virus-hiv-infection-screening)" June 2019.
41. All non-grandfathered private plans, including those sold in both the individual and group markets are required to cover. Grandfathered plans, plans that were in place prior to the ACA and that have not undergone significant changes, are not required to cover preventive services without cost sharing. Per KFF's Employer Health Benefit Survey, in 2018, 20% of firms offering health benefits offer at least one grandfathered health plan, and 16% of covered workers are enrolled in a grandfathered plan. The share of plans with grandfathered status is expected to decline over time.
42. KFF, Preventive Services Covered by Private Health Plans under the Affordable Care Act (http://kff.org/health-reform/fact-sheet/preventive-services-covered-by-private-health-plans/); June 2015.
43. Each state Medicaid program determines its own definition of medical necessity, although it generally refers to procedures recommended by a physician. In the case of HIV, for example, HIV testing is clinically indicated based on a patient's risk factors and/or signs of HIV infection.
44. KFF, *State Medicaid Coverage of Routine HIV Screening* (https://www.kff.org/hivaids/state-indicator/hiv-testing/? currentTimeframe=0&sortModel=%7B%22colId%22:%22Location%22,%22sort%22:%22asc%22%7D); 2015.
45. Personal communications with HHS, June 2019.
46. KFF. Status of State Action on the Medicaid Expansion Decision, as of May 2019. https://www.kff.org/health-reform/state-indicator/state-activity-around-expanding-medicaid-under-the-affordable-care-act/
47. Centers for Medicare & Medicaid Services, "Decision Memo for Screening for the Human Immunodeficiency Virus (HIV) Infection (CAG-00409R) (http://www.cms.gov/medicare-coverage-database/details/nca-decision-memo.aspx?NCAId=276);" April 2015.
48. Centers for Medicare & Medicaid Services, "Decision Memo for Screening for the Human Immunodeficiency Virus (HIV) Infection (CAG-00409R) (http://www.cms.gov/medicare-coverage-database/details/nca-decision-memo.aspx?NCAId=276);" April 2015.
49. CDC, *CDC-Funded HIV Testing, United States, Puerto Rico, and the U.S. Virgin Islands, 2017* (https://www.cdc.gov/hiv/pdf/library/reports/cdc-hiv-funded-hiv-testing-report-2017.pdf); 2018.
50. CDC, *CDC-Funded HIV Testing, United States, Puerto Rico, and the U.S. Virgin Islands, 2017* (https://www.cdc.gov/hiv/pdf/library/reports/cdc-hiv-funded-hiv-testing-report-2017.pdf); 2018.
51. CDC, *CDC-Funded HIV Testing, United States, Puerto Rico, and the U.S. Virgin* https://www.cdc.gov/hiv/pdf/library/reports/cdc-hiv-funded-hiv-testing-report-2017.pdf Islands, *2017; 2018.*
52. CDC, HIV Basics: Testing (http://www.cdc.gov/hiv/basics/testing.html); updated March 2018.
53. FDA Consumer Information, "Fourth Generation HIV Diagnostic Test Approved, permitting earlier detection of infection;" June 2010.
54. FDA Consumer Information, "First rapid diagnostic test to detect both HIV-1 antigen and HIV-1/2 antibodies approved."
55. CDC, HIV Basics: Testing (http://www.cdc.gov/hiv/basics/testing.html); updated March 2018.
56. Jeffrey L. Greenwald et al., "A Rapid Review of Rapid HIV Antibody Tests," *Clinical Infectious Diseases* 8(2); March 2006.

57. FDA, Complete List of Donor Screening Assays for Infectious Agents and HIV Diagnostic Assays (http://www.fda.gov/BiologicsBloodVaccines/BloodBloodProducts/ApprovedProducts/LicensedProductsBLAs/BloodDonorScreening/InfectiousDisease/ucm080466.htm).
58. Jeffrey L. Greenwald et al., "A Rapid Review of Rapid HIV Antibody Tests," *Clinical Infectious Diseases* 8(2); March 2006. FDA, Complete List of Donor Screening Assays for Infectious Agents and HIV Diagnostic Assays (http://www.fda.gov/BiologicsBloodVaccines/BloodBloodProducts/ApprovedProducts/LicensedProductsBLAs/BloodDonorScreening/InfectiousDisease/ucm080466.htm).
59. FDA Approval Letter, July 3, 2012 Approval Letter, OraQuick In-Home HIV Test (http://www.fda.gov/BiologicsBloodVaccines/BloodBloodProducts/ApprovedProducts/PremarketApprovalsPMAs/ucm310592.htm).
60. U.S. Department of Health and Human Services, *Guidelines for the Use of Antiretroviral Agents in Adults and Adolescents with HIV;* (https://aidsinfo.nih.gov/guidelines/html/1/adult-and-adolescent-arv/0) updated October 2018.
61. CDC. HIV Basics: Prevention (https://www.cdc.gov/hiv/basics/prevention.html); updated January 2019.
62. CDC, HIV Basics: PrEP [...]; updated May 2019.

12.2

HIV Testing

U.S. Center for Disease Control and Prevention

Test Today. Don't Delay.

1 in 2 people with HIV have had the virus at least 3 years before diagnosis.

About **40%** of new HIV infections come from people who don't know they have HIV.

7 in 10 people at high risk for HIV who weren't tested last year saw a healthcare provider during that year.

Now available

[...]

IT IS IMPORTANT FOR EVERYONE TO know their HIV status. Getting an HIV test is the first step for people living with HIV to get care and treatment and control the infection.* Taking HIV medicine as prescribed helps people living with HIV to live a long, healthy life and protect their sex partners from HIV. About 85% of people with HIV in the US know they have the virus. However, 15% (162,500) of people with HIV don't know they have the virus, and about 40% of new HIV infections come from them. Half of people with HIV have had the virus 3 years or more before diagnosis. Most people at high risk who didn't get tested last year saw a healthcare provider during the year. Everyone should get tested at least once, and people at high risk should be tested at least once a year. Healthcare providers can diagnose HIV sooner if they test more people and test people at high risk more often.

Healthcare providers can:

- Routinely provide HIV testing to all people aged 13 to 64, according to CDC guidelines. [...].

* Take HIV medicine as prescribed so the amount of HIV in the body gets and stays extremely low (less than 200 copies per milliliter of blood or undetectable level).

Source: https://www.cdc.gov/vitalsigns/hiv-testing/index.html.

- Screen all teens and adults for HIV risk, and test people at high risk at least once a year. This includes some gay and bisexual men who may benefit from more frequent testing (for example, every 3 to 6 months).
- Start people on HIV treatment as quickly as possible after diagnosis.
- Discuss prevention tools with patients. Provide or refer to prevention services, including pre-exposure prophylaxis (PrEP) and services for people who inject drugs. www.cdc.gov/hiv/risk

Problem

Many people have HIV for years before they know it.

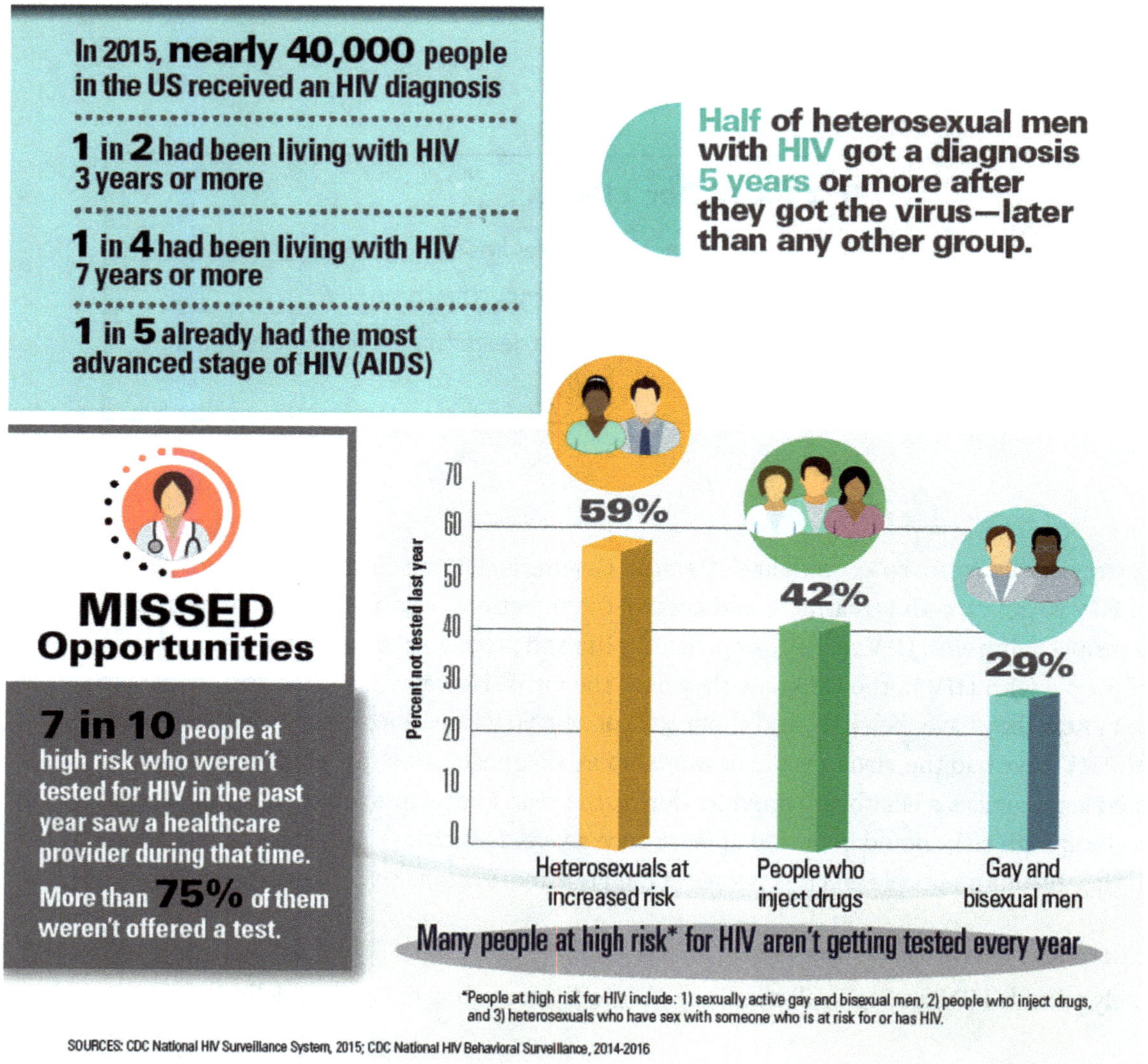

12.3

HIV Testing in Health Care Settings—California Law

IN CALIFORNIA, CHANGES TO HIV TESTING law have supported the effort to bring "opt-out" (routine offering with the option to decline to take an HIV test) HIV testing to the state's health care facilities.

As of January 1, 2008, Assembly Bill (AB) 682 (PDF) (Berg, Chapter 550, Statutes of 2007), added California Health and Safety (H&S) Code Section 120990, which eliminated the requirement for written consent for an HIV test when ordered by a medical care provider.

Medical care providers ordering HIV tests under H&S Code Section 120990(a) are not required to obtain written consent for an HIV test, nor are laboratories processing HIV tests ordered by medical care providers under H&S Code Section 120990(a) required to obtain either written or oral consent to process the ordered test. Furthermore:

Continued requirements for written consent under H&S Code Section 120990(c) refer to HIV testing provided and/or processed in non-medical settings (such as OA-funded confidential HIV test sites).

Instead of required written consent, H&S Code Section 120990(a) requires medical care providers to do the following before they order an HIV test:

1. Inform the patient that an HIV test is planned;
2. Provide information about the HIV test;
3. Inform the patient that there are numerous treatment options available for a patient who tests positive for HIV and that a person who tests negative for HIV should continue to be routinely tested;
4. Advise the patient that he or she has the right to decline the HIV test; and
5. If the patient declines the HIV test, document that fact in the patient's medical file.

AB 682 also amended H&S Code Section 125090, which eliminated the requirement for written consent for HIV testing for pregnant women. H&S Code Section 125090 states that if a woman does not have an HIV test documented in her prenatal record during prenatal care or at the time of labor and delivery, the physician and surgeon or other person engaged in the prenatal care or attending the woman shall ensure that the woman is informed about the:

1. Intent to perform an HIV test,
2. Routine nature of the test,
3. Purpose of the test,

Source: https://www.cdph.ca.gov/Programs/CID/DOA/Pages/OA_prev_hivhcv.aspx.

4. Risks and benefits of the test,
5. Risk of transmission of HIV, that approved treatments are known to decrease the risk of perinatal transmission of HIV, and
6. Right to decline HIV testing.

pregnant women

If the woman verbally accepts testing, she must then receive an HIV test "by a method that will ensure the earliest possible results." Currently, there are several HIV tests available that can provide preliminary results within 20 minutes; therefore, hospitals should be able to provide rapid HIV testing in labor and delivery. If a woman receives appropriate HIV treatment during labor and delivery, she can decrease the chances of transmitting HIV to her infant by approximately one-half.

As of January 1, 2009, AB 1894 (PDF) (Krekorian, Chapter 631, Statutes of 2008) added H&S Code Section 1367.46 and Insurance Code Section 10123.91 to require individual and group health care service plans and health insurers to provide coverage for testing for HIV in medical care settings regardless of whether the testing is related to the primary diagnosis. Insurance Code Section 10123.91 further states that reimbursement shall be provided according to the respective principles and policies of the health insurer. This statute does not cover reimbursement through all public funding.

12.4

Recommended Laboratory HIV Testing Algorithm for Serum or Plasma Specimens

U.S. Center for Disease Control and Prevention

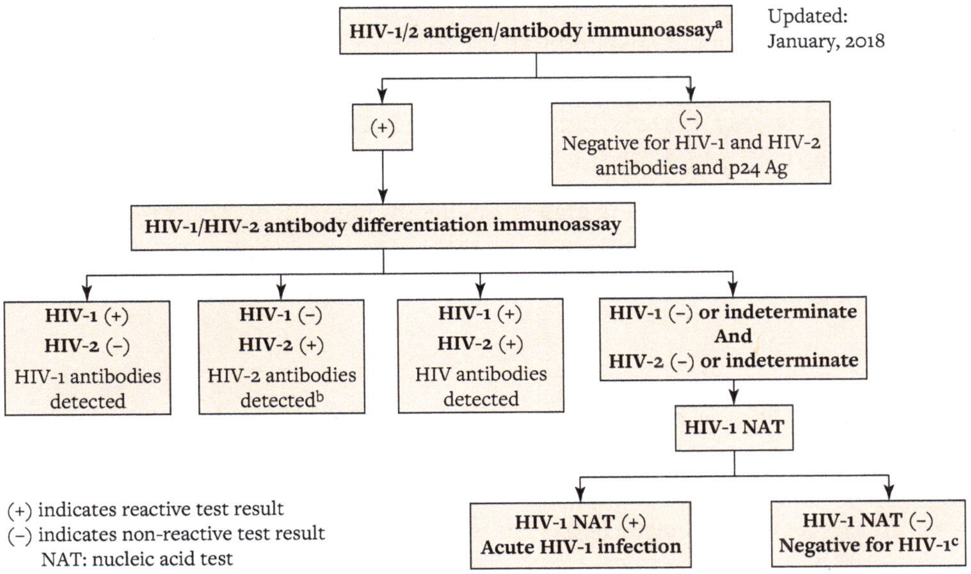

1. Laboratories should conduct initial testing for HIV with an FDA-approved antigen/antibody immunoassay[a1] that detects HIV-1 and HIV-2 antibodies and HIV-1 p24 antigen to test for established HIV-1 and HIV-2 infection and for acute HIV-1 infection, respectively. No further testing is required for specimens that are non-reactive on the initial immunoassay. However, if there is a possibility of very early infection leading to a non-reactive initial antigen/antibody immunoassay, such as when recent HIV exposure is suspected or reported, then conduct an HIV-1 nucleic acid test (NAT), or request a new specimen and repeat the algorithm according to CDC guidance (1,4,5,6).

---

a The FDA-approved single-use rapid HIV-1/HIV-2 antigen/antibody immunoassay can be used as the initial assay in the laboratory HIV testing algorithm for serum or plasma. If any instrumented antigen/antibody test is available, it is preferred due to its superior sensitivity for detecting HIV during acute infection (1,2).

Source: https://stacks.cdc.gov/view/cdc/50872.

2. Specimens with a reactive antigen/antibody immunoassay result (or repeatedly reactive, if repeat testing is recommended by the manufacturer or required by regulatory authorities) should be tested with an FDA-approved supplemental antibody immunoassay that differentiates HIV-1 antibodies from HIV-2 antibodies. Reactive results on the initial antigen/antibody immunoassay and the HIV-1/HIV-2 antibody differentiation immunoassay should be interpreted as positive for HIV-1 antibodies, HIV-2 antibodies[b2], or HIV antibodies, untypable (undifferentiated).
3. Specimens that are reactive on the initial antigen/antibody immunoassay and non-reactive or indeterminate on the HIV-1/HIV-2 antibody differentiation immunoassay should be tested with an FDA-approved HIV-1 NAT.
   - A reactive HIV-1 NAT result and non-reactive or indeterminate HIV-1/HIV-2 antibody differentiation immunoassay result indicates laboratory evidence of acute HIV-1 infection.
   - A negative HIV-1 NAT result and non-reactive or HIV-1 indeterminate antibody differentiation immunoassay result indicates an HIV-1 false-positive result on the initial immunoassay.
   - A negative HIV-1 NAT result and repeatedly HIV-2 indeterminate or HIV indeterminate antibody differentiation immunoassay result should be referred for testing with a different validated supplemental HIV-2 test (antibody test or NAT) or repeat the algorithm in 2 to 4 weeks, starting with an antigen/antibody immunoassay (3).
4. Laboratories should use this same testing algorithm, beginning with an antigen/antibody immunoassay on all serum or plasma specimens submitted for testing after a preliminary positive result from any rapid HIV test conducted in a CLIA-waived setting (7).

References

1. Laboratory Testing for the Diagnosis of HIV Infection: Updated Recommendations https://stacks.cdc.gov/view/cdc/23447
2. Use of the Determine HIV 1/2 Ag/Ab Combo Test with Serum or Plasma in the Laboratory Algorithm for HIV Diagnosis https://stacks.cdc.gov/view/cdc/48472
3. Technical Update on HIV-1/2 Differentiation Assays https://stacks.cdc.gov/view/cdc/40790
4. Suggested Reporting Language for the HIV Laboratory Diagnostic Testing Algorithm https:/stacks.cdc.gov/view/cdc/45930
5. Updated Guidelines for Antiretroviral Postexposure Prophylaxis After Sexual, Injection Drug Use, or Other Nonoccupational Exposure to HIV-United States, 2016 https://stacks.cdc.gov/view/cdc/38856
6. Web content: How Soon Can Clinicians Rule Out Infection? https://www.cdc.gov/hiv/testing/clinical/index.html
7. Web content: Clinical Laboratory Improvement Amendments https://wwwn.cdc.gov/clia/

b This includes specimens reported as HIV-2 positive with HIV-1 cross-reactivity (3).

GUIDANCE FOR reporting results from the HIV laboratory diagnostic algorithm for use with serum and plasma specimens (4)

Guidance for Reporting Results from the HIV Laboratory Diagnostic Testing Algorithm for Serum and Plasma Specimens[a]

Test Outcomes: Test Sequence — Step 1: HIV-1/HIV-2 Ag/Ab IA[b]	Step 2: HIV-1/HIV-2 Antibody Differentiation IA[c]	Step 3: HIV-1 NAT	Final Algorithm Interpretation[d]	Interpretation for Provider[e] (Sample should be reported as:)	Further Actions[f]
Nonreactive	n/a	n/a	HIV-1 antigen and HIV-1/HIV-2 antibodies were not detected. No laboratory evidence of HIV infection.	HIV negative	If recent HIV exposure is suspected or reported, conduct HIV-1 NAT or request a new specimen and repeat the algorithm according to CDC guidance.[g]
Reactive	HIV-1 Positive	n/a	Positive for HIV-1 antibodies. Laboratory evidence of HIV-1 infection is present.	HIV-1 Positive	Link patient to HIV medical care and provide appropriate prevention counseling.[h]
Reactive	HIV-2 Positive	n/a	Positive for HIV-2 antibodies. Laboratory evidence of HIV-2 infection is present.	HIV-2 Positive	Link patient to HIV medical care and provide appropriate prevention counseling.[h]
Reactive	HIV-2 Positive with HIV-1 Cross reactivity	n/a	Positive for HIV-2 antibodies. Laboratory evidence of HIV-2 infection is present.	HIV-2 Positive. This result is distinct from HIV positive untypable (undifferentiated).	Link patient to HIV medical care and provide appropriate prevention counseling.[h]
Reactive	HIV Positive untypable (undifferentiated)	n/a	Positive for HIV-1 and HIV-2 antibodies. Laboratory evidence of HIV-1 and/or HIV-2 infection is present.	HIV Positive	Link patient to HIV medical care and provide appropriate prevention counseling.[h] Provider may consider additional testing for HIV-1 RNA or DNA and HIV-2 RNA or DNA to verify or rule out HIV-1/HIV-2 dual infection. Request additional specimen if original specimen volume is insufficient.
Reactive	HIV-1 indeterminate, HIV-2 indeterminate[i], HIV indeterminate	Detected	Positive for HIV-1. Laboratory evidence of HIV-1 infection consistent with an acute HIV-1 infection.	Acute HIV-1 Positive	Link patient to HIV medical care and provide appropriate prevention counseling immediately[h] to expedite prevention practices.
Reactive	HIV-1 indeterminate	Not detected	HIV-1 antibodies were not confirmed and HIV-1 RNA was not detected.	HIV Negative	If recent HIV exposure is suspected or reported, request a new specimen and repeat the algorithm according to CDC guidance.[g]

(continue)

Guidance for Reporting Results from the HIV Laboratory Diagnostic Testing Algorithm for Serum and Plasma Specimens[a]

Test Outcomes	Reactive	HIV-2 indeterminate[i]	Not detected	HIV antibodies were not confirmed and HIV-1 RNA was not detected. HIV-2 inconclusive.	HIV-1 Negative, HIV-2 inconclusive	Refer sample for testing with a different validated supplemental HIV-2 test (antibody test or NAT) if available. Alternatively, redraw and repeat algorithm 2–4 weeks to assess HIV-2 infection.
	Reactive	HIV Indeterminate	Not detected	HIV-1 antibodies were not confirmed and HIV-1 RNA was not detected. HIV-2 inconclusive.	HIV-1 Negative, HIV-2 inconclusive	Refer sample for testing with a different validated supplemental HIV-2 test (antibody test or NAT) if available. Alternatively, redraw and repeat algorithm in 2–4 weeks to assess HIV-2 infection.
	Reactive	Negative	Detected	Positive for HIV-1. Laboratory evidence of HIV-1 infection consistent with an acute HIV-1 infection.	Acute HIV-1 Positive	Link patient to HIV medical care and provide appropriate prevention counseling immediately[h] to expedite prevention practices.
	Reactive	Negative	Not detected	HIV antibodies were not confirmed and HIV-1 RNA was not detected.	HIV Negative	If recent HIV exposure is suspected or reported, request a new specimen and repeat the algorithm according to CDC guidance.[g]
	Reactive	Negative or Indeterminate	Invalid or not performed	Inconclusive	Inconclusive	Request an additional specimen and repeat the algorithm. Ensure HIV-1 NAT is performed, if indicated by results of HIV-1/HIV-2 Ag/Ab IA and HIV-1/HIV-2 Ab differentiation IA.

a. The tests outlined in this table are not FDA approved for oral fluid or dried blood spots. **b.** The need for repeating screening IA on an initial reactive test is assay dependent, refer to product package insert. **c.** This column contains the Final Assay interpretation per the Geenius package insert, the only FDA approved test for this step. We recommend excluding the individual HIV-1 and HIV-2 results on the laboratory report. If they are used, the final assay interpretation or final assay result should also be included. **d.** This column contains suggested language to be used for the laboratory report and it can be directly used for reporting from LIMS systems. **e.** This column contains simplified language of the previous column, "Final Algorithm interpretation," and is included here for healthcare providers or other non-laboratorians that may also use this table as a reference document. This does not need to be included on the laboratory report. **f.** Comments under "Further Action" can be included as language in the laboratory report or can be used as guidance for laboratorians to discuss test results with healthcare providers or health department staff. **g.** Please refer to Centers for Disease Control and Prevention guidance. Available at: https://www.cdc.gov/hiv/testing/laboratorytests.html, https://stacks.cdc.gov/view/cdc/38856 and https://www.cdc.gov/hiv/testing/clinical/index.html **h.** Please refer to the Centers for Disease Control and Prevention HIV Guidelines and Recommendations to find the most appropriate information by age and risk group for the patient in question. Available at: http://www.cdc.gov/hiv/guidelines/ **i.** Follow Geenius package insert and refer to the CDC Technical Update. Available at: https://stacks.cdc.gov/view/cdc/40790

Section XIII

Transmission and Prevention

13.1

HIV Transmission

U.S. Center for Disease Control and Prevention

MYTHS PERSIST ABOUT HOW HIV IS transmitted. This section provides the facts about HIV risk from different types of sex, injection drug use, and other activities.

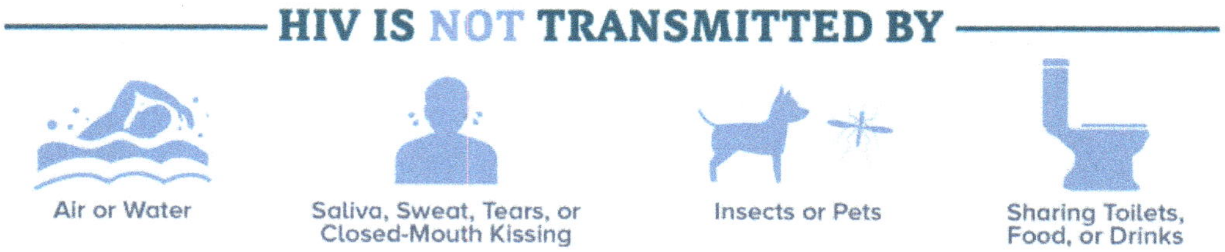

How is HIV passed from one person to another?

You can get or transmit HIV only through specific activities. Most commonly, people get or transmit HIV through sexual behaviors and needle or syringe use.

Only certain body fluids—blood, semen (*cum*), pre-seminal fluid (*pre-cum*), rectal fluids, vaginal fluids, and breast milk—from a person who has HIV can transmit HIV. These fluids must come in contact with a mucous membrane or damaged tissue or be directly injected into the bloodstream (from a needle or syringe) for transmission to occur. Mucous membranes are found inside the rectum, vagina, penis, and mouth.

In the United States, HIV is spread mainly by

- Having anal or vaginal sex with someone who has HIV without using a condom or taking medicines to prevent or treat HIV.
    - For the HIV-negative partner, receptive anal sex (bottoming) is the highest-risk sexual behavior, but you can also get HIV from insertive anal sex (topping).
    - Either partner can get HIV through vaginal sex, though it is less risky for getting HIV than receptive anal sex.
- Sharing needles or syringes, rinse water, or other equipment (works) used to prepare drugs for injection with someone who has HIV. HIV can live in a used needle up to 42 days depending on temperature and other factors.

Source: http://www.cdc.gov/hiv/resources/qa/transmission.htm.

Less commonly, HIV may be spread

- From mother to child during pregnancy, birth, or breastfeeding. Although the risk can be high if a mother is living with HIV and not taking medicine, recommendations to test all pregnant women for HIV and start HIV treatment immediately have lowered the number of babies who are born with HIV.
- By being stuck with an HIV-contaminated needle or other sharp object. This is a risk mainly for health care workers.

In extremely rare cases, HIV has been transmitted by

- Oral sex—putting the mouth on the penis (fellatio), vagina (cunnilingus), or anus (rimming). In general, there's little to no risk of getting HIV from oral sex. But transmission of HIV, though extremely rare, is theoretically possible if an HIV-positive man ejaculates in his partner's mouth during oral sex. [...]
- Receiving blood transfusions, blood products, or organ/tissue transplants that are contaminated with HIV. This was more common in the early years of HIV, but now the risk is extremely small because of rigorous testing of the US blood supply and donated organs and tissues.

TABLE 13.1.1

Disease	Test	Year Implemented
HIV/AIDS	HIV-1 antibody test	1985
	HIV-1/2 antibody test	1992
	HIV-1 P24 antigen test	1996
	Nucleic acid test (NAT)	1999
Hepatitis B	Hepatitis B surface antigen test	1971
	Hepatitis B core antibody test	1986
	Nucleic acid test (NAT)	2009
Heptatitis C	Hepatitis C antibody test	1990
	Nucleic acid test (NAT)	1999
Syphilis (Treponema pallidum)	Syphilis serologic test	1948
HTLV	HTLV-I antibody test	1989
	HTLV-I/II antibody test	1998
West Nile Fever	Nucleic acid testing (NAT)	2003
Chagas disease	Trypanosom cruzi antibody test	2007
Babesiosis	Babesia microti antibody test	2012
	Nucleic acid testing (NAT)	2012
Zika fever	Nucleic acid test (NAT)	2016

Source: American Red Cross
More information on testing of blood donations can be found here:
https://www.redcrossblood.org/biomedical-services/blood-diagnostic-testing/blood-testing.html

- Eating food that has been pre-chewed by a person with HIV. The contamination occurs when infected blood from a caregiver's mouth mixes with food while chewing. The only known cases are among infants.
- Being bitten by a person with HIV. Each of the very small number of documented cases has involved severe trauma with extensive tissue damage and the presence of blood. There is no risk of transmission if the skin is not broken.
- Contact between broken skin, wounds, or mucous membranes and HIV-infected blood or blood-contaminated body fluids.
- Deep, open-mouth kissing if both partners have sores or bleeding gums and blood from the HIV-positive partner gets into the bloodstream of the HIV-negative partner. HIV is not spread through saliva.

[...]

How well does HIV survive outside the body?

HIV does not survive long outside the human body (such as on surfaces), and it cannot reproduce outside a human host. It **is not** spread by

- Mosquitoes, ticks, or other insects.
- Saliva, tears, or sweat that is not mixed with the blood of an HIV-positive person.
- Hugging, shaking hands, sharing toilets, sharing dishes, or closed-mouth or "social" kissing with someone who is HIV-positive.
- Other sexual activities that don't involve the exchange of body fluids (for example, touching).

[...]

Sexual Transmission

Can I get HIV from anal sex?

Yes. In fact, anal sex is the riskiest type of sex for getting or transmitting HIV.

HIV can be found in certain body fluids—blood, semen (*cum*), pre-seminal fluid (*pre-cum*), or rectal fluids—of a person who has HIV. Although receptive anal sex (bottoming) is much riskier for getting HIV than insertive anal sex (topping), it's possible for either partner—the top or the bottom—to get HIV. The bottom's risk is very high because the lining of the rectum is thin and may allow HIV to enter the body during anal sex. The top is also at risk because HIV can enter the body through the opening at the tip of the penis (or urethra); the foreskin if the penis isn't circumcised; or small cuts, scratches, or open sores anywhere on the penis. [...]

Can I get HIV from vaginal sex?

Yes. Either partner can get HIV through vaginal sex, though it is less risky for getting HIV than receptive anal sex.

When a woman has vaginal sex with a partner who's HIV-positive, HIV can enter her body through the mucous membranes that line the vagina and cervix. Most women who get HIV get it from vaginal sex.

Men can also get HIV from having vaginal sex with a woman who's HIV-positive. This is because vaginal fluid and blood can carry HIV. Men get HIV through the opening at the tip of the penis (or urethra); the foreskin if they're not circumcised; or small cuts, scratches, or open sores anywhere on the penis.

[...]

Can I get HIV from oral sex?

The chance that an HIV-negative person will get HIV from oral sex with an HIV-positive partner is extremely low.

Oral sex involves putting the mouth on the penis (fellatio), vagina (cunnilingus), or anus (anilingus). In general, there's little to no risk of getting or transmitting HIV through oral sex.

Factors that may increase the risk of transmitting HIV through oral sex are ejaculation in the mouth with oral ulcers, bleeding gums, genital sores, and the presence of other sexually transmitted diseases (STDs), which may or may not be visible.

You can get other STDs from oral sex. And, if you get feces in your mouth during anilingus, you can get hepatitis A and B, parasites like *Giardia*, and bacteria like *Shigella*, *Salmonella*, *Campylobacter*, and *E. coli*.

[...]

Is there a connection between HIV and other sexually transmitted diseases?

Yes. Having another sexually transmitted disease (STD) can increase the risk of getting or transmitting HIV.

If you have another STD, you're more likely to get or transmit HIV to others. Some of the most common STDs include gonorrhea, chlamydia, syphilis, trichomoniasis, human papillomavirus (HPV), genital herpes, and hepatitis. The only way to know for sure if you have an STD is to get tested. If you're sexually active, you and your partners should get tested for STDs (including HIV if you're HIV-negative) regularly, even if you don't have symptoms.

If you are HIV-negative but have an STD, you are about 3 times as likely to get HIV if you have unprotected sex with someone who has HIV. There are two ways that having an STD can increase the likelihood of getting HIV. If the STD causes irritation of the skin (for example, from syphilis, herpes, or human papillomavirus), breaks or sores may make it easier for HIV to enter the body during sexual contact. Even STDs that cause no breaks or open sores (for example, chlamydia, gonorrhea, trichomoniasis) can increase your risk by causing inflammation that increases the number of cells that can serve as targets for HIV.

If you are HIV-positive and also have another STD, you are about 3 times as likely as other people with HIV to transmit HIV through sexual contact. This appears to happen because there is an increased concentration of HIV in the semen and genital fluids of HIV-positive people who also have another STD.

[...]

Are lesbians or other women who have sex with women at risk for HIV?

Case reports of female-to-female transmission of HIV are rare. The well-documented risk of female-to-male transmission shows that vaginal fluids and menstrual blood may contain the virus and that exposure to these fluids through mucous membranes (in the vagina or mouth) could potentially lead to HIV infection.

[...]

Does my HIV-positive partner's viral load affect my risk of getting HIV?

Yes. As an HIV-positive person's viral load goes down, the chance of transmitting HIV can go down dramatically.

Viral load is the amount of HIV in the blood of someone who has HIV. Taking HIV medicine (called antiretroviral therapy or ART) as prescribed can make the viral load very low—so low that a test can't detect it (called an *undetectable viral load*). People with HIV who take HIV medicine as prescribed and get and keep an undetectable viral load have effectively no risk of transmitting HIV to an HIV-negative partner through sex.

If you're HIV positive, getting into care and taking HIV medicine as prescribed will give you the greatest chance to get and keep an undetectable viral load; live a longer, healthier life; and protect your partners.

If you're HIV-negative and have an HIV-positive partner, encourage your partner to get into care and to take HIV medicine as prescribed.

Treatment is a powerful tool for preventing sexual transmission of HIV. But it works only as long as the HIV-positive partner gets and keeps an undetectable viral load. Here are some things to consider when deciding whether treatment as prevention is right for you and your partner:

- Not everyone taking HIV medicine has an undetectable viral load. **Up to one-third of people in HIV care don't keep an undetectable viral load**. To stay undetectable, people with HIV must take HIV medicine every day as prescribed.
- Missing some doses can increase the viral load and the risk of transmitting HIV. People who have trouble taking medicine as prescribed can talk with their health care provider about the challenges

they are facing and develop a plan to ensure they take their medicine every day. They should also consider using other prevention strategies like condoms.

- We don't know how often people living with HIV need to have their viral load tested if they are using their undetectable viral load status as their only prevention method. But to stay healthy and protect their partners, they need to visit their provider regularly and get a viral load test as recommended.
- Some people who take HIV medicine daily can get an undetectable viral load very quickly, but it can take some people up to six months. The only way to know if you are undetectable is by getting your viral load tested.
- People taking HIV medicine sometimes have small increases or "blips" in their viral load. These blips usually go back down by the next viral load test. But people who experience blips may benefit from using other prevention strategies (condoms) until their viral load is undetectable again.
- HIV medicine does not protect against other STDs.
- Both partners should learn about all their options for preventing HIV, as well as other STDs, so they can make the decisions that are best for them.

Consider other actions to prevent HIV, like using condoms or a negative partner being on pre-exposure prophylaxis (PrEP), especially if the person with HIV

- Has trouble regularly taking HIV medicine,
- Has an increased viral load, or a load of 200 copies/ml of blood or greater,
- Hasn't had a recent test (last 6 months) that shows the viral load is undetectable,
- Missed some doses since the last viral load test, or
- Has stopped taking HIV medicine in the past and may choose to do so again.

Important Note: Consider using condoms if either partner is concerned about getting or transmitting other STDs.

[...]

Can I get HIV from injecting drugs?

Yes. Your risk for getting HIV is very high if you use needles or works (such as cookers, cotton, or water) after someone with HIV has used them.

People who inject drugs, hormones, steroids, or silicone can get HIV by sharing needles or syringes and other injection equipment. The needles and equipment may have someone else's blood in them, and blood can transmit HIV. Likewise, you're at risk for getting hepatitis B and C if you share needles and works because these infections are also transmitted through blood.

Another reason people who inject drugs can get HIV (and other sexually transmitted diseases) is that when people are high, they're more likely to have risky sex.

Stopping injection and other drug use can lower your chances of getting HIV a lot. You may need help to stop or cut down using drugs, but many resources are available.

[...]

If you keep injecting drugs, you can lower your risk for getting HIV by using only new, sterile needles and works each time you inject. Never share needles or works.

[...]

Can I get HIV from using other kinds of drugs?

When you're drunk or high, you're more likely to make decisions that put you at risk for HIV, such as having sex without a condom.

Drinking alcohol, particularly binge drinking, and using "club drugs" like Ecstasy, ketamine, GHB, and poppers can alter your judgment, lower your inhibitions, and impair your decisions about sex or other drug use. You may be more likely to have unplanned and unprotected sex, have a harder time using a condom the right way every time you have sex, have more sexual partners, or use other drugs, including injection drugs or meth. Those behaviors can increase your risk of exposure to HIV. If you have HIV, they can also increase your risk of spreading HIV to others. Being drunk or high affects your ability to make safe choices.

If you're going to a party or another place where you know you'll be drinking or using drugs, you can bring a condom so that you can reduce your risk if you have vaginal or anal sex.

[...]

If I already have HIV, can I get another kind of HIV?

Yes. This is called HIV superinfection.

HIV superinfection is when a person with HIV gets infected with another strain of the virus. The new strain of HIV can replace the original strain or remain along with the original strain.

The effects of superinfection differ from person to person. Superinfection may cause some people to get sicker faster because they become infected with a new strain of the virus that is resistant to the medicine (antiretroviral therapy or ART) they're taking to treat their original infection.

Research suggests that a hard-to-treat superinfection is rare. Taking medicine to treat HIV (ART) may reduce someone's chance of getting a superinfection.

[...]

Health Care and the US Blood Supply

Are health care workers at risk of getting HIV on the job?

The risk of health care workers being exposed to HIV on the job (occupational exposure) is very low, especially if they use protective practices and personal protective equipment to prevent HIV and other blood-borne infections. For health care workers on the job, the main risk of HIV transmission is from being stuck with an HIV-contaminated needle or other sharp object. However, even this risk is small. Scientists estimate that the risk of HIV infection from being stuck with a needle used on a person with HIV is less than 1%.

[...]

Can I get HIV from receiving medical care?

Although HIV transmission is possible in health care settings, it is extremely rare.

Careful practice of infection control, including universal precautions (using protective practices and personal protective equipment to prevent HIV and other blood-borne infections), protects patients as well as health care providers from possible HIV transmission in medical and dental offices and hospitals.

The risk of getting HIV from receiving blood transfusions, blood products, or organ/tissue transplants that are contaminated with HIV is extremely small because of rigorous testing of the US blood supply and donated organs and tissues.

It is important to know that **you cannot get HIV from donating blood**. Blood collection procedures are highly regulated and safe.

[...]

Other Modes of Transmission

Can I get HIV from casual contact ("social kissing," shaking hands, hugging, using a toilet, drinking from the same glass, or the sneezing and coughing of a person with HIV)?

No. HIV isn't transmitted

- By hugging, shaking hands, sharing toilets, sharing dishes, or closed-mouth or "social" kissing with someone who is HIV-positive.
- Through saliva, tears, or sweat that is not mixed with the blood of an HIV-positive person.
- By mosquitoes, ticks or other blood-sucking insects.
- Through the air.

Only certain body fluids—blood, semen (*cum*), pre-seminal fluid (*pre-cum*), rectal fluids, vaginal fluids, and breast milk—from a person with HIV can transmit HIV. Most commonly, people get or transmit HIV through sexual behaviors and needle or syringe use. Babies can also get HIV from an HIV-positive mother during pregnancy, birth, or breastfeeding.

[...]

Can I get HIV from a tattoo or a body piercing?

There are no known cases in the United States of anyone getting HIV this way. However, it is possible to get HIV from a reused or not properly sterilized tattoo or piercing needle or other equipment, or from contaminated ink.

It's possible to get HIV from tattooing or body piercing if the equipment used for these procedures has someone else's blood in it or if the ink is shared. The risk of getting HIV this way is very low, but the risk increases when the person doing the procedure is unlicensed, because of the potential for unsanitary practices such as sharing needles or ink. If you get a tattoo or a body piercing, be sure that the person doing the procedure is properly licensed and that they use only new or sterilized needles, ink, and other supplies.

[...]

Can I get HIV from being spit on or scratched by a person with HIV?

No. HIV isn't spread through saliva, and there is no risk of transmission from scratching because no body fluids are transferred between people.

[...]

Can I get HIV from mosquitoes?

No. HIV is not transmitted by mosquitoes, ticks, or any other insects.

From the onset of the HIV epidemic, there has been concern about transmission of the virus by biting and bloodsucking insects. However, studies conducted by researchers at CDC and elsewhere have shown no evidence of HIV transmission through insects—even in areas where there are many cases of AIDS and large populations of insects such as mosquitoes. Lack of such outbreaks, despite intense efforts to detect them, supports the conclusion that HIV is not transmitted by insects.

The results of experiments and observations of insect biting behavior indicate that when an insect bites a person, it does not inject its own or a previously bitten person's or animal's blood into the next person bitten. Rather, it injects saliva, which acts as a lubricant or anticoagulant so the insect can feed efficiently. Such diseases as yellow fever and malaria are transmitted through the saliva of specific species of mosquitoes. However, HIV lives for only a short time inside an insect and, unlike organisms that are transmitted via insect bites, HIV does not reproduce (and does not survive) in insects. Thus, even if the virus enters a mosquito or another sucking or biting insect, the insect does not become infected and cannot transmit HIV to the next human it feeds on or bites. HIV is not found in insect feces.

There is also no reason to fear that a biting or bloodsucking insect, such as a mosquito, could transmit HIV from one person to another through HIV-infected blood left on its mouth parts. Two factors serve to explain why this is so—first, infected people do not have constant, high levels of HIV in their bloodstreams and, second, insect mouth parts do not retain large amounts of blood on their surfaces.

Further, scientists who study insects have determined that biting insects normally do not travel from one person to the next immediately after ingesting blood. Rather, they fly to a resting place to digest this blood meal.

[...]

Can I get HIV from food?

You can't get HIV from consuming food handled by someone with HIV. Even if the food contained small amounts of HIV-infected blood or semen, exposure to the air, heat from cooking, and stomach acid would destroy the virus.

Though it is very rare, HIV can be spread by eating food that has been pre-chewed by someone with HIV. The contamination occurs when infected blood from a caregiver's mouth mixes with food while chewing. The only known cases are among infants.

[...]

Is the risk of HIV different for different people?

Some groups of people in the United States are more likely to get HIV than others because of many factors, including the status of their sex partners, their risk behaviors, and where they live.

When you live in a community where many people have HIV infection, the chances of having sex or sharing needles or other injection equipment with someone who has HIV are higher. You can use CDC's HIV, STD, hepatitis, and tuberculosis atlas to see the percentage of people with HIV ("prevalence") in different US communities. Within any community, the prevalence of HIV can vary among different populations.

Gay and bisexual men have the largest number of new diagnoses in the United States. Blacks/African Americans and Hispanics/Latinos are disproportionately affected by HIV compared to other racial and ethnic groups. Also, transgender women who have sex with men are among the groups at highest risk for HIV infection, and injection drug users remain at significant risk for getting HIV.

Risky behaviors, like having anal or vaginal sex without using a condom or taking medicines to prevent or treat HIV, and sharing needles or syringes play a big role in HIV transmission. Anal sex is the highest-risk sexual behavior. If you don't have HIV, being a receptive partner (or bottom) for anal sex is the highest-risk sexual activity for getting HIV. If you do have HIV, being the insertive partner (or top) for anal sex is the highest-risk sexual activity for transmitting HIV.

But there are more tools available today to prevent HIV than ever before. Choosing less risky sexual behaviors, taking medicines to prevent and treat HIV, and using condoms with lubricants are all highly effective ways to reduce the risk of getting or transmitting HIV.

[...]

13.2

HIV Risk Behaviors

U.S. Center for Disease Control and Prevention

THE RISK OF GETTING HIV VARIES widely depending on the type of exposure or behavior (such as sharing needles or having sex without a condom). Some exposures to HIV carry a much higher risk of transmission than other exposures. For some exposures, while transmission is biologically possible, the risk is so low that it is not possible to put a precise number on it. But risks do add up over time. Even relatively small risks can add up over time and lead to a high lifetime risk of getting HIV. In other words, there may be a relatively small chance of acquiring HIV when engaging in a risk behavior with an infected partner *only once*; but, if *repeated many times*, the overall likelihood of becoming infected after repeated exposures is actually much higher.

The table below lists the risk of transmission per 10,000 exposures for various types of exposures.

ESTIMATED PER-ACT Probability of Acquiring HIV from an Infected Source, by Exposure Act*

Type of Exposure	Risk per 10,000 Exposures
Parenteral	
Blood Transfusion	9,250
Needle-Sharing During Injection Drug Use	63
Percutaneous (Needle-Stick)	23
Sexual	
Receptive Anal Intercourse	138
Insertive Anal Intercourse	11
Receptive Penile-Vaginal Intercourse	8
Insertive Penile-Vaginal Intercourse	4
Receptive Oral Intercourse	Low
Insertive Oral Intercourse	Low
Other^	
Biting	Negligible
Spitting	Negligible
Throwing Body Fluids (Including Semen or Saliva)	Negligible
Sharing Sex Toys	Negligible

Source: https://www.cdc.gov/hiv/risk/estimates/riskbehaviors.html.

* Factors that may increase the risk of HIV transmission include sexually transmitted diseases, acute and late-stage HIV infection, and high viral load. Factors that may decrease the risk include condom use, male circumcision, antiretroviral treatment, and pre-exposure prophylaxis. None of these factors are accounted for in the estimates presented in the table.
^ HIV transmission through these exposure routes is technically possible but unlikely and not well documented.

Source

Patel P., Borkowf C.B., Brooks J.T. Et al. Estimating per-act HIV transmission risk: a systematic review. AIDS. 2014. doi: 10.1097/QAD.0000000000000298.

Pretty L.A., Anderson G.S., Sweet D.J.. Human bites and the risk of human immunodeficiency virus transmission. Am J Forensic Med Pathol 1999; 20(3): 232–239.

13.3

How Can HIV Be Prevented?

U.S. Center for Disease Control and Prevention

TODAY, MORE TOOLS THAN EVER ARE available to prevent HIV. You can use strategies such as abstinence (not having sex), limiting your number of sexual partners, never sharing needles, and using condoms the right way every time you have sex. You may also be able to take advantage of newer HIV prevention medicines such as pre-exposure prophylaxis (PrEP) and post-exposure prophylaxis (PEP).

If you have HIV, there are many actions you can take to prevent transmitting it to others. The most important is taking HIV medicine (called antiretroviral therapy, or ART) as prescribed. If you take HIV medicine as prescribed and get and keep an undetectable viral load (or stay virally suppressed), you can stay healthy and have effectively no risk of transmitting HIV to an HIV-negative sex partner.

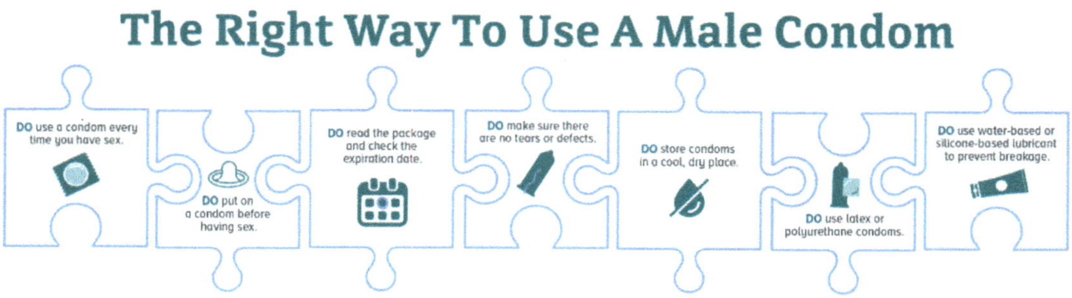

Is Abstinence the only 100% Effective HIV Prevention Option?

Yes. Abstinence means not having oral, vaginal, or anal sex. An abstinent person is someone who's never had sex or someone who's had sex but has decided not to continue having sex for some period of time. Abstinence is the only 100% effective way to prevent HIV, other sexually transmitted diseases (STDs), and pregnancy. The longer you wait to start having oral, vaginal, or anal sex, the fewer sexual partners you are likely to have in your lifetime. Having fewer partners lowers your chances of having sex with someone who has HIV or another STD.

[...]

Source: http://www.cdc.gov/hiv/topics/basic/.

How can I prevent getting HIV from oral sex?

In general, there is little to no risk of getting or transmitting HIV from oral sex. Theoretically, transmission of HIV is possible if an HIV-positive man ejaculates in his partner's mouth during oral sex. However, the risk is still very low, and much lower than with anal or vaginal sex.

Oral sex involves putting the mouth on the penis (fellatio), vagina (cunnilingus), or anus (anilingus). There's little to no risk of getting or transmitting HIV through oral sex. Factors that may increase the risk of transmitting HIV through oral sex are oral ulcers, bleeding gums, genital sores, and the presence of other sexually transmitted diseases (STDs), which may or may not be visible.

While there is little to no risk of getting HIV from oral sex, using a barrier (for example, a condom, dental dam, or cut-open nonlubricated condom) can further reduce your risk of getting or transmitting HIV and protect you and your partner from some other STDs, including gonorrhea of the throat and hepatitis.

The risk is also lower if the HIV-positive partner is taking medicine to treat HIV (called antiretroviral therapy or ART), or if the HIV-negative partner is taking medicine to prevent HIV (called pre-exposure prophylaxis or PrEP). Both PrEP and ART need to be taken as prescribed in order to work.

Because your mouth may come into contact with feces or other body fluids during oral sex, it is important that you talk to a health care provider about your chances of getting hepatitis A and B. If you've never had hepatitis A or B, there are vaccines to prevent them. Your provider can help you decide if vaccination is right for you.

[...]

How can I prevent getting HIV from anal or vaginal sex?

Use condoms the right way every time you have sex, take medicines to prevent or treat HIV if appropriate, choose less risky sexual behaviors, get tested for other sexually transmitted diseases (STDs), and limit your number of sex partners. The more of these actions you take, the safer you can be.

Specifically, you can:

- Use condoms the right way every time you have sex [...]. Learn the right way to use a male condom.
- Reduce your number of sexual partners. This can lower your chances of having a sex partner who will transmit HIV to you. The more partners you have, the more likely you are to have a partner with HIV whose viral load is not suppressed or to have a sex partner with a sexually transmitted disease. Both of these factors can increase the risk of HIV transmission.
- Talk to your doctor about pre-exposure prophylaxis (PrEP), taking HIV medicines daily to prevent HIV infection, if you are at very high risk for HIV. PrEP should be considered if you are HIV-negative and in an ongoing sexual relationship with an HIV-positive partner. PrEP also should be considered if you aren't in a mutually monogamous relationship with a partner who recently tested HIV-negative, *and* you are a:
    - o gay or bisexual man who has had anal sex without a condom or been diagnosed with an STD in the past 6 months;

- o man who has sex with both men and women; or
- o heterosexual man or woman who does not regularly use condoms during sex with partners of unknown HIV status who are at very high risk of HIV infection (for example, people who inject drugs or women who have bisexual male partners).

- Post-exposure prophylaxis (PEP) means taking HIV medicines after being potentially exposed to HIV to prevent becoming infected. If you're HIV-negative or don't know your HIV status and think you have recently been exposed to HIV during sex (for example, if the condom breaks), talk to your health care provider or an emergency room doctor about PEP right away (within 3 days). The sooner you start PEP, the better; every hour counts. If you're prescribed PEP, you'll need to take it once or twice daily for 28 days. Keep in mind that your chance of getting HIV is lower if your HIV-positive partner is taking medicine to treat HIV infection (called antiretroviral therapy, or ART) as prescribed and his or her viral load stays undetectable [...].
- If you're HIV-negative and your partner is HIV-positive, encourage your partner to get and stay on treatment. If taken as prescribed, HIV medicine (ART) can make the amount of HIV in the blood (viral load) very low—so low that a test can't detect it (called an *undetectable viral load*). People with HIV who get and keep an undetectable viral load can stay healthy for many years and have effectively no risk of transmitting HIV to an HIV-negative partner through sex.
- Choose less risky sexual behaviors. HIV is mainly spread by having anal or vaginal sex without a condom or without taking medicines to prevent or treat HIV.

Receptive anal sex is the riskiest type of sex for getting HIV. It's possible for either partner—the partner inserting the penis in the anus (the top) or the partner receiving the penis (the bottom)—to get HIV, but it is much riskier for an HIV-negative partner to be the receptive partner. That's because the lining of the rectum is thin and may allow HIV to enter the body during anal sex.

Vaginal sex also carries a risk for getting HIV, though it is less risky than receptive anal sex. Most women who get HIV get it from vaginal sex, but men can also get HIV from vaginal sex.

In general, there is little to no risk of getting or transmitting HIV from **oral sex**. Theoretically, transmission of HIV is possible if an HIV-positive man ejaculates in his partner's mouth during oral sex. However, the risk is still very low, and much lower than with anal or vaginal sex. Factors that may increase the risk of transmitting HIV through oral sex are oral ulcers, bleeding gums, genital sores, and the presence of other STDs, which may or may not be visible. [...]

Sexual activities that **don't involve contact with body fluids** (semen, vaginal fluid, or blood) carry no risk of HIV transmission but may pose a risk for other STDs.

[...]

How well do condoms prevent HIV?

If you use them the right way every time you have sex, condoms are highly effective in preventing HIV infection. But it's important to educate yourself about how to use them the right way.

Condoms can also help prevent other sexually transmitted diseases (STDs) you can get through body fluids, like gonorrhea and chlamydia. However, they provide less protection against STDs spread through skin-to-skin contact, like human papillomavirus or HPV (genital warts), genital herpes, and syphilis.

There are two main types of condoms: male and female.

Male Condoms

- A male condom is a thin layer of latex, polyurethane, polyisoprene, or natural membrane worn over the penis during sex. Male Condom Dos and Don'ts.
- Latex condoms provide the best protection against HIV. Polyurethane (plastic) or polyisoprene (synthetic rubber) condoms are good options for people with latex allergies, but plastic ones break more often than latex ones. Natural membrane (such as lambskin) condoms have small holes in them, so they don't block HIV and other STDs.
- Use water- or silicone-based lubricants to lower the chances that a condom will break or slip during sex. Don't use oil-based lubricants (for example, Vaseline, shortening, mineral oil, massage oils, body lotions, and cooking oil) with latex condoms because they can weaken the condom and cause it to break. Don't use lubricants containing nonoxynol-9. It irritates the lining of the vagina and anus and increases the risk of getting HIV.

Female Condoms

- A female condom is a thin pouch made of a synthetic latex product called nitrile. It's designed to be worn by a woman in her vagina during sex. Female Condom Dos and Don'ts.
- When worn in the vagina, female condoms are comparable to male condoms at preventing HIV, other STDs, and pregnancy. Some people use female condoms for anal sex. We don't currently know how well female condoms prevent HIV and other STDs when used by men or women for anal sex. But we do know that HIV can't travel through the nitrile barrier.
- It is safe to use any kind of lubricant with nitrile female condoms.

Even if you use condoms the right way every time you have sex, there's still a chance of getting HIV. For some individuals at high risk of getting or transmitting HIV, adding other prevention methods, like taking medicines to prevent and treat HIV, can further reduce their risk.

[...]

Can using a lubricant help reduce my HIV risk?

Yes, because lubricants can help prevent condoms from breaking or slipping.

Water-based and silicon-based lubricants are safe to use with all condoms. Oil-based lubricants and products containing oil, such as hand lotion, Vaseline, or Crisco, should not be used with latex condoms because they can weaken the condom and cause it to break. It is safe to use any kind of lubricant with nitrile female condoms. But lubricants containing nonoxynol-9 should not be used because nonoxynol-9 irritates the lining of the vagina and anus and increases the risk of getting HIV.

[...]

Can Male Circumcision Prevent HIV?

Circumcised men are less likely than uncircumcised men to get HIV from HIV-positive female partners, but circumcision doesn't decrease their risk as much as other prevention options. There is no evidence that male circumcision decreases a woman's risk of getting HIV, and the evidence about the benefits of circumcision among gay and bisexual men is inconclusive.

Circumcised men should take other actions, like using condoms the right way every time they have sex or taking medicine to prevent or treat HIV, to further reduce their risk of getting HIV or to protect their partners.

[...]

Can I Take Medicines to Prevent Getting HIV?

If you are at very high risk for HIV from sex or injecting drugs, taking HIV medicines daily, called pre-exposure prophylaxis (or PrEP), can greatly reduce your risk of HIV infection. You can combine additional strategies with PrEP to reduce your risk even further.

Federal guidelines recommend that PrEP be considered for people who are HIV-negative and at very high risk for HIV. This includes anyone who is in an ongoing sexual relationship with an HIV-positive partner. It also includes anyone who:

1. Is not in a mutually monogamous* relationship with a partner who recently tested HIV-negative, *and*
2. Is a
   - gay or bisexual man who has had anal sex without a condom or been diagnosed with an STD in the past 6 months;
   - man who has sex with both men and women; or
   - heterosexual man or woman who does not regularly use condoms during sex with partners of unknown HIV status who are at substantial risk of HIV infection (for example, people who inject drugs or women who have bisexual male partners).

PrEP is also recommended for people who've injected drugs in the past 6 months and have shared needles or works or been in drug treatment in the past 6 months.

If you have a partner who is HIV-positive and are considering getting pregnant, talk to your doctor about PrEP. It may be an option to help protect you and your baby.

PrEP involves daily medication and regular visits to a health care provider.

[...]

* Mutually monogamous means that you and your partner only have sex with each other and do not have sex outside the relationship.

Can I take medicines to prevent HIV after exposure?

Yes. Taking medicine after being potentially exposed to HIV, called post-exposure prophylaxis (or PEP), can keep you from becoming infected. But PEP must be started within 72 hours after a possible exposure.

If you think you've recently been exposed to HIV during sex (for example, if the condom breaks) or through sharing needles and works to prepare drugs (for example, cotton, cookers, water), talk to your health care provider or an emergency room doctor about PEP right away. The sooner you start PEP, the better; every hour counts. If you're prescribed PEP, you'll need to take it once or twice daily for 28 days.

Someone who is on PEP should continue to use condoms with sex partners and safe injection practices while taking PEP.

[...]

Can I get vaccinated to prevent HIV?

No. There is currently no vaccine that will prevent HIV infection or treat those who have it.

[...]

Can I use microbicides to prevent HIV?

No. Microbicides are gels, films, or suppositories that can kill or neutralize viruses and bacteria. Researchers are studying both vaginal and rectal microbicides to see if they can prevent sexual transmission of HIV, but none are currently available for use.

[...]

If I am living with HIV, how can I prevent passing it to others?

There are many actions you can take to lower your risk of transmitting HIV to a partner. The more actions you take, the safer you can be.

- The most important thing you can do is to take medicine to treat HIV infection, called antiretroviral therapy (ART), as prescribed. Taking HIV medicine as prescribed can make the amount HIV in your blood (viral load) very low—so low that a test can't detect it (called an *undetectable viral load*). Getting and keeping an undetectable viral load is the best thing you can do to stay healthy. If your viral load stays undetectable, you have effectively no risk of transmitting HIV to an HIV-negative partner through sex.

- If you're taking ART, follow your health care provider's advice. Visit your health care provider regularly and always take your medicines as prescribed. Find Ryan White HIV/AIDS Program medical care providers who help people living with HIV access the HIV primary medical care, medications, and essential support services they need (from HRSA).
- Use condoms the right way every time you have sex. Learn the right way to use a male condom.
- Choose less risky sexual behaviors. Anal sex is the highest-risk sexual activity for HIV transmission. If your partner is HIV-negative, it's less risky if they're the insertive partner (top) and you're the receptive partner (bottom) during anal sex. Oral sex is much less risky than anal or vaginal sex. Sexual activities that don't involve contact with body fluids (semen, vaginal fluid, or blood) carry no risk of HIV transmission.
- If you inject drugs, never share your needles or works with anyone.
- Talk to your partners about pre-exposure prophylaxis (PrEP), taking HIV medicines the right way, every day to prevent HIV infection. [...]
- Talk to your partners about post-exposure prophylaxis (PEP) if you think they've recently had a possible exposure to HIV (for example, if they had anal or vaginal sex without a condom or if the condom broke during sex). Your partners should talk to a health care provider right away (within 72 hours) after a possible exposure. Starting PEP immediately and taking it daily for 28 days will reduce their chance of getting HIV.
- Get tested and treated for other STDs and encourage your partners to do the same. If you are sexually active, get tested at least once a year. STDs can have long-term health consequences. They can also increase the risk of getting or transmitting HIV. Find an STD testing site.

Also, encourage your partners who are HIV-negative to get tested for HIV so they are sure about their status and can take action to keep themselves healthy. [...]

My viral load is not undetectable. How can I prevent HIV transmission?

Getting and keeping an undetectable viral load is the best thing you can do to stay healthy. If you keep an undetectable viral load, you have effectively no risk of transmitting HIV to an HIV-negative sex partner.

Most people can get the virus under control within six months. But some people face challenges that make it hard to stick to a treatment plan, and a few people cannot get an undetectable viral load even though they take HIV medicine as prescribed.

If your viral load is not undetectable—or does not stay undetectable—you can still protect your partner by using other prevention methods. The following actions are highly effective for preventing HIV:

- Use condoms the right way every time you have anal or vaginal sex.
- Choose sexual activities with little to no risk, like oral sex. You could also use condoms or dental dams with oral sex to lower the risk even more.

- Your partner can take medicine to prevent HIV, called pre-exposure prophylaxis (PrEP). Your partner will need to take PrEP every day for around 7 days before it becomes as effective as it can be for receptive anal sex and around 20 days for receptive vaginal sex,* and they'll need to keep taking PrEP every day.
- Never share syringes or works to inject drugs.

If your partner or you have other sexually transmitted diseases (STDs), getting treatment for those STDs can also help lower your risk of transmitting HIV. People who are HIV-positive and have another STD may have an increased concentration of HIV in their semen and genital fluids, which might make them more likely to transmit HIV. People who are HIV-negative and have another STD may have irritation that makes it easier for HIV to enter their body during sex, or inflammation in their body may increase the number of cells that HIV can target.

Keep in mind that your greatest chance of transmitting HIV is when you are the insertive partner (top) during anal sex. But it's also possible to transmit HIV when you are the receptive partner during anal sex or either partner during vaginal sex.

[...]

How can I prevent getting HIV from drug use?

Stopping injection and other drug use can lower your chances of getting or transmitting HIV a lot. If you keep injecting drugs, use only sterile needles and works. Never share needles or works.

You are at very high risk for getting HIV if you use a needle or works after someone with HIV has used them. Also, when people are high, they're more likely to have risky sex, which increases the chance of getting or transmitting HIV.

The best way to reduce your risk of HIV is to stop using drugs. You may need help to stop or cut down using drugs, but many resources are available. Talk with a counselor, doctor, or other health care provider about substance abuse treatment. [...]

If you keep injecting drugs, here are some things you can do to lower your risk for getting HIV and other infections:

- Use only new, sterile needles and works each time you inject. Many communities have needle exchange programs where you can get new needles and works, and some pharmacies may sell needles without a prescription.
- Never share needles or works.
- Clean used needles with bleach only when you can't get new ones. Bleaching a needle may reduce the risk of HIV but doesn't eliminate it.
- Use sterile water to fix drugs.
- Clean your skin with a new alcohol swab before you inject.

---

* The number of days depends on the person's HIV risk behaviors: For **receptive anal sex**, an HIV-negative person needs to take PrEP **7 days** in a row (and keep taking it) to get the most protection. For **receptive vaginal sex** and **injection drug use**, they need to take PrEP **20 days** in a row (and keep taking it) to get the most protection. We don't know yet how long it takes to get the most protection for **insertive anal or insertive vaginal sex**. [...]

- Be careful not to get someone else's blood on your hands or your needle or works.
- Dispose of needles safely after one use. Use a sharps container, or keep used needles away from other people.
- Get tested for HIV at least once a year.
- Ask your doctor about taking daily medicine to prevent HIV (called pre-exposure prophylaxis or PrEP).
- Don't have sex if you're high. If you do have sex, use a condom the right way every time. Learn the right way to use a male condom.

[...]

How can I prevent passing HIV to my baby?

If you have HIV, the most important thing you can do is to take medicine to treat HIV infection (called antiretroviral therapy or ART) as prescribed.

If you're pregnant, talk to your health care provider about getting tested for HIV and other ways to keep you and your child from getting HIV. Women in their third trimester should be tested again if they engage in behaviors that put them at risk for HIV.

If you are HIV-negative but you have an HIV-positive partner and are considering getting pregnant, talk to your doctor about taking pre-exposure prophylaxis (PrEP) to help keep you from getting HIV. Encourage your partner to take medicine to treat HIV (ART). People with HIV who take HIV medicine as prescribed and get and keep an undetectable viral load have effectively no risk of transmitting HIV to an HIV-negative partner through sex.

If you have HIV, take ART as prescribed. If you are treated for HIV early in your pregnancy, your risk of transmitting HIV to your baby can be 1% or less. After delivery, you can prevent transmitting HIV to your baby by avoiding breastfeeding, since breast milk contains HIV. A woman living with HIV should avoid breastfeeding even if she has an undetectable viral load.

[...]

13.4

HIV Infection

Epidemiology, Pathogenesis, Treatment, and Prevention

Gary Maartens, Connie Celum, Sharon R. Lewin

HIV PREVALENCE IS INCREASING WORLDWIDE BECAUSE people on antiretroviral therapy are living longer, although new infections decreased from 3.3 million in 2002, to 2.3 million in 2012. Global AIDS-related deaths peaked at 2.3 million in 2005, and decreased to 1.6 million by 2012. An estimated 9.7 million people in low-income and middle-income countries had started antiretroviral therapy by 2012. New insights into the mechanisms of latent infection and the importance of reservoirs of infection might eventually lead to a cure. The role of immune activation in the pathogenesis of non-AIDS clinical events (major causes of morbidity and mortality in people on antiretroviral therapy) is receiving increased recognition. Breakthroughs in the prevention of HIV important to public health include male medical circumcision, antiretrovirals to prevent mother-to-child transmission, antiretroviral therapy in people with HIV to prevent transmission, and antiretrovirals for pre-exposure prophylaxis. Research into other prevention interventions, notably vaccines and vaginal microbicides, is in progress.

Epidemiology

The HIV epidemic arose after zoonotic infections with simian immunodeficiency viruses from African primates; bushmeat hunters were probably the first group to be infected with HIV.[1] HIV-1 was transmitted from apes and HIV-2 from sooty mangabey monkeys.[1] Four groups of HIV-1 exist and represent three separate transmission events from chimpanzees (M, N, and O), and one from gorillas (P). Groups N, O, and P are restricted to west Africa. Group M, which is the cause of the global HIV pandemic, started about 100 years ago and consists of nine subtypes: A–D, F–H, J, and K. Subtype C predominates in Africa and India, and accounted for 48% of cases of HIV-1 in 2007 worldwide.[2] Subtype B predominates in western Europe, the Americas, and Australia. Circulating recombinant subtypes are becoming more common.[2] The marked genetic diversity of HIV-1 is a consequence of the error-prone function of reverse transcriptase, which results in a high mutation rate. HIV-2 is largely confined to west Africa and causes a similar illness to HIV-1, but immunodeficiency progresses more slowly and HIV-2 is less transmissible.[1]

In 2012 an estimated 35.3 million people were living with HIV.[3] Sub-Saharan Africa, especially southern Africa, has the highest global burden of HIV (70.8%; Figure 13.4.1). The global epidemiology of HIV

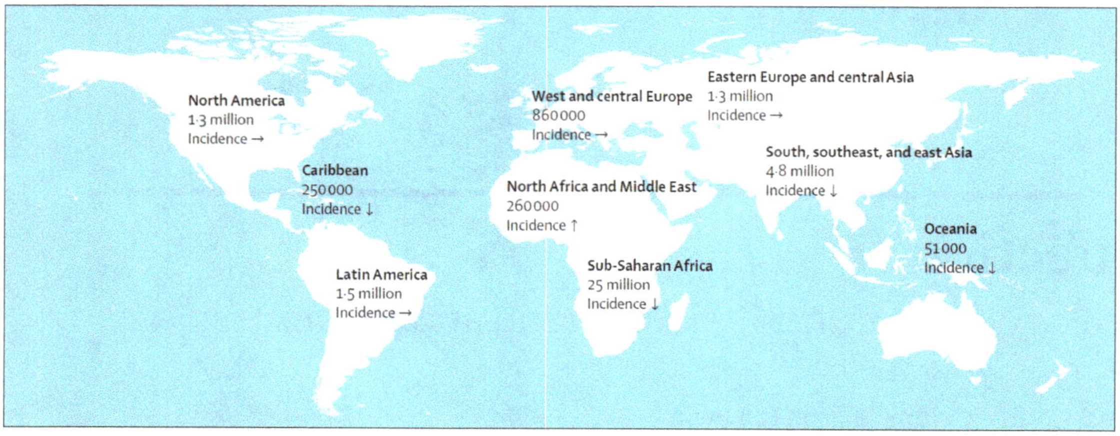

FIGURE 13.4.1 Estimated number of people living with HIV in 2012 and trends in the incidence of new infections from 2001 to 2012 by global region

Data from UNAIDS 2013 report.[3]

infection has changed markedly as a result of the expanding access to antiretroviral therapy; by 2012, 9.7 million people in low-income and middle-income countries had started antiretroviral therapy.[4] The global prevalence of HIV has increased from 31.0 million in 2002, to 35.3 million in 2012, because people on antiretroviral therapy are living longer,[5] whereas global incidence has decreased from 3.3 million in 2002, to 2.3 million in 2012.[3] The reduction in global HIV incidence is largely due to reductions in heterosexual transmission. Punitive attitudes towards people who inject drugs (especially in eastern Europe) restrict the implementation of opioid substitution treatment and needle and syringe programmes, which are effective prevention strategies that reduce HIV transmission.[6] In regions where the main route of transmission is men who have sex with men (eg, western and central Europe and the Americas), incidence is stable despite high antiretroviral therapy coverage (eg, 75% in Latin America in 2012,[3] and 80% in the UK in 2010).[7] The drivers of the HIV epidemic in men who have sex with men are complex, and include increasing risk behaviour since the introduction of effective antiretroviral therapy (a phenomenon termed therapeutic optimism[8]), high transmission risk of receptive anal intercourse, sexual networks, and stigma restricting access to care.[9]

[...]

The number of new infections in children in the 21 priority African countries in the UN Programme on HIV/AIDS (UNAIDS) global plan[10] decreased by 38% between 2009 and 2012, because of increased access to antiretrovirals to prevent mother-to-child transmission. However, access to antiretroviral therapy is much lower in children than adults.[3]

HIV is a major contributor to the global burden of disease. In 2010, HIV was the leading cause of disability-adjusted life years worldwide for people aged 30–44 years, and the fifth leading cause for all ages.[11] Global AIDS-related deaths peaked at 2.3 million in 2005, and decreased to 1.6 million by 2012.[3] About 50% of all deaths in people on antiretroviral therapy in high-income countries are not due to AIDS.[12] In one study, major causes of non-AIDS-related deaths were non-AIDS-defining cancers (23.5%), cardiovascular disease (15.7%), and liver disease (14.1%).[12] People with HIV have a 50% increased risk of myocardial infarctions than do people without HIV after adjustment for vascular risk factors.[13] Liver disease is common, mainly because of co-infection with hepatitis B and C, which share similar routes of transmission with HIV.[14]

Tuberculosis continues to be a major cause of morbidity and mortality in low-income and middle-income countries, especially in Africa.[15] Findings of a study[16] done in South Africa in the pre-antiretroviral therapy era showed that tuberculosis doubled within a year after HIV infection, thereafter incidence increased as immunity decreased, and reached a very high incidence of 25·7 per 100 person-years in patients with CD4 T-cell counts lower than 50 cells per µL.[17] Worldwide, HIV-related tuberculosis mortality is decreasing,[15] but many people with HIV in Africa die of undiagnosed tuberculosis.[18]

HIV-1 Transmission

The most important factor that increases the risk of sexual transmission of HIV-1 is the number of copies per mL of plasma HIV-1 RNA (viral load), with a 2·4 times increased risk of sexual transmission for every 1 $\log_{10}$ increase.[19] Acute HIV infection, which causes very high plasma viral loads in the first few months, is an important driver of HIV epidemics.[20] A reduction in plasma viral load of 0·7 $\log_{10}$ is estimated to reduce HIV-1 transmission by 50%.[21] Seminal and endocervical viral load independently predict risk of HIV-1 sexual transmission, after adjustment for plasma viral load.[22] Other factors associated with increased risk of sexual transmission of HIV include sexually transmitted infections (notably genital ulcers of any cause,[23] herpes simplex type-2 infection,[24] and bacterial vaginosis[25]), pregnancy,[26] and receptive anal intercourse.[27] Male circumcision is associated with a reduced risk of sexual transmission of HIV.[28]

Findings of some observational studies showed an increased risk of HIV-1 acquisition in women who used long-acting injectable progestogens for contraception, but not with combined oral contraceptives.[29] A health priority in eastern and southern Africa, where the incidence of HIV-1 in young women is very high,[30] is to find out whether long-acting injectable progestogens (the commonest form of contraception used in this region) increase HIV-1 transmission.

Behavioural factors that increase HIV-1 sexual transmission include many sexual partners,[31] and concurrent partnerships.[32] Findings of a study[33] of African heterosexual serodiscordant couples showed that self-reported condom use reduced the per-coital act risk of HIV-1 transmission by 78%.[33] Sex inequality is an important driver of the HIV epidemic, especially in sub-Saharan Africa where women account for 57% of people living with HIV.[3] Injection and non-injection drug use, including alcohol, are associated with increased sexual risk behaviour, whereas injection drug use causes HIV transmission by shared needles.[34] Women who reported intimate partner violence had an increased incidence of HIV infection in a South African study.[35] UNAIDS have identified stigma against HIV, and discrimination and punitive laws against high-risk groups (eg, men who have sex with men, people who inject drugs, and commercial sex workers) as barriers for people to undergo HIV testing, access care, and access prevention measures.[3]

Pathogenesis

HIV Life Cycle and Host Immune Responses

Figure 13.4.2 shows the virus life cycle. The main target of HIV is activated CD4 T lymphocytes; entry is via interactions with CD4 and the chemokine coreceptors, CCR5 or CXCR4. Other cells bearing CD4 and chemokine receptors are also infected, including resting CD4 T cells, monocytes and macrophages, and dendritic cells. CD4-independent HIV infection of cells can happen, notably in astrocytes[37] and renal epithelial cells,[38] and subsequent HIV gene expression has an important role in the pathogenesis of HIV-associated neurocognitive disorder (related to astrocytes) and nephropathy (related to epithelial cells). A range of host proteins interact with HIV proteins or HIV DNA to either restrict or promote virus replication in specific cell types (Table 13.4.1).

TABLE 13.4.1 Host proteins that interact with HIV proteins or DNA and either restrict or help with HIV infection in human cells

	Action	HIV target
APOBEC-3G[39]	RNA editing protein	vif
TRIM-5α[40]	E3 ubiquitin ligase tripartite motif targets viral capsid	Capsid
Tetherin (BST-2)[41]	Immunomodulatory membrane protein that inhibits virus budding	vpu
SAMHD1[42,43]	Hydrolyses dNTPs and restricts efficient reverse transcription of HIV	vpx*
TREX-1[44]	Cytosolic exonuclease that inhibits the immune recognition of viral products such as HIV DNA	HIV DNA
LEDGF/p75[45]	Brings HIV DNA in close proximity to chromatin	integrase

APOBEC-3G=apolipoprotein B mRNA-editing enzyme-catalytic polypeptide-like-3G. TRIM=tripartide motif. SAM=sterile α motif. HD1=histidine aspartic acid domain-containing protein 1. LEDGF=lens epithelium-derived growth factor. *Expressed by HIV-2 only.

Transmission of HIV across mucosal membranes is usually established by one founder virus, which has unique phenotypic properties including usage of CCR5 rather than CXR4 for entry,[46] enhanced interaction with dendritic cells, and resistance to interferon-α.[47] Transmission of the founder virus is followed by a rapid increase in HIV replication and then a striking induction of inflammatory cytokines and chemokines, which is in stark contrast to the minimum initial response to other chronic viral infections such as hepatitis B or hepatitis C.[48]

Viral load then decreases to a so-called setpoint, the level of which is established largely by innate and adaptive immune responses (Figure 13.4.2). HIV-specific CD8 killing of productively infected cells mediated by T cells happens soon after infection, and the potent adaptive immune response to HIV selects for the emergence of mutations in key epitopes, often leading to immune escape.[49] In some HLA types, such as individuals with *HLA-B27* allele infected with clade B, an effective immune response can arise, characterised by HIV-specific T cells with high avidity, polyfunctionality, and capacity to proliferate[50] against both the immunodominant and escaped peptides.[51] However, in nearly all individuals, progressive exhaustion of HIV-specific T cells happens, characterised by high expression of programmed death 1 (PD-1) on both total and HIV-specific T cells and a loss of effector function.[52]

Neutralising antibodies arise roughly 3 months after transmission and select for viral escape mutants.[53] Broadly neutralising antibodies, which can neutralise many HIV-1 subtypes, are produced by

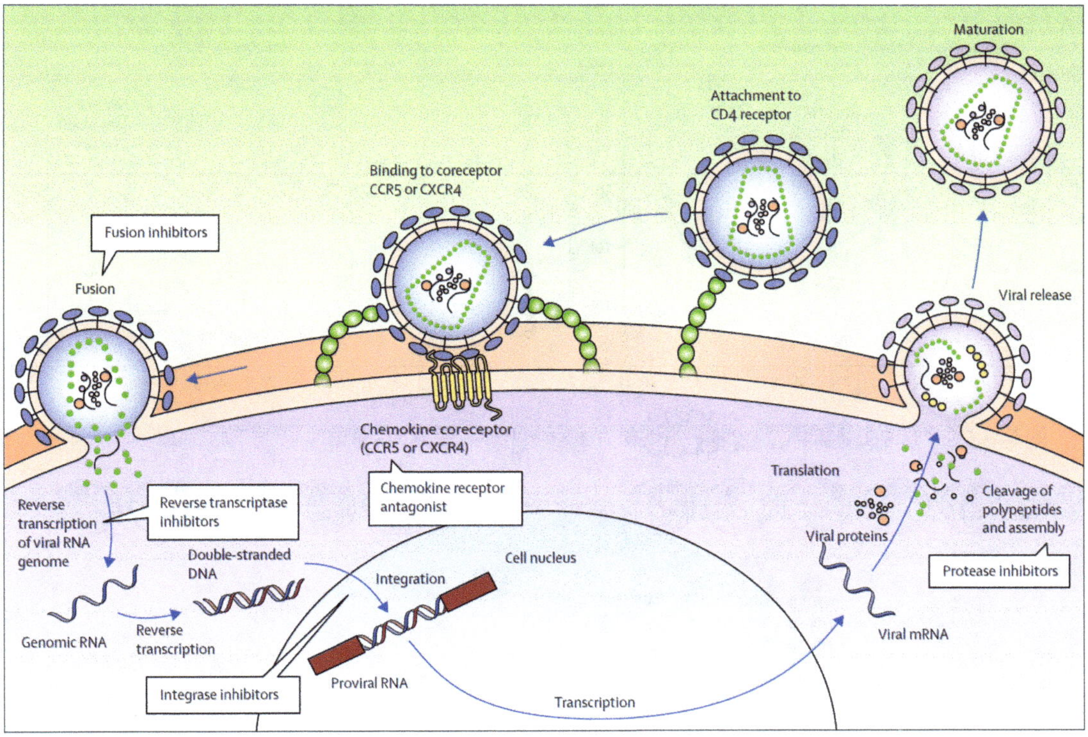

FIGURE 13.4.2 HIV life cycle showing the sites of action of different classes of antiretroviral drugs

Adapted from Walker and colleagues,[36] by permission of Elsevier.

about 20% of patients.[54] These antibodies are characterised by a high frequency of somatic mutations that often take years to develop.[55] Broadly neutralising antibodies do not usually provide benefit to the patient because of the development of viral escape mutants.[56] The production of broadly neutralising antibodies by use of new immunogen design strategies is a major focus of vaccine research.[57]

The innate immune response to HIV is largely mediated by natural killer cells, and is also crucial for virus control. Viral escape mutants also emerge, and restrict the antiviral effects of natural killer cells.[58]

Immune Dysfunction

The hallmark of HIV infection is the progressive depletion of CD4 T cells because of reduced production and increased destruction. CD4 T cells are eliminated by direct infection,[59] and bystander effects of syncitia formation, immune activation, proliferation, and senescence. In early infection, a transient reduction in circulating CD4 T cells is followed by recovery to near normal concentrations, which then slowly decrease by about 50–100 cells per μL (Figure 13.4.2).

The most important effect on T-cell homoeostasis happens very early in the gastrointestinal tract, which has a massive depletion of activated CD4 T cells with minimum recovery after antiretroviral therapy.[60] In addition to loss of total CD4 T cells, profound changes in T-cell subsets happen, including preferential loss of T-helper-17 cells,[61] and mucosal-associated invariant T cells, which are crucial for defence against bacteria.[62] The profound depletion of lymphoid cells in the gastrointestinal tract, together with enterocyte apoptosis, and enhanced gastrointestinal tract permeability,

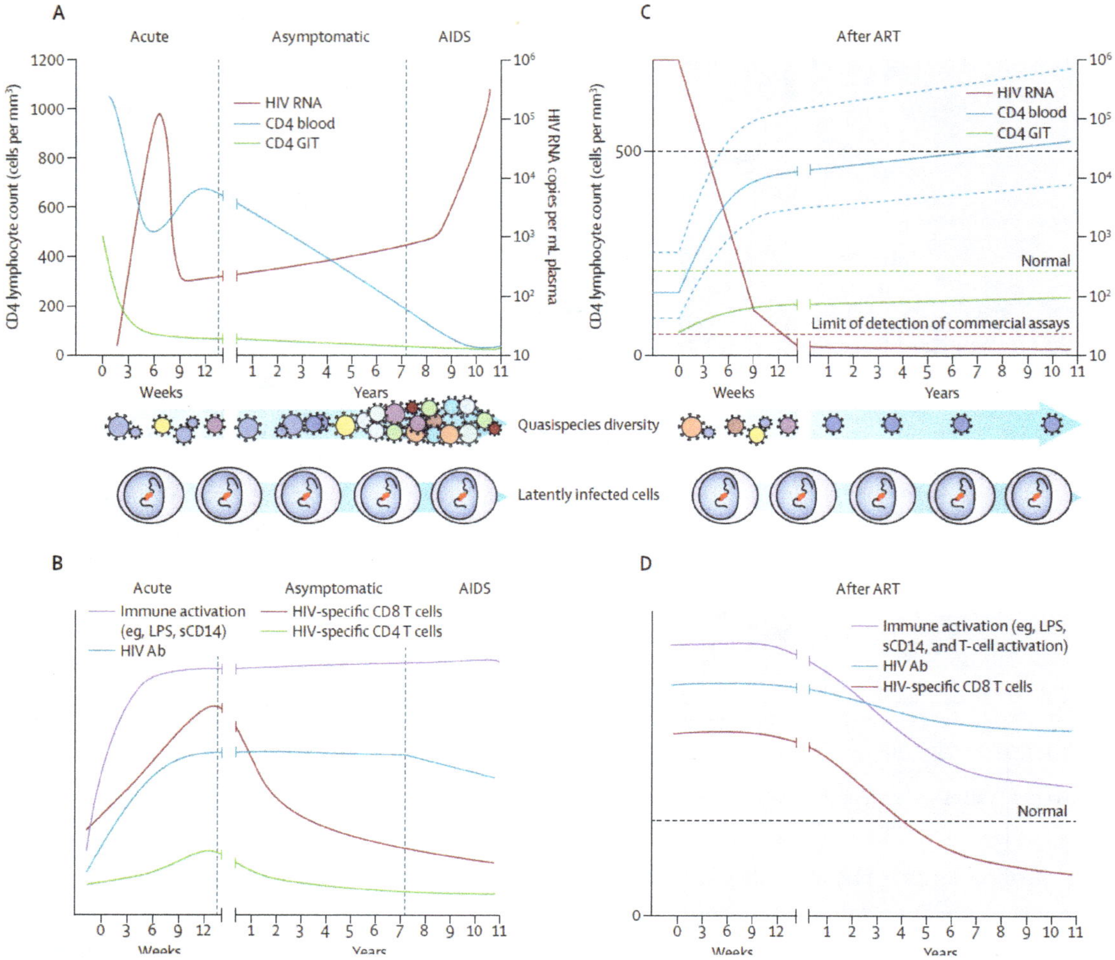

FIGURE 13.4.3 Natural history of untreated HIV infection and changes after antiretroviral therapy

(A) In untreated HIV infection, CD4 T cells are progressively lost in blood but CD4 T cells in the gastrointestinal tract are rapidly depleted early on. (B) The acute response to HIV infection includes a dramatic increase in markers of immune activation and production of non-neutralising antibodies and HIV-specific CD4 and CD8 T cells that are associated temporally with a decrease in HIV RNA in blood. (C) After antiretroviral therapy, HIV RNA significantly decreases followed by recovery of CD4 T cells, which varies between individuals (panel). By contrast, recovery of CD4 T cells in the gastrointestinal tract is reduced. (D) With reduction of HIV RNA and viral antigen, HIV-specific T cells decrease after antiretroviral therapy, whereas antibody persists in all patients. Immune activation decreases after antiretroviral therapy but in most patients remains significantly increased compared with healthy controls. GIT=gastrointestinal tract. LPS=lipopolysaccharide.

leads to increased plasma concentration of microbial products such as lipopolysaccharides.[63] Finally, destruction of the fibroblastic reticular cell network, collagen deposition, and restricted access to the T-cell survival factor interleukin 7 in the lymphoid tissue further contribute to depletion of both CD4-naive and CD8-naive T cells.[64]

Immune Activation

HIV infection is also characterised by a marked increase in immune activation, which includes both the adaptive and innate immune systems, and abnormalities in coagulation.[65] The drivers for immune activation include the direct effects of HIV as a ligand for the Toll-like receptor (TLR7 and

TLR 8) expressed on plasmacytoid dendritic cells, leading to production of interferon-α;[66] microbial translocation, with lipopolysaccharide as a potent activator or TLR4 leading to the production of pro-inflammatory cytokines such as interleukin 6 and tumour necrosis factor α (TNFα);[63] co-infection with viruses such as cyto megalovirus that induce profound expansion of activated cytomegalovirus-specific T cells;[67] and a reduced ratio of T-helper-17 and regulatory T cells, especially in the gastrointestinal tract.[61]

Evidence of residual inflammation or increased immune activation exists, even in patients with HIV with adequate CD4 T-cell restoration on antiretroviral therapy (Figure 13.4.3c). Markers of residual inflammation in patients with HIV on antiretroviral therapy have been significantly associated with mortality,[68] cardiovascular disease,[69] cancer,[70] neurological disease,[71] and liver disease.[72] Intensification of antiretroviral therapy in participants with virological suppression with the addition of the integrase inhibitor raltegravir reduced T-cell activation in about a third of participants.[73] These data suggest that low-level HIV replication might contribute to persistent inflammation. Treatment of co-infections, such as cytomegalovirus and hepatitis C, reduces T-cell activation too.[74,75]

Although many studies have identified associations between different biomarkers of inflammation and adverse clinical events, causation in studies in people has been difficult to establish. So far, strategies aimed to reduce residual inflammation in patients with HIV have consisted of small observational studies with surrogate endpoints.[76] Several drugs that are available for other indications (eg, statins, aspirin, angiotensin-converting enzyme inhibitors, and hydroxychloroquine) have the potential to reduce HIV-associated inflam mation.[76] Randomised controlled studies are needed to establish whether targeting of inflammation in people with virological suppression on antiretroviral therapy will have a significant clinical effect.

Antiretroviral Therapy

Combination antiretroviral therapy regimens that were able to suppress viral replication were developed in the late 1990s and transformed HIV from a progressive illness with a fatal outcome into a chronic manageable disease. More than 25 licensed drugs that block HIV replication at many steps in the virus lifecycle are available (Figure 13.4.3b). Recommended antiretroviral therapy regimens are less toxic, more effective, have a lower pill burden, and are dosed less frequently than the initial protease inhibitor-based regimens. Standard anti retroviral therapy regimens combine two nucleoside reverse transcriptase inhibitors (emtricitabine or lamivudine together with one of abacavir, tenofovir, or zidovudine) with a non-nucleoside reverse transcriptase inhibitor, protease inhibitor, or integrase inhibitor. Several effective nucleoside reverse transcriptase inhibitor-sparing regimens can be used if intolerance or resistance to nucleoside reverse transcriptase inhibitors develops.

After initiation of antiretroviral therapy, the plasma viral load decreases to concentrations below the lower limit of detection of available commercial assays in most people, usually within 3 months (Figure 13.4.3c). By contrast, the recovery of CD4 T cells in individuals on antiretroviral therapy is variable. In one study[77] of responses to antiretroviral therapy at 6 months in low-income countries, 56% of patients had a successful virological and CD4 response, 19% a virological response without a CD4 response, and 15% a CD4 response without a virological response. Individuals with impaired CD4 T-cell recovery despite virological suppression, which is associated with several risk factors (panel),[78] are at increased risk of adverse outcomes, including serious non-AIDS events.[79] Adjunctive interleukin

2 significantly increases CD4 T-cell counts, but does not result in clinical benefit.[80] Interleukin 7, which enhances proliferation of both naive and memory T cells, also increases CD4 T-cell counts, although whether this results in enhanced clinical benefit is unknown.[81] However, interleukin 7 might have the undesirable effect of expanding the pool of T cells that are latently infected with HIV.[82]

Panel: Factors associated with poor CD4 T-cell recovery after antiretroviral therapy

Host factors

- Older age, low CD4 nadir, high baseline HIV RNA
- HLA type
- Genetic polymorphisms in:
  - Chemokine/chemokine receptors—eg, CCR5D32,
  - Cytokine/cytokine receptors—eg, interleukin 7 receptor
  - Fas/Fas ligand

Viral factors

- CXCR4 using virus
- Co-infection with cytomegalovirus, hepatitis C virus, or GB virus C

Immunological factors

- Low thymic output
- Poor bone marrow function
- Increased immune activation
- Proliferation
- Senescence
- Increased PD-1 expression
- Increased apoptosis

Guidelines in high-income countries allow clinicians to choose a starting regimen of dual nucleoside reverse transcriptase inhibitors combined with either a non-nucleoside reverse transcriptase inhibitor, a ritonavir-boosted protease inhibitor, or an integrase inhibitor, because these three regimens have similar efficacy and tolerability.[83] Subsequent antiretroviral therapy regimen switches for virological failure are guided by the results of resistance testing. For low-income and middle-income countries, WHO recommends a public health approach to use of antiretroviral therapy with standardised first-line (non-nucleoside reverse transcriptase inhibitor plus dual nucleoside reverse transcriptase inhibitors) and second-line (ritonavir-boosted protease inhibitor plus dual nucleoside reverse transcriptase inhibitors) regimens, and restricted monitoring for both efficacy and toxic effects.[84] Resistance testing is seldom available. Clinical and CD4 count monitoring is used in many low-income countries where viral load monitoring is unavailable, but this monitoring strategy[85] results in both unnecessary switches to second-line therapy and continuation of failing first-line antiretroviral therapy regimens, which will increase the number of resistance mutations. Viral load monitoring would be cost effective in resource-limited settings if low-cost tests, which are available, were used.[86]

Investigators of a study[87] that compared a public health approach with individualised approaches to antiretroviral therapy in people starting treatment in South Africa and Switzerland, reported similar virological outcomes, but the switching rate for toxic effects in Switzerland was higher than in South Africa. Early mortality rates after initiation of antiretroviral therapy are much higher in resource-limited settings than in high-income countries after adjustment for baseline CD4 count, but the difference attenuates after 6 months.[88] Near-normal life expectancy is estimated for patients (other than people who inject drugs) who achieve a normal CD4 count and a suppressed viral load on antiretroviral therapy.[89]

Increasing data suggest that short-course antiretroviral therapy started in early HIV infection might slow disease progression, but further studies of patients presenting with acute infection need to be done.[90] Most international guidelines, including those for low-income and middle-income countries,[84] have increased the CD4 criterion for initiation of antiretroviral therapy to 500 cells per µL or higher, despite no good evidence that antiretroviral therapy initiation at CD4 counts higher than 350 cells per µL provides individual benefit.[91] Increased access to antiretroviral therapy is expected to reduce HIV transmission, but the durability of this effect is unknown, and starting antiretroviral therapy early exposes patients to toxic effects of drugs and the development of resistance before they derive clinical benefit.[92] Retention of patients in care in low-income and middle income countries will be a major challenge because the number of people eligible for antiretroviral therapy will increase from 16·7 million to 25·9 million in 2013, if the WHO 2013 guidelines are introduced.[4] In sub-Saharan Africa, 57% of people are expected to complete eligibility assessment for antiretroviral therapy, and only 65% of people who start treatment remain in care after 3 years.[93] Loss to follow-up increased with increasing population size in a large antiretroviral therapy programme in South Africa.[94] Low rates of retention care are not restricted to low-income and middle-income countries, as shown by a US report[95] that noted that only 51% of patients who were diagnosed with HIV were retained in care in 2010.

Antiretroviral therapy taken in the presence of continuing viral replication will result in the selection of sub-populations of HIV with mutations conferring resistance to antiretroviral drugs. Suboptimum adherence is the major factor associated with the development of resistance.[96] Antiretroviral drugs differ in their ability to select for resistant mutations. Some drugs (eg, emtricitabine, lamivudine, efavirenz, nevirapine, and raltegravir) rapidly select for one mutation conferring high-level resistance, whereas most other antiretrovirals select for resistance mutations slowly and need several resistant mutations before loss of drug efficacy. Patients who develop antiretroviral resistance can transmit resistant virus to others. The prevalence of antiretroviral resistance in antiretroviral therapy-naive people in high-income countries has reached a plateau of 10–17% with resistance to one or more antiretroviral drugs, whereas the prevalence is steadily increasing in low-income and middle-income countries, reaching 6·6% in 2009.[97] Guidelines for high-income countries recommend a resistance test before initiation of antiretroviral therapy, but this strategy is too expensive to implement in resource-limited settings.

Immune Reconstitution Disease

Immune reconstitution disease, also called immune reconstitution inflammatory syndrome, is an immunopathological response resulting from the rapid restoration of pathogen-specific immune responses to pre-existing antigens combined with immune dysregulation, which happens shortly after initiation of antiretroviral therapy.[98] Most commonly, the antigens triggering immune reconstitution disease are from opportunistic infections, notably tuberculosis, cryptococcal meningitis, and cytomegalovirus retinitis.[99] Immune reconstitution disease is common, with an overall incidence of 16.1% reported in a systematic review.[99] The disease causes high morbidity, but mortality is low (4.5%), except with cryptococcal meningitis immune reconstitution disease (20.8% mortality). Findings of a small randomised controlled trial[100] showed benefit of adjunctive prednisone in participants with tuberculosis-associated immune reconstitution disease. Immune reconstitution disease happens more commonly when antiretroviral therapy is started in patients with low CD4 counts or soon after starting treatment for the opportunistic infection. Strategies to reduce immune reconstitution disease include initiation of antiretroviral therapy at high CD4 counts, delayed initiation of antiretroviral therapy in patients with an infection (especially if infection includes the CNS), and screening for and prevention of opportunistic infections before initiation of antiretroviral therapy.[98]

Latency, Reservoirs, and Potential Cure

Despite great successes of antiretroviral therapy in the control of HIV replication and significant reduction of morbidity and mortality, antiretroviral therapy is unable to cure HIV and life-long treatment is needed. HIV can persist in patients on antiretroviral therapy because of resting memory T cells that are long-lived and latently infected,[101] residual replication in some individuals,[73] and anatomical reservoirs such as the gastrointestinal tract,[102] lymphoid tissue, and the CNS.[103]

Latency is defined as integration of HIV DNA into the host genome in the absence of virus production. Latency can be established in vitro via direct infection of resting CD4 T cells in the presence of specific chemokines,[104] or after reversion of an activated infected T cell to a resting state (Figure 13.4.3d).[105] Latency has been shown in vivo in central and transitional memory T cells,[101,106] and in naive T cells.[107] Latency can also be established in monocyte-macrophages[108] and astrocytes,[109] but the importance of these cells to virus persistence in patients on antiretroviral therapy is unclear.

Many factors restrict efficient HIV transcription from the integrated provirus in latently infected resting CD4 T cells including the sub-nuclear localisation of the provirus, the absence of transcription factors such as NF-kB and nuclear factor of activated T cells, the presence of transcriptional repressors, the epigenetic control of the HIV promoter (including histone modification by acetylation and methylation, and DNA modification), and sub-optimum concentrations of the virus protein *tat*.[110] Additionally, post-transcriptional blocks including microRNAs restrict viral translation in resting T cells.[111] Finally, latently infected T cells can undergo homoeostatic proliferation[106] via stimulation from homoeostatic cytokines such as interleukin 7,[82] which further contribute to ther long half-life and persistence.

Much interest surrounds the discovery of either a functional cure (long-term control of HIV without antiretroviral therapy) or a sterilising cure (complete elimination of all HIV-infected cells). Hopes that a cure might be possible have been raised by a case report of a man who underwent stem cell transplants for leukaemia,[112] and an infant who started antiretroviral therapy soon after delivery.[113] The best documented report of cure is the Berlin patient,[112] a man with HIV on antiretroviral therapy who had acute myeloid leukaemia and received two bone marrow transplants from a donor with a homozygous defect in CCR5, a key coreceptor needed by HIV for cell entry. Shortly after transplantation, the patient ceased antiretroviral therapy and minimum or no virus has been detected in plasma or tissue for more than 6 years.[114] This case has inspired the development of gene therapy to eliminate CCR5 in patient-derived T cells and stem cells with new technologies such as zinc finger nucleases that can effectively eliminate CCR5 expression.[115]

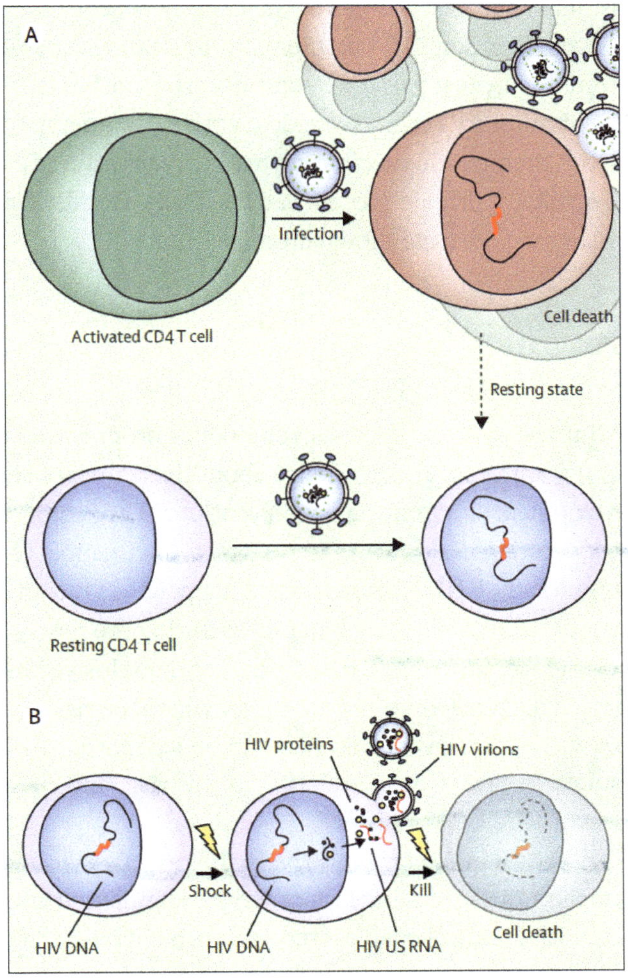

FIGURE 13.4.4 Latency and activation of cellular HIV infection

(A) Latency can be established via survival of an activated infected T cell, which reverts to a memory state, or after direct infection of a resting CD4 T cell in the presence of appropriate signalling mediated by either chemokines or cell-to-cell signalling. (B) Activating transcription from latency will induce HIV transcription (with an increase in cell associated unspliced RNA), HIV protein, and virion production with the aim of cell death induction by either virus-induced cytolysis or stimulation of HIV-specific cytotoxic T cells. Additional interventions that kill the cell might also be needed

Early initiation of antiretroviral therapy alone might have a substantial effect on reduction of the reservoir and preservation of effective immune function. Long-term control of low-level viraemia after cessation of antiretroviral therapy has been reported in 1–15% of individuals who initiated antiretroviral therapy in acute infection.[116,117] Very early initiation of antiretroviral therapy might restrict infection of long-lived central memory T cells that have been latently infected.[118]

Another approach to cure HIV is to eliminate latently infected T cells. One strategy under investigation is the activation of latent HIV, which will induce expression of viral proteins leading to immune-mediated clearance or cytolysis of infected cells (Figure 13.4.3d). In vitro, many compounds can activate HIV production from latency, including histone deacetylase inhibitors, methylation inhibitors, activators of NF-kB such as prostratin, and other compounds including disulfiram.[119]

Results of the first studies of the histone deacetylase inhibitor vorinostat, showed an increase in HIV transcription,[120,121] but it remains unclear whether activation alone effectively eliminates latently infected cells, as suggested by one in-vitro model of HIV latency.[122] Additionally, boost of HIV-specific T-cell immunity might be needed, with either therapeutic vaccination or immuno-modulation. Up to now, therapeutic vaccination to allow cessation of antiretroviral therapy has yielded disappointing results,[123] although recent vaccine trials with dendritic cells[124] and a cytomegalovirus vector in a simian model[125] have shown promise.[126]

Prevention

Mother-to-Child HIV-1 Transmission

During the past two decades, remarkable progress has been made in the risk reduction of perinatal HIV-1 transmission. Knowledge about the timing of HIV-1 transmission to infants has allowed the development of appropriate interventions. The risk of HIV-1 transmission to the infant is about 25% at delivery in the absence of interventions, with most of the risk arising after 36 weeks and especially intrapartum.[127] HIV-1 transmission happens at a rate of 8·9 per 100 child-years of breastfeeding after the fourth week,[128] with higher rates during the first 4 weeks.[119] Mixed feeding roughly doubles the risk of HIV-1 transmission compared with exclusive breastfeeding.[127] Prolonged breastfeeding is the norm in most resource-poor settings, where the risk of transmitting HIV-1 to children reached about 40% without interventions. Recommended mother-to-child HIV-1 transmission interventions have resulted in a ten times reduction in this risk, and complete elimination of mother-to-child HIV-1 transmission is now feasible.

Antiretroviral therapy is the mainstay of prevention of mother-to-child HIV-1 transmission. Antepartum zidovudine monotherapy, augmented with one dose of nevirapine during labour, was an effective and affordable intervention, but it has been superseded by standard combination antiretroviral therapy for women who do not qualify for continuing antiretroviral therapy. Combination antiretroviral therapy is more effective at prevention of mother-to-child HIV-1 transmission than zidovudine plus one dose of nevirapine,[129] and has the additional advantages of reducing sexual HIV transmission and reducing HIV-associated morbidity and mortality. Antiretroviral therapy should ideally be started after the first trimester, provided that women are well enough to wait. In resource-limited settings the reduction in infant HIV transmission by formula feeding is offset by a higher infant mortality,[130] which shows the crucial role that breastfeeding has in child health. Strategies to reduce HIV transmission from breastfeeding in resource-limited settings include the use of antiretroviral monotherapy to infants,[131] or continuing combination antiretroviral therapy until weaning in mothers who do not qualify for ongoing antiretroviral therapy.[129,132] WHO recommends either continuing combination antiretroviral therapy until weaning or for life in pregnant women with HIV who do not qualify for continuing antiretroviral therapy.[84]

Antiretrovirals alone will not reach the goal of elimination of prevention of mother-to-child HIV-1 transmission. Access to antenatal care, HIV testing, and mother-to-child HIV-1 transmission interventions will need to be substantially increased in regions with high HIV prevalence.[133] In Africa, uptake of mother-to-child HIV-1 transmission interventions was improved if the male partner was included, but this is often difficult to achieve.[133] In low-income and middle-income countries, many women present late for antenatal care or deliver without antenatal care; therefore, HIV transmission to infants will be higher than when antiretroviral therapy is started at the optimum time of about 14 weeks. A further challenge to the implementation of antiretroviral therapy for mothers to prevent transmission from breastfeeding is that antiretroviral therapy adherence post partum has been found to be significantly lower than antepartum in a recent meta-analysis.[134] Studies of interventions to improve post-partum adherence to antiretroviral therapy are urgently needed. Last, in view of the annual HIV-1 incidence rates of up to 10% in some areas of southern Africa, a crucial priority for prevention of mother-to-child HIV-1 transmission is to reduce new HIV infections in young women, which would lead to fewer HIV-1 infected pregnant women and infants.

Sexual HIV Transmission

Prevention of sexual HIV transmission has been a priority since the beginning of the epidemic. No one prevention intervention is effective enough on its own, and many interventions are necessary to control the epidemic. Several major advances have been made in research on prevention intervention in the past 5 years, especially including the use of antiretrovirals. The most potent intervention to reduce sexual transmission of HIV is antiretroviral therapy, as shown by findings of the landmark HPTN 052 study.[135] In this study the partner with HIV from a serodiscordant couple with CD4 counts of 350–550 cells per μL were randomised to receive immediate antiretroviral therapy or deferred antiretroviral therapy (when two CD4 counts were <250 cells per μL). Immediate antiretroviral therapy was associated with a 96% reduction in HIV transmission events, in the context of almost universal viral suppression. Results of HPTN 052 also showed the need for complementary prevention interventions, because 25% of HIV transmissions were not from the infected partner. The public health effect of antiretroviral therapy coverage was assessed in rural KwaZulu-Natal, South Africa, an area with very high HIV prevalence.[136] The risk of HIV acquisition was associated with antiretroviral therapy coverage in the local community. HIV acquisition was 38% lower in communities with high antiretroviral therapy coverage, defined as 30–40% among all HIV-infected people, than in communities with antiretroviral therapy coverage of less than 10%.[136] The population-level effect of earlier antiretroviral therapy initiation at all CD4 counts, the so-called test and treat strategy, is being studied in randomised trials.

TABLE 13.4.2 Association between adherence and efficacy of oral tenofovir-emtricitabine for the prevention of HIV-1 acquisition in trials of preexposure prophylaxis

	Efficacy of tenofovir-emtricitabine compared with placebo	Adherence*
Partners PrEP[144]	75%	82%
Botswana TDF2[145]	62%	79%
Bangkok Tenofovir Study[146]	49%	67%
iPrEx[147]	44%	51%
Fem-PrEP[148]	6%	26%
VOICE[149]	−4·2%	29%

*Assessed by plasma tenofovir concentrations.

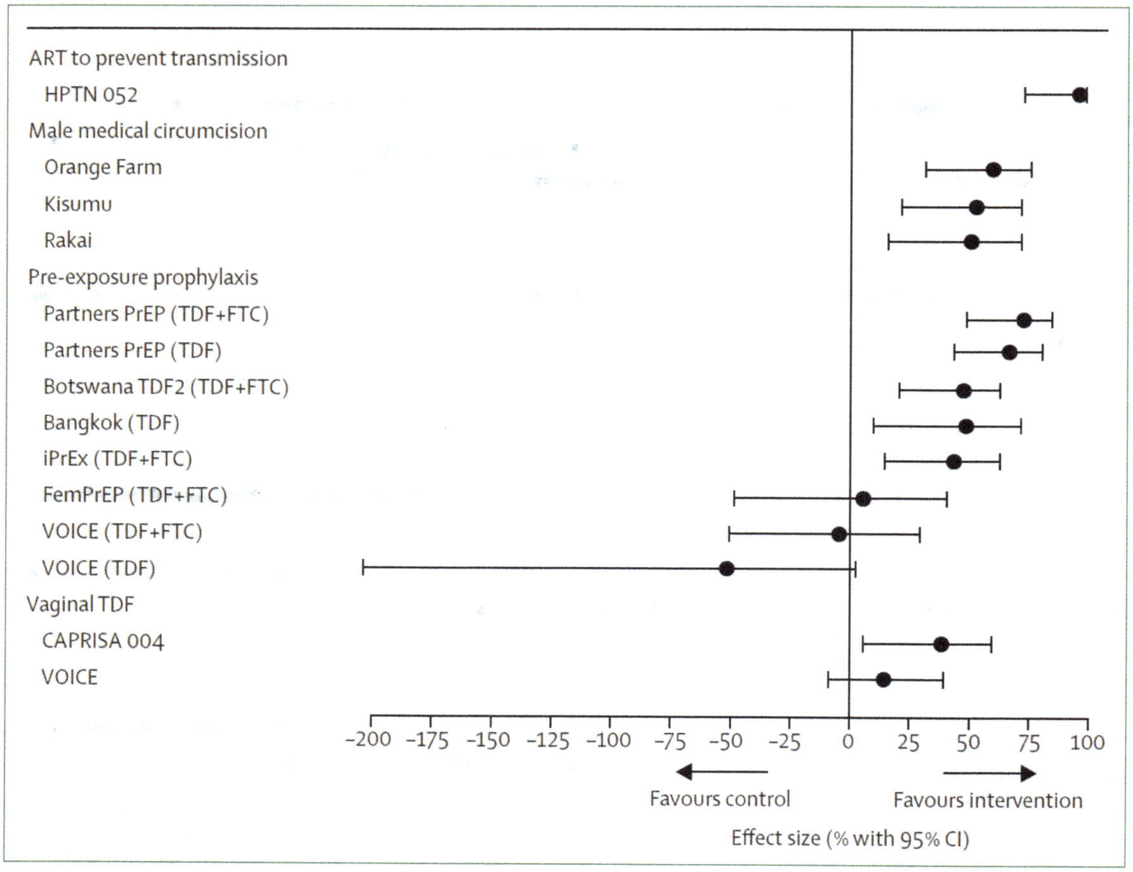

FIGURE 13.4.5 Clinical trials of interventions to prevent sexual transmission of HIV-1

TDF=tenofovir. FTC=emtricitabine. References for studies: HPTN052;[135] Orange Farm;[141] Kisumu;[142] Rakai;[143] Partners PrEP;[144] Botswana TDF2;[145] Bangkok;[146] iPrEX;[147] FemPrEP;[148] VOICE;[149] CAPRISA 004.150

The feasibility of achievement of the benefits of antiretroviral therapy will need effective interventions to greatly increase knowledge of HIV status (achieved in Project Accept[137] through community mobilisation and mobile HIV testing), and near universal testing (accomplished through home-based HIV testing).[138] Effective messaging will be needed to motivate people to initiate antiretroviral therapy when they are asymptomatic and at high CD4 counts, and to address barriers to linkages between HIV care and retention in care.[139] A cautionary point about the introduction of the test and treat strategy is that it could increase antiretroviral resistance.[140]

Pre-exposure prophylaxis with daily oral tenofovir or tenofovir plus emtricitabine effectively reduced HIV acquisition in four of six trials (Figure 13.4.5). The efficacy of pre-exposure prophylaxis ranged from 44% to 75%, and was strongly associated with adherence (Table 13.4.2). Factors that affect risk perception, uptake of pre-exposure prophylaxis, and adherence to pre-exposure prophylaxis need to be studied in different populations at high risk for HIV.

Vaginal and, more recently, rectal microbicides are attractive interventions because, unlike condoms, they are under the control of the receptive partner. Findings of 12 clinical trials of vaginal microbicides with non-specific activity against HIV and sexually transmitted infections failed to show efficacy.[151] The emphasis has shifted to vaginal microbicides that target different stages of the HIV life cycle.[152] Results of the CAPRISA 004 trial[150] in South Africa showed that pericoital use of 1% tenofovir gel reduced HIV acquisition by 39%. By contrast, in the VOICE trial[149] the daily 1% tenofovir gel group was stopped early because of absence of efficacy. The results of the FACTS 001 study (NCT01386294), a confirmatory trial of pericoital use of 1% tenofovir gel, are awaited. In recognition of the challenges with daily or pericoital dosing of topical microbicides, novel delivery strategies are being assessed with slow drug-eluting delivery devices, such as intra-vaginal rings containing antiretrovirals.[153]

Medical male circumcision is an effective HIV prevention intervention, which significantly decreased HIV acquisition in men (incidence risk ratio 0·5 at 12 months compared with men randomised to the control group who were not circumcised) in a meta-analysis of three randomised controlled trials done in Africa.[154] In high-risk communities in Africa, for every eight operations done, one HIV infection is expected to be averted, and the rate of male-to-female HIV transmission after medical male circumcision is reduced by 46%.[155] Medical male circumcision is cost-saving in sub-Saharan Africa.[156] Task shifting of medical male circumcision from doctors to non-physician clinicians is safe,[157] and would help scale up in low-income countries. Despite the potential public health benefits of medical male circumcision, the past 5 years have shown several scale-up challenges.[158] Many strategies are needed to increase demand for medical male circumcision, including promotion of benefits of circumcision to men and their female partners, and supply-side interventions to provide medical male circumcision through mobile clinics and devices that reduce procedure time.[158] Findings of meta-analyses of studies in several different risk groups and regions have shown that behavioural interventions reduce self-reported risk behaviour.[126,159–162] Findings of some studies of behavioural interventions showed that condom use reduced the incidence of HIV infection.[160,163] Voluntary counselling and testing for HIV reduces the number of self-reported sexual partners, but the benefit is largely confined to people with HIV.[164]

Other interventions to reduce HIV infectiousness have focused on treatment of co-infections, notably herpes simplex type-2 infection, which causes genital herpes. Aciclovir and valaciclovir decrease plasma and genital HIV concentrations.[165] To establish whether the magnitude of HIV suppression was sufficient to reduce HIV transmission, a placebo-controlled trial was done in African HIV serodiscordant couples, aciclovir reduced plasma HIV concentrations by 0·25 $\log_{10}$, which was not associated with decreased HIV transmission,[166] but delayed HIV disease progression slightly.[167] Increased doses of valaciclovir achieved significantly higher reductions in plasma HIV concentrations.[168] Additional research is needed to define the role of other interventions to treat co-infections.[169] The first trial of population-based interventions to control sexually transmitted infections showed a reduction in HIV incidence,[170] but three subsequent trials and a meta-analysis reported no significant effect on HIV incidence.[171]

Vaccines

Big challenges face the development of an effective HIV vaccine, including the genetic diversity of HIV, uncertainty about what constitutes protective immunity, and difficulty in the development of antigens that are highly immunogenic. Findings of clinical trials of HIV vaccines have eliminated several candidate vaccines that have not shown efficacy. One trial[172] of a prime-boost HIV vaccine strategy that used an adenovirus vector resulted in an increased rate of HIV infections in the active group in uncircumcised men and men who had pre-existing antibodies to the adenovirus vector serotype. The RV144 trial[173] done in Thailand, provided the only evidence up to now that vaccine protection could be achieved with a 31% reduction in HIV acquisition. Immune correlates of protection from the RV144 trial,[174] together with new vector approaches that improve the breadth of T-cell responses and identify targets for broadly neutralising antibodies, will hopefully result in the development of more effective vaccines.[175]

Conclusions

HIV continues to be a major contributor to the global burden of disease, especially in sub-Saharan Africa. Antiretroviral therapy is changing the global epidemiology of HIV by increasing prevalence because of reductions in AIDS deaths, and is contributing to decreasing HIV incidence by reduction of the risk of transmission. HIV incidence in men who have sex with men is not decreasing despite high antiretroviral therapy coverage. The drivers of the HIV epidemic in men who have sex with men include increasing risk behaviour since the introduction of effective antiretroviral therapy, the high transmission risk of receptive anal intercourse, sexual networks, and stigma restricting access to care. In injection drug users stigma plays a major part in restriction of access to interventions that prevent HIV and care for those who are HIV-positive. Immune activation, which is reduced but not abolished by antiretroviral therapy, plays an important part in the pathogenesis of vascular disease, the risk of which is increased in HIV infection. Improved understanding of viral latency and reservoirs might result in a cure. Recent advances in the prevention of HIV have been dominated by the role of antiretroviral drugs in reduction of mother-to-child transmission and as pre-exposure prophylaxis in high risk groups. The use of antiretroviral therapy in early HIV infection to reduce transmission is being studied in randomised controlled trials, but there will be implementation challenges in countries with a generalised HIV epidemic. An effective vaccine remains elusive despite two decades of effort.

Contributors

All authors contributed equally.

Declaration of Interests

SL's institution has received funding from Merck Sharp and Dohme, Gilead, Janssen, Bristol-Myers Squibb, and ViiV Healthcare for her participation in investigator initiated research, preparation of educational materials, presentations at symposia, and consultancy work. GM and CC declare no competing interests. There was no funding source for this Seminar.

References

1. Sharp PM, Hahn BH. Origins of HIV and the AIDS pandemic. *Cold Spring Harb Perspect Med* 2011; **1**: 006841.

2. Hemelaar J, Gouws E, Ghys PD, Osmanov S, for the WHO-UNAIDS Network for HIV Isolation and Characterisation. Global trends in molecular epidemiology of HIV-1 during 2000–2007. *AIDS* 2011; **25**: 679–89.
3. UNAIDS. Report on the global AIDS epidemic 2013. http://www.unaids.org/en/media/unaids/ contentassets/documents/epidemiology/2013/gr2013/UNAIDS_Global_Report_2013_en.pdf (accessed Nov 9, 2013).
4. WHO. Global update on HIV treatment 2013: results, impact and opportunities. June 2013. Geneva, Switzerland; World Health Organization, 2013.
5. Zaidi J, Grapsa E, Tanser F, Newell ML, Barnighausen T. Dramatic increases in HIV prevalence after scale-up of antiretroviral treatment: a longitudinal population-based HIV surveillance study in rural kwazulu-natal. *AIDS* 2013; **27**: 2301–05.
6. Degenhardt L, Mathers B, Vickerman P, Rhodes T, Latkin C, Hickman M. Prevention of HIV infection for people who inject drugs: why individual, structural, and combination approaches are needed. *Lancet* 2010; **376**: 285–301.
7. Birrell PJ, Gill ON, Delpech VC, et al. HIV incidence in men who have sex with men in England and Wales 2001–10: a nationwide population study. *Lancet Infect Dis* 2013; **13**: 313–18.
8. Mayer KH, Mimiaga MJ. Past as prologue: the refractory and evolving HIV epidemic among men who have sex with men. *Clin Infect Dis* 2011; **52**: 1371–73.
9. Beyrer C, Sullivan P, Sanchez J, et al. The global HIV epidemics in MSM: time to act. *AIDS* 2013; 27: 2665–78.
10. UNAIDS. 2013 progress report on the global plan towards the elimination of new HIV infections among children by 2015 and keeping their mothers alive. Nov, 2013. http://www.unaids.org/en/media/ unaids/contentassets/documents/unaidspublication/2013/20130625_progress_global_plan_en.pdf (accessed Jan 30, 2014).
11. Ortblad KF, Lozano R, Murray CJ. The burden of HIV: insights from the GBD 2010. *AIDS* 2013; **27**: 2003–17.
12. Antiretroviral Therapy Cohort Collaboration. Causes of death in HIV-1-infected patients treated with antiretroviral therapy, 1996–2006: collaborative analysis of 13 HIV cohort studies. *Clin Infect Dis* 2010; **50**: 1387–96.
13. Freiberg MS, Chang CC, Kuller LH, et al. HIV infection and the risk of acute myocardial infarction. *JAMA Intern Med* 2013; **173**: 614–22.
14. Joshi D, O'Grady J, Dieterich D, Gazzard B, Agarwal K. Increasing burden of liver disease in patients with HIV infection. *Lancet* 2011; **377**: 1198–209.
15. Glaziou P, Falzon D, Floyd K, Raviglione M. Global epidemiology of tuberculosis. *Semin Respir Crit Care Med* 2013; **34**: 3–16.
16. Sonnenberg P, Glynn JR., Fielding K, Murray J, Godfrey-Faussett P, Shearer S. How soon after infection with HIV does the risk of tuberculosis start to increase? A retrospective cohort study in South African gold miners. *J Infect Dis* 2005; **191**: 150–58.
17. Holmes CB, Wood R, Badri M, et al. CD4 decline and incidence of opportunistic infections in Cape Town, South Africa: implications for prophylaxis and treatment. *J Acquir Immune Defic SynDr.* 2006; **42**: 464–69.
18. Cohen T, Murray M, Wallengren K, Alvarez GG, Samuel EY, Wilson D. The prevalence and drug sensitivity of tuberculosis among patients dying in hospital in KwaZulu-Natal, South Africa: a postmortem study. *PLoS Med* 2010; **7**: e1000296.

19. Quinn TC, Wawer MJ, Sewankambo N, et al, and the Rakai Project Study Group. Viral load and heterosexual transmission of human immunodeficiency virus type 1. *N Engl J Med* 2000; **342**: 921–29.
20. Cohen MS, Shaw GM, McMichael AJ, Haynes BF. Acute HIV-1 Infection. *N Engl J Med* 2011; **364**: 1943–54.
21. Lingappa JR., Hughes JP, Wang RS, et al, and the Partners in Prevention HSV/HIV Transmission Study Team. Estimating the impact of plasma HIV-1 RNA reductions on heterosexual HIV-1 transmission risk. *PLoS One* 2010; **5**: e12598.
22. Baeten JM, Kahle E, Lingappa JR., et al, and the Partners in Prevention HSV/HIV Transmission Study Team. Genital HIV-1 RNA predicts risk of heterosexual HIV-1 transmission. *Sci Transl Med* 2011; **3**: 77ra29.
23. Røttingen JA, Cameron DW, Garnett GP. A systematic review of the epidemiologic interactions between classic sexually transmitted diseases and HIV: how much really is known? *Sex Transm Dis* 2001; **28**: 579–97.
24. Glynn JR., Biraro S, Weiss HA. Herpes simplex virus type 2: a key role in HIV incidence. *AIDS* 2009; **23**: 1595–98.
25. Atashili J, Poole C, Ndumbe PM, Adimora AA, Smith JS. Bacterial vaginosis and HIV acquisition: a meta-analysis of published studies. *AIDS* 2008; **22**: 1493–501.
26. Mugo NR, Heffron R, Donnell D, et al, and the Partners in Prevention HSV/HIV Transmission Study Team. Increased risk of HIV-1 transmission in pregnancy: a prospective study among African HIV-1-serodiscordant couples. *AIDS* 2011; **25**: 1887–95.
27. Baggaley RF, White RG, Boily MC. HIV transmission risk through anal intercourse: systematic review, meta-analysis and implications for HIV prevention. *Int J Epidemiol* 2010; **39**: 1048–63.
28. Weiss HA, Quigley MA, Hayes RJ. Male circumcision and risk of HIV infection in sub-Saharan Africa: a systematic review and meta-analysis. *AIDS* 2000; **14**: 2361–70.
29. Polis CB, Curtis KM. Use of hormonal contraceptives and HIV acquisition in women: a systematic review of the epidemiological evidence. *Lancet Infect Dis* 2013; **13**: 797–808.
30. Butler AR, Smith JA, Polis CB, Gregson S, Stanton D, Hallett TB. Modelling the global competing risks of a potential interaction between injectable hormonal contraception and HIV risk. *AIDS* 2013; **27**: 105–13.
31. Tanser F, Bärnighausen T, Hund L, Garnett GP, McGrath N, Newell ML. Effect of concurrent sexual partnerships on rate of new HIV infections in a high-prevalence, rural South African population: a cohort study. *Lancet* 2011; **378**: 247–55.
32. Epstein H, Morris M. Concurrent partnerships and HIV: an inconvenient truth. *J Int AIDS Soc* 2011; **14**: 13.
33. Hughes JP, Baeten JM, Lingappa JR., et al, and the Partners in Prevention HSV/HIV Transmission Study Team. Determinants of per-coital-act HIV-1 infectivity among African HIV-1-serodiscordant couples. *J Infect Dis* 2012; **205**: 358–65.
34. Crawford ND, Vlahov D. Progress in HIV reduction and prevention among injection and noninjection drug users. *J Acquir Immune Defic SynDr.* 2010; **55** (suppl 2): S84–87.
35. Jewkes RK, Dunkle K, Nduna M, Shai N. Intimate partner violence, relationship power inequity, and incidence of HIV infection in young women in South Africa: a cohort study. *Lancet* 2010; **376**: 41–48.
36. Davidson's Principles and Practice of Medicine, 22nd edn. Walker BR, Colledge NR, Ralston SH, Penman I, eds. London, UK: Churchill Livingstone. 2014.
37. Liu Y, Liu H, Kim BO, et al. CD4-independent infection of astrocytes by human immunodeficiency virus type 1: requirement for the human mannose receptor. *J Virol* 2004; **78**: 4120–33.

38. Chen P, Chen BK, Mosoian A, et al. Virological synapses allow HIV-1 uptake and gene expression in renal tubular epithelial cells. *J Am Soc Nephrol* 2011; **22**: 496–507.
39. Sheehy AM, Gaddis NC, Malim MH. The antiretroviral enzyme APOBEC3G is degraded by the proteasome in response to HIV-1 Vif. *Nat Med* 2003; **9**: 1404–07.
40. Stremlau M, Owens CM, Perron MJ, Kiessling M, Autissier P, Sodroski J. The cytoplasmic body component TRIM5alpha restricts HIV-1 infection in Old World monkeys. *Nature* 2004; **427**: 848–53.
41. Neil SJ, Zang T, Bieniasz PD. Tetherin inhibits retrovirus release and is antagonized by HIV-1 Vpu. *Nature* 2008; **451**: 425–30.
42. Hrecka K, Hao C, Gierszewska M, et al. Vpx relieves inhibition of HIV-1 infection of macrophages mediated by the SAMHD1 protein. *Nature* 2011; **474**: 658–61.
43. Laguette N, Sobhian B, Casartelli N, et al. SAMHD1 is the dendritic- and myeloid-cell-specific HIV-1 restriction factor counteracted by Vpx. *Nature* 2011; **474**: 654–57.
44. Yan N, Regalado-Magdos AD, Stiggelbout B, Lee-Kirsch MA, Lieberman J. The cytosolic exonuclease TREX1 inhibits the innate immune response to human immunodeficiency virus type 1. *Nat Immunol* 2010; **11**: 1005–13.
45. Maertens G, Cherepanov P, Pluymers W, et al. LEDGF/p75 is essential for nuclear and chromosomal targeting of HIV-1 integrase in human cells. *J Biol Chem* 2003; **278**: 33528–39.
46. Keele BF, Giorgi EE, Salazar-Gonzalez JF, et al. Identification and characterization of transmitted and early founder virus envelopes in primary HIV-1 infection. *Proc Natl Acad Sci USA* 2008; **105**: 7552–57.
47. Parrish NF, Gao F, Li H, et al. Phenotypic properties of transmitted founder HIV-1. *Proc Natl Acad Sci USA* 2013; **110**: 6626–33.
48. Stacey AR, Norris PJ, Qin L, et al. Induction of a striking systemic cytokine cascade prior to peak viremia in acute human immunodeficiency virus type 1 infection, in contrast to more modest and delayed responses in acute hepatitis B and C virus infections. *J Virol* 2009; **83**: 3719–33.
49. Goonetilleke N, Liu MK, Salazar-Gonzalez JF, et al, and the CHAVI Clinical Core B. The first T cell response to transmitted/founder virus contributes to the control of acute viremia in HIV-1 infection. *J Exp Med* 2009; **206**: 1253–72.
50. Almeida JR., Price DA, Papagno L, et al. Superior control of HIV-1 replication by CD8+ T cells is reflected by their avidity, polyfunctionality, and clonal turnover. *J Exp Med* 2007; **204**: 2473–85.
51. Ladell K, Hashimoto M, Iglesias MC, et al. A molecular basis for the control of preimmune escape variants by HIV-specific CD8+ T cells. *Immunity* 2013; **38**: 425–36.
52. Trautmann L, Janbazian L, Chomont N, et al. Upregulation of PD-1 expression on HIV-specific CD8+ T cells leads to reversible immune dysfunction. *Nat Med* 2006; **12**: 1198–202.
53. Richman DD, Wrin T, Little SJ, Petropoulos CJ. Rapid evolution of the neutralizing antibody response to HIV type 1 infection. *Proc Natl Acad Sci USA* 2003; **100**: 4144–49.
54. Walker LM, Huber M, Doores KJ, et al, and the Protocol G Principal Investigators. Broad neutralization coverage of HIV by multiple highly potent antibodies. *Nature* 2011; **477**: 466–70.
55. Klein F, Diskin R, Scheid JF, et al. Somatic mutations of the immunoglobulin framework are generally required for broad and potent HIV-1 neutralization. *Cell* 2013; **153**: 126–38.
56. Liao HX, Lynch R, Zhou T, et al, and the NISC Comparative Sequencing Program. Co-evolution of a broadly neutralizing HIV-1 antibody and founder virus. *Nature* 2013; **496**: 469–76.

57. Jardine J, Julien JP, Menis S, et al. Rational HIV immunogen design to target specific germline B cell receptors. *Science* 2013; 340: 711–16.
58. Alter G, Heckerman D, Schneidewind A, et al. HIV-1 adaptation to NK-cell-mediated immune pressure. *Nature* 2011; **476**: 96–100.
59. Cooper A, García M, Petrovas C, Yamamoto T, Koup RA, Nabel GJ. HIV-1 causes CD4 cell death through DNA-dependent protein kinase during viral integration. *Nature* 2013; **498**: 376–79.
60. Mehandru S, Poles MA, Tenner-Racz K, et al. Mechanisms of gastrointestinal CD4+ T-cell depletion during acute and early human immunodeficiency virus type 1 infection. *J Virol* 2007; **81**: 599–612.
61. Prendergast A, Prado JG, Kang YH, et al. HIV-1 infection is characterized by profound depletion of CD161+ Th17 cells and gradual decline in regulatory T cells. *AIDS* 2010; **24**: 491–502.
62. Cosgrove C, Ussher JE, Rauch A, et al. Early and nonreversible decrease of CD161++/MAIT cells in HIV infection. *Blood* 2013; **121**: 951–61.
63. Brenchley JM, Price DA, Schacker TW, et al. Microbial translocation is a cause of systemic immune activation in chronic HIV infection. *Nat Med* 2006; **12**: 1365–71.
64. Zeng M, Southern PJ, Reilly CS, et al. Lymphoid tissue damage in HIV-1 infection depletes naïve T cells and limits T cell reconstitution after antiretroviral therapy. *PLoS Pathog* 2012; **8**: e1002437.
65. Lichtfuss GF, Hoy J, Rajasuriar R, Kramski M, Crowe SM, Lewin SR. Biomarkers of immune dysfunction following combination antiretroviral therapy for HIV infection. *Biomarkers Med* 2011; **5**: 171–86.
66. Meier A, Chang JJ, Chan ES, et al. Sex differences in the Toll-like receptor-mediated response of plasmacytoid dendritic cells to HIV-1. *Nat Med* 2009; **15**: 955–59.
67. Hsue PY, Hunt PW, Sinclair E, et al. Increased carotid intima-media thickness in HIV patients is associated with increased cytomegalovirus-specific T-cell responses. *AIDS* 2006; **20**: 2275–83.
68. Kuller LH, Tracy R, Belloso W, et al, and the INSIGHT SMART Study Group. Inflammatory and coagulation biomarkers and mortality in patients with HIV infection. *PLoS Med* 2008; **5**: e203.
69. Hsue PY, Scherzer R, Hunt PW, et al. Carotid intima-media thickness progression in HIV-infected adults occurs preferentially at the carotid bifurcation and is predicted by inflammation. *J Am Heart Assoc* 2012; 1.
70. Marks MA, Rabkin CS, Engels EA, et al. Markers of microbial translocation and risk of AIDS-related lymphoma. *AIDS* 2013; **27**: 469–74.
71. Ancuta P, Kamat A, Kunstman KJ, et al. Microbial translocation is associated with increased monocyte activation and dementia in AIDS patients. *PLoS One* 2008; **3**: e2516.
72. Andrade BB, Hullsiek KH, Boulware DR, et al, and the INSIGHT Study Group. Biomarkers of inflammation and coagulation are associated with mortality and hepatitis flares in persons coinfected with HIV and hepatitis viruses. *J Infect Dis* 2013; **207**: 1379–88.
73. Buzón MJ, Massanella M, Llibre JM, et al. HIV-1 replication and immune dynamics are affected by raltegravir intensification of HAART-suppressed subjects. *Nat Med* 2010; **16**: 460–65.
74. Hunt PW, Martin JN, Sinclair E, et al. Valganciclovir reduces T cell activation in HIV-infected individuals with incomplete CD4+ T cell recovery on antiretroviral therapy. *J Infect Dis* 2011; **203**: 1474–83.
75. Gonzalez VD, Falconer K, Blom KG, et al. High levels of chronic immune activation in the T-cell compartments of patients coinfected with hepatitis C virus and human immunodeficiency virus type 1 and on highly active antiretroviral therapy are reverted by alpha interferon and ribavirin treatment. *J Virol* 2009; **83**: 11407–11.

76. Rajasuriar R, Khoury G, Kamarulzaman A, French MA, Cameron PU, Lewin SR. Persistent immune activation in chronic HIV infection: do any interventions work? *AIDS* 2013; **27**: 1199–208.
77. Tuboi SH, Brinkhof MW, Egger M, et al. Discordant responses to potent antiretroviral treatment in previously naive HIV-1-infected adults initiating treatment in resource-constrained countries: the antiretroviral therapy in low-income countries (ART-LINC) collaboration. *J Acquir Immune Defic SynDr.* 2007; **45**: 52–59.
78. Rajasuriar R, Gouillou M, Spelman T, et al. Clinical predictors of immune reconstitution following combination antiretroviral therapy in patients from the Australian HIV Observational Database. *PLoS One* 2011; **6**: e20713.
79. Helleberg M, Kronborg G, Larsen CS, et al. Causes of death among Danish HIV patients compared with population controls in the period 1995–2008. *Infection* 2012; **40**: 627–34.
80. Abrams D, Lévy Y, Losso MH, et al, and the INSIGHT-ESPRIT Study Group, and the SILCAAT Scientific Committee. Interleukin-2 therapy in patients with HIV infection. *N Engl J Med* 2009; **361**: 1548–59.
81. Sereti I, Dunham RM, Spritzler J, et al, and the ACTG 5214 Study Team. IL-7 administration drives T cell-cycle entry and expansion in HIV-1 infection. *Blood* 2009; **113**: 6304–14.
82. Vandergeeten C, Fromentin R, DaFonseca S, et al. Interleukin-7 promotes HIV persistence during antiretroviral therapy. *Blood* 2013; **121**: 4321–29.
83. Thompson MA, Aberg JA, Hoy JF, et al. Antiretroviral treatment of adult HIV infection: 2012 recommendations of the International Antiviral Society-USA panel. *JAMA* 2012; **308**: 387–402.
84. World Health Organization. Consolidated guidelines on the use of antiretroviral drugs for treating and preventing HIV infection. Recommendations for a public health approach. June 2013. http://www.who.int/hiv/pub/guidelines/arv2013/download/en/index.html (accessed Aug 30, 2013).
85. Sigaloff KC, Hamers RL, Wallis CL, et al, and the PharmAccess African Studies to Evaluate Resistance (PASER). Unnecessary antiretroviral treatment switches and accumulation of HIV resistance mutations; two arguments for viral load monitoring in Africa. *J Acquir Immune Defic SynDr.* 2011; **58**: 23–31.
86. Boyer S, March L, Kouanfack C, et al, and the Stratall ANRS 12110/ESTHER Study Group. Monitoring of HIV viral load, CD4 cell count, and clinical assessment versus clinical monitoring alone for antiretroviral therapy in low-resource settings (Stratall ANRS 12110/ESTHER): a cost-effectiveness analysis. *Lancet Infect Dis* 2013; **13**: 577–86.
87. Keiser O, Orrell C, Egger M, et al, and the Swiss HIV Cohort Study (SHCS) and the International Epidemiologic Databases to Evaluate AIDS in Southern Africa (IeDEA-SA). Public-health and individual approaches to antiretroviral therapy: township South Africa and Switzerland compared. *PLoS Med* 2008; **5**: e148.
88. Boulle A, Schomaker M, May M, Egger M, Sterne JA. Mortality after starting ART in treatment-naïve adults in 3 continents: collaborative analysis of international epidemiologic databases to evaluate AIDS in southern Africa and ART cohort collaboration cohorts. 20th Conference on Retroviruses and Opportunistic Infections. Atlanta, Georgia; 2013.
89. Rodger AJ, Lodwick R, Schechter M, et al, and the INSIGHT SMART, ESPRIT Study Groups. Mortality in well controlled HIV in the continuous antiretroviral therapy arms of the SMART and ESPRIT trials compared with the general population. *AIDS* 2013; **27**: 973–79.
90. Walker BD, Hirsch MS. Antiretroviral therapy in early HIV infection. *N Engl J Med* 2013; **368**: 279–81.

91. Sabin CA, Cooper DA, Collins S, Schechter M. Rating evidence in treatment guidelines: a case example of when to initiate combination antiretroviral therapy (cART) in HIV-positive asymptomatic persons. *AIDS* 2013; **27**: 1839–46.
92. Kulkarni SP, Shah KR, Sarma KV, Mahajan AP. Clinical uncertainties, health service challenges, and ethical complexities of HIV "test-and-treat": a systematic review. *Am J Public Health* 2013; **103**: e14–23.
93. Kranzer K, Govindasamy D, Ford N, Johnston V, Lawn SD. Quantifying and addressing losses along the continuum of care for people living with HIV infection in sub-Saharan Africa: a systematic review. *J Int AIDS Soc* 2012; **15**: 17383.
94. Boulle A, Van Cutsem G, Hilderbrand K, et al. Seven-year experience of a primary care antiretroviral treatment programme in Khayelitsha, South Africa. *AIDS* 2010; **24**: 563–72.
95. Centers for Disease Control and Prevention. Vital signs: HIV prevention through care and treatment—United States2011. http://www.cdc.gov/mmwr/preview/mmwrhtml/ mm6047a4.htm (accessed June 3, 2014).
96. Gardner EM, Burman WJ, Steiner JF, Anderson PL, Bangsberg DR. Antiretroviral medication adherence and the development of class-specific antiretroviral resistance. *AIDS* 2009; **23**: 1035–46.
97. World Health Organization. WHO HIV drug resistance report 2012. 2012.
98. Lawn SD, Meintjes G. Pathogenesis and prevention of immune reconstitution disease during antiretroviral therapy. *Expert Rev Anti Infect Ther* 2011; **9**: 415–30.
99. Müller M, Wandel S, Colebunders R, Attia S, Furrer H, Egger M, and the IeDEA Southern and Central Africa. Immune reconstitution inflammatory syndrome in patients starting antiretroviral therapy for HIV infection: a systematic review and meta-analysis. *Lancet Infect Dis* 2010; **10**: 251–61.
100. Meintjes G, Wilkinson RJ, Morroni C, et al. Randomized placebo-controlled trial of prednisone for paradoxical tuberculosis-associated immune reconstitution inflammatory syndrome. *AIDS* 2010; **24**: 2381–90.
101. Finzi D, Blankson J, Siliciano JD, et al. Latent infection of CD4+ T cells provides a mechanism for lifelong persistence of HIV-1, even in patients on effective combination therapy. *Nat Med* 1999; **5**: 512–17.
102. Chun TW, Nickle DC, Justement JS, et al. Persistence of HIV in gut-associated lymphoid tissue despite long-term antiretroviral therapy. *J Infect Dis* 2008; **197**: 714–20.
103. Cusini A, Vernazza PL, Yerly S, et al, and the Swiss HIV Cohort Study. Higher CNS penetration-effectiveness of long-term combination antiretroviral therapy is associated with better HIV-1 viral suppression in cerebrospinal fluid. *J Acquir Immune Defic SynDr.* 2013; **62**: 28–35.
104. Saleh S, Solomon A, Wightman F, Xhilaga M, Cameron PU, Lewin SR. CCR7 ligands CCL19 and CCL21 increase permissiveness of resting memory CD4+ T cells to HIV-1 infection: a novel model of HIV-1 latency. *Blood* 2007; **110**: 4161–64.
105. Yang HC, Xing S, Shan L, et al. Small-molecule screening using a human primary cell model of HIV latency identifies compounds that reverse latency without cellular activation. *J Clin Invest* 2009; **119**: 3473–86.
106. Chomont N, El-Far M, Ancuta P, et al. HIV reservoir size and persistence are driven by T cell survival and homeostatic proliferation. *Nat Med* 2009; **15**: 893–900.
107. Wightman F, Solomon A, Khoury G, et al. Both CD31(+) and CD31 naive CD4(+) T cells are persistent HIV type 1-infected reservoirs in individuals receiving antiretroviral therapy. *J Infect Dis* 2010; **202**: 1738–48.

108. Ellery P, Sonza S, Paukovics G, et al. CD14lo/CD16hi monocytes are more permissive to HIV infection in vitro and may selectively harbour HIV-1 in patients on highly active antiretroviral therapy. 11th Conference on Retroviruses and Opportunistic Infections; 2004; San Francisco, CA; 2004. p. Abstract 426.
109. Gorry P, Purcell D, Howard J, McPhee D. Restricted HIV-1 infection of human astrocytes: potential role of nef in the regulation of virus replication. *J Neurovirol* 1998; **4**: 377–86.
110. Van Lint C, Bouchat S, Marcello A. HIV-1 transcription and latency: an update. *Retrovirology* 2013; **10**: 67.
111. Huang J, Wang F, Argyris E, et al. Cellular microRNAs contribute to HIV-1 latency in resting primary CD4+ T lymphocytes. *Nat Med* 2007; **13**: 1241–47.
112. Hütter G, Nowak D, Mossner M, et al. Long-term control of HIV by CCR5 Delta32/Delta32 stem-cell transplantation. *N Engl J Med* 2009; **360**: 692–98.
113. Persaud D, Gay H, Ziemniak C, et al. Absence of detectable HIV-1 viremia after treatment cessation in an infant. *N Engl J Med* 2013; **369**: 1828–35.
114. Yukl SA, Boritz E, Busch M, et al. Challenges in detecting HIV persistence during potentially curative interventions: a study of the Berlin patient. *PLoS Pathog* 2013; **9**: e1003347.
115. Li L, Krymskaya L, Wang J, et al. Genomic Editing of the HIV-1 Coreceptor CCR5 in Adult Hematopoietic Stem and Progenitor Cells Using Zinc Finger Nucleases. *Mol Ther JAm Soc Gene Ther* 2013; **21**: 1259–69.
116. Sáez-Cirión A, Bacchus C, Hocqueloux L, et al, and the ANRS VISCONTI Study Group. Post-treatment HIV-1 controllers with a long-term virological remission after the interruption of early initiated antiretroviral therapy ANRS VISCONTI Study. *PLoS Pathog* 2013; **9**: e1003211.
117. Lodi S, Meyer L, Kelleher AD, et al. Immunovirologic control 24 months after interruption of antiretroviral therapy initiated close to HIV seroconversion. *Arch Intern Med* 2012; **172**: 1252–55.
118. Ananworanich J, Schuetz A, Vandergeeten C, et al, and the RV254/SEARCH 010 Study Group. Impact of multi-targeted antiretroviral treatment on gut T cell depletion and HIV reservoir seeding during acute HIV infection. *PLoS One* 2012; **7**: e33948.
119. Lewin SR, Rouzioux C. HIV cure and eradication: how will we get from the laboratory to effective clinical trials? *AIDS* 2011; **25**: 885–97.
120. Archin NM, Liberty AL, Kashuba AD, et al. Administration of vorinostat disrupts HIV-1 latency in patients on antiretroviral therapy. *Nature* 2012; **487**: 482–85.
121. Elliott J, Solomon A, Wightman F, et al. The Safety and Effect of Multiple Doses of Vorinostat on HIV Transcription in HIV+ Patients Receiving cART. 20th Conference on Retroviruses and Opportunistic Infections. Atlanta, GA; 2013. p. 50LB.
122. Shan L, Deng K, Shroff NS, et al. Stimulation of HIV-1-specific cytolytic T lymphocytes facilitates elimination of latent viral reservoir after virus reactivation. *Immunity* 2012; **36**: 491–501.
123. Papagno L, Alter G, Assoumou L, et al, and the ORVACS Study Group. Comprehensive analysis of virus-specific T-cells provides clues for the failure of therapeutic immunization with ALVAC-HIV vaccine. *AIDS* 2011; **25**: 27–36.
124. Garcia F, Climent N, Guardo AC, et al. A dendritic cell-based vaccine elicits T cell responses associated with control of HIV-1 replication. *Science Transl Med* 2013; **5**: 166ra2.
125. Hansen SG, Piatak M Jr., Ventura AB, et al. Immune clearance of highly pathogenic SIV infection. *Nature* 2013; **502**: 100–04.

126. Dutta A, Wirtz AL, Baral S, Beyrer C, Cleghorn FR. Key harm reduction interventions and their impact on the reduction of risky behavior and HIV incidence among people who inject drugs in low-income and middle-income countries. *Curr Opin HIV AIDS* 2012; **7**: 362–68.
127. Kourtis AP, Lee FK, Abrams EJ, Jamieson DJ, Bulterys M. Mother-to-child transmission of HIV-1: timing and implications for prevention. *Lancet Infect Dis* 2006; **6**: 726–32.
128. Breastfeeding, Group HIVITS, Coutsoudis A, et al. Late postnatal transmission of HIV-1 in breast-fed children: an individual patient data meta-analysis. *J Infect Dis* 2004; **189**: 2154–66.
129. de Vincenzi I, and the Kesho Bora Study Group. Triple antiretroviral compared with zidovudine and single-dose nevirapine prophylaxis during pregnancy and breastfeeding for prevention of mother-to-child transmission of HIV-1 (Kesho Bora study): a randomised controlled trial. *Lancet Infect Dis* 2011; **11**: 171–80.
130. Thior I, Lockman S, Smeaton LM, et al, and the Mashi Study Team. Breastfeeding plus infant zidovudine prophylaxis for 6 months vs formula feeding plus infant zidovudine for 1 month to reduce mother-to-child HIV transmission in Botswana: a randomized trial: the Mashi Study. *JAMA* 2006; **296**: 794–805.
131. Coovadia HM, Brown ER, Fowler MG, et al, and the HPTN 046 protocol team. Efficacy and safety of an extended nevirapine regimen in infant children of breastfeeding mothers with HIV-1 infection for prevention of postnatal HIV-1 transmission (HPTN 046): a randomised, double-blind, placebo-controlled trial. *Lancet* 2012; **379**: 221–28.
132. Thomas TK, Masaba R, Borkowf CB, et al, and the KiBS Study Team. Triple-antiretroviral prophylaxis to prevent mother-to-child HIV transmission through breastfeeding—the Kisumu Breastfeeding Study, Kenya: a clinical trial. *PLoS Med* 2011; **8**: e1001015.
133. Wettstein C, Mugglin C, Egger M, et al, and the IeDEA Southern Africa Collaboration. Missed opportunities to prevent mother-to-child-transmission: systematic review and meta-analysis. *AIDS* 2012; **26**: 2361–73.
134. Nachega JB, Uthman OA, Anderson J, et al. Adherence to antiretroviral therapy during and after pregnancy in low-income, middle-income, and high-income countries: a systematic review and meta-analysis. *AIDS* 2012; **26**: 2039–52.
135. Cohen MS, Chen YQ, McCauley M, et al, and the HPTN 052 Study Team. Prevention of HIV-1 infection with early antiretroviral therapy. *N Engl J Med* 2011; **365**: 493–505.
136. Tanser F, Bärnighausen T, Grapsa E, Zaidi J, Newell ML. High coverage of ART associated with decline in risk of HIV acquisition in rural KwaZulu-Natal, South Africa. *Science* 2013; **339**: 966–71.
137. Coates T, Eshleman S, Chariyalertsak S, et al. Community-level reductions in estimated HIV incidence: HIV Prevention Trials Network 043, Project Accept. 20th Conference on Retroviruses and Opportunistic Infections (CROI). Atlanta, GA; 2013. p. Abstract 30.
138. Sabapathy K, Van den Bergh R, Fidler S, Hayes R, Ford N. Uptake of home-based voluntary HIV testing in sub-Saharan Africa: a systematic review and meta-analysis. *PLoS Med* 2012; **9**: e1001351.
139. Gardner EM, McLees MP, Steiner JF, Del Rio C, Burman WJ. The spectrum of engagement in HIV care and its relevance to test-and-treat strategies for prevention of HIV infection. *Clin Infect Dis* 2011; **52**: 793–800.
140. Sood N, Wagner Z, Jaycocks A, Drabo E, Vardavas R. Test-and-treat in Los Angeles: a mathematical model of the effects of test-and-treat for the population of men who have sex with men in Los Angeles County. *Clin Infect Dis* 2013; **56**: 1789–96.

141. Auvert B, Taljaard D, Lagarde E, Sobngwi-Tambekou J, Sitta R, Puren A. Randomized, controlled intervention trial of male circumcision for reduction of HIV infection risk: the ANRS 1265 Trial. *PLoS Med* 2005; **2**: e298.
142. Bailey RC, Moses S, Parker CB, et al. Male circumcision for HIV prevention in young men in Kisumu, Kenya: a randomised controlled trial. *Lancet* 2007; **369**: 643–56.
143. Gray RH, Kigozi G, Serwadda D, et al. Male circumcision for HIV prevention in men in Rakai, Uganda: a randomised trial. *Lancet* 2007; **369**: 657–66.
144. Baeten JM, Donnell D, Ndase P, et al, and the Partners PrEP Study Team. Antiretroviral prophylaxis for HIV prevention in heterosexual men and women. *N Engl J Med* 2012; **367**: 399–410.
145. Thigpen MC, Kebaabetswe PM, Paxton LA, et al, and the TDF2 Study Group. Antiretroviral preexposure prophylaxis for heterosexual HIV transmission in Botswana. *N Engl J Med* 2012; **367**: 423–34.
146. Choopanya K, Martin M, Suntharasamai P, et al, and the Bangkok Tenofovir Study Group. Antiretroviral prophylaxis for HIV infection in injecting drug users in Bangkok, Thailand (the Bangkok Tenofovir Study): a randomised, double-blind, placebo-controlled phase 3 trial. *Lancet* 2013; **381**: 2083–90.
147. Grant RM, Lama JR., Anderson PL, et al, and the iPrEx Study Team. Preexposure chemoprophylaxis for HIV prevention in men who have sex with men. *N Engl J Med* 2010; **363**: 2587–99.
148. Van Damme L, Corneli A, Ahmed K, et al, and the FEM-PrEP Study Group. Preexposure prophylaxis for HIV infection among African women. *N Engl J Med* 2012; **367**: 411–22.
149. Marrazzo J, Ramjee G, Nair G, et al. Pre-exposure prophylaxis for HIV in women: daily oral tenofovir, oral tenofovir/embricitabine, or vaginal tenofovir gel in the VOICE study (MTN 003). 20th Conference on Retroviruses and Opportunistic Infections (CROI). Atlanta, GA; 2013. p. Abstract 26LB.
150. Abdool Karim Q, Abdool Karim SS, Frohlich JA, et al, and the CAPRISA 004 Trial Group. Effectiveness and safety of tenofovir gel, an antiretroviral microbicide, for the prevention of HIV infection in women. *Science* 2010; **329**: 1168–74.
151. Obiero J, Mwethera PG, Hussey GD, Wiysonge CS. Vaginal microbicides for reducing the risk of sexual acquisition of HIV infection in women: systematic review and meta-analysis. *BMC Infect Dis* 2012; **12**: 289.
152. Herrera C, Shattock RJ. Candidate Microbicides and Their Mechanisms of Action. *Curr Top Microbiol Immunol* 2013 [Epub ahead of print].
153. Ball C, Krogstad E, Chaowanachan T, Woodrow KA. Drug-eluting fibers for HIV-1 inhibition and contraception. *PLoS One* 2012; **7**: e49792.
154. Siegfried N, Muller M, Deeks JJ, Volmink J. Male circumcision for prevention of heterosexual acquisition of HIV in men. *Cochrane Database Syst Rev* 2009; **2**: CD003362.
155. Hallett TB, Alsallaq RA, Baeten JM, et al. Will circumcision provide even more protection from HIV to women and men? New estimates of the population impact of circumcision interventions. *Sex Transm Infect* 2011; **87**: 88–93.
156. Uthman OA, Popoola TA, Yahaya I, Uthman MM, Aremu O. The cost-utility analysis of adult male circumcision for prevention of heterosexual acquisition of HIV in men in sub-Saharan Africa: a probabilistic decision model. *Value Health* 2011; **14**: 70–79.
157. Ford N, Chu K, Mills EJ. Safety of task-shifting for male medical circumcision: a systematic review and meta-analysis. *AIDS* 2012; **26**: 559–66.
158. Gray RH, Wawer MJ, Kigozi G. Programme science research on medical male circumcision scale-up in sub-Saharan Africa. *Sex Transm Infect* 2013; **89**: 345–49.

159. Lorimer K, Kidd L, Lawrence M, McPherson K, Cayless S, Cornish F. Systematic review of reviews of behavioural HIV prevention interventions among men who have sex with men. *AIDS Care* 2013; 25: 133–50.
160. Wariki WM, Ota E, Mori R, Koyanagi A, Hori N, Shibuya K. Behavioral interventions to reduce the transmission of HIV infection among sex workers and their clients in low- and middle-income countries. *Cochrane Database Syst Rev* 2012; **2**: CD005272.
161. Kerrigan DL, Fonner VA, StroM.D.ahl S, Kennedy CE. Community empowerment among female sex workers is an effective HIV prevention intervention: a systematic review of the peer-reviewed evidence from low- and middle-income countries. *AIDS Behav* 2013; **17**: 1926–40.
162. Kennedy CE, Medley AM, Sweat M.D., O'Reilly KR. Behavioural interventions for HIV positive prevention in developing countries: a systematic review and meta-analysis. *Bull World Health Organ* 2010; **88**: 615–23.
163. Scott-Sheldon LA, Huedo-Medina TB, Warren MR, Johnson BT, Carey MP. Efficacy of behavioral interventions to increase condom use and reduce sexually transmitted infections: a meta-analysis, 1991 to 2010. *J Acquir Immune Defic SynDr.* 2011; **58**: 489–98.
164. Fonner VA, Denison J, Kennedy CE, O'Reilly K, Sweat M. Voluntary counseling and testing (VCT) for changing HIV-related risk behavior in developing countries. *Cochrane Database Syst Rev* 2012; **9**: CD001224.
165. Barnabas RV, Celum C. Infectious co-factors in HIV-1 transmission herpes simplex virus type-2 and HIV-1: new insights and interventions. *Curr HIV Res* 2012; **10**: 228–37.
166. Celum C, Wald A, Lingappa JR., et al, and the Partners in Prevention HSV/HIV Transmission Study Team. Acyclovir and transmission of HIV-1 from persons infected with HIV-1 and HSV-2. *N Engl J Med* 2010; **362**: 427–39.
167. Lingappa JR., Baeten JM, Wald A, et al, and the Partners in Prevention HSV/HIV Transmission Study Team. Daily acyclovir for HIV-1 disease progression in people dually infected with HIV-1 and herpes simplex virus type 2: a randomised placebo-controlled trial. *Lancet* 2010; **375**: 824–33.
168. Mugwanya K, Baeten JM, Mugo NR, Irungu E, Ngure K, Celum C. High-dose valacyclovir HSV-2 suppression results in greater reduction in plasma HIV-1 levels compared with standard dose acyclovir among HIV-1/HSV-2 coinfected persons: a randomized, crossover trial. *J Infect Dis* 2011; 204: 1912–17.
169. Barnabas RV, Webb EL, Weiss HA, Wasserheit JN. The role of coinfections in HIV epidemic trajectory and positive prevention: a systematic review and meta-analysis. *AIDS* 2011; **25**: 1559–73.
170. Grosskurth H, Mosha F, Todd J, et al. Impact of improved treatment of sexually transmitted diseases on HIV infection in rural Tanzania: randomised controlled trial. *Lancet* 1995; **346**: 530–36.
171. Ng BE, Butler LM, Horvath T, Rutherford GW. Population-based biomedical sexually transmitted infection control interventions for reducing HIV infection. *Cochrane Database Syst Rev* 2011; **3**: CD001220.
172. Buchbinder SP, Mehrotra DV, Duerr A, et al, and the Step Study Protocol Team. Efficacy assessment of a cell-mediated immunity HIV-1 vaccine (the Step Study): a double-blind, randomised, placebo-controlled, test-of-concept trial. Lancet 2008; 372: 1881–93.
173. Rerks-Ngarm S, Pitisuttithum P, Nitayaphan S, et al, and the MOPH-TAVEG Investigators. Vaccination with ALVAC and AIDSVAX to prevent HIV-1 infection in Thailand. *N Engl J Med* 2009; **361**: 2209–20.
174. Haynes BF, Gilbert PB, McElrath MJ, et al. Immune-correlates analysis of an HIV-1 vaccine efficacy trial. *N Engl J Med* 2012; **366**: 1275–86.
175. Haynes BF, McElrath MJ. Progress in HIV-1 vaccine development. *Curr Opin HIV AIDS* 2013; **8**: 326–32.

13.5

Know Your Epidemic, Know Your Response

David Wilson and Daniel Halperin

LED BY UNAIDS, *KNOW YOUR EPIDEMIC, know your response* has become a rallying cry for an intensified focus on HIV prevention, spurred by the sobering realisation that for every person enrolled on antiretroviral treatment, many more become newly infected.[1] The quest to better understand epidemics reflects growing recognition that there is no single global HIV epidemic, but rather a multitude of diverse epidemics. No single prescription can apply to countries as diverse as South Africa, Egypt, Russia, Thailand, or Papua New Guinea. The era of standard global prevention guidance is over.

However, there is a globally useful distinction between concentrated and generalised epidemics, which are fundamentally different—not because of arbitrary prevalence thresholds, but about who gets infected and how. Epidemics are concentrated if transmission occurs largely in defined vulnerable groups—typically sex workers, men who have sex with men, and injecting drug users, and their sexual partners—and if protecting them would protect wider society. Conversely, epidemics are generalised if transmission is sustained by sexual behaviour in the general population and would persist despite effective programmes for vulnerable groups. For too long, the global HIV-prevention community has pursued generalised responses in concentrated epidemics, concentrated approaches in generalised epidemics, or hedged their bets and done a bit of everything.[2–7]

At the extremes, the differences between concentrated and generalised epidemics are stark. Those in Latin America, the Middle East, Europe, and Asia—ie, most of the world—are and undoubtedly will remain concentrated, while most of southern and parts of eastern Africa are generalised.[2–9] Between these extremes, it is less clear whether some epidemics of the Caribbean, central and west Africa, and parts of the Pacific are concentrated, low-grade generalised, or mixed (table).

While the global quest to know your epidemic is welcome, there are pitfalls to avoid. First, we must understand, but not overcomplicate. Broad, rapid brush strokes are sufficient for action. We can build our ships as we sail, guided by an overarching question: are our epidemics essentially concentrated, generalised, or (in some cases) substantially mixed? And where, in broad categories, are most new infections occurring: in sex workers, men who have sex with men, or injecting drug users (and their sexual partners), or through multiple concurrent partnerships in the general population?

David Wilson and Daniel Halperin, "Know Your Epidemic, Know Your Response," *The Lancet*, vol. 372, no. 9637, pp. 423–426.

HIV EPIDEMIC Characteristics and Priorities

Factor	Concentrated epidemics	Generalised epidemics	Potentially mixed epidemics
Geographic areas	North, Central and South America, Europe, Middle East, Asia, Australasia	Most of southern Africa and parts of east Africa	Parts of the Caribbean, west Africa, horn of Africa, and the Pacific region
Priorities needed for surveillance, monitoring, and evaluation	Far greater emphasis on biological and behavioural surveillance of vulnerable groups (sex workers, men who have sex with men, injecting drug users)	Antenatal and episodic population-based surveillance	Both vulnerable group and antenatal/general population surveillance
Analysis	HIV prevalence, mapping, population-size estimation, behavioural interactions within vulnerable groups and between vulnerable groups, and their sexual or injecting partners	Greater focus on understanding how to fundamentally change societal norms of sexual behaviour	Greater focus on understanding transmission dynamics, including behavioural interactions between vulnerable groups and general population
Investments	Invest in surveillance, targeted interventions for vulnerable groups, and stigma-reduction campaigns for general population	Investments should focus on promoting normative and social change to reduce multiple and concurrent partnerships, and to greatly increase availability of safe and affordable male circumcision services	Investments should be matched to sources of transmission, which may vary across subnational regions and overtime
Interventions	Goal is saturation coverage of vulnerable groups	Goal is to help change community norms, values, and sexual behaviour at population level, and to frame male circumcision within broader rubric of male reproductive health and HIV prevention/behavior change	Goal is to relate interventions to transmission sources and maintain objective balance between targeted and general population activities
Key research questions	How to reach vulnerable groups with high coverage of high-quality targeted interventions	How to change fundamental community norms and to de-norm multiple and concurrent partnerships at population level	How to more accurately estimate relative proportion of infections from different transmission sources, and how to combine vulnerable group and general population interventions to reflect transmission patterns

Second, although mathematical modelling of incident infections may be helpful, such models are in their infancy, make several major assumptions, and require better data than are generally available. Therefore the seductively precise graphs produced by such models must be carefully triangulated against other sources, including empirical risk-factor and incidence studies and rigorously grounded epidemiological syntheses.

Third, while participatory consultative approaches to "know your epidemic, know your response" are laudable, these may compromise rigour if they are not grounded in evidence. For example, after three decades the global community is only beginning to accept that there is no simple direct association between income, education, gender inequality, and HIV. Population-based surveys show that wealthier African countries have the highest, not lowest, infection levels in Africa, and more educated, upper-income people are generally more likely to be infected with HIV.[6,7,10] And whilst it is clearly necessary to address gender inequality and age discordance in relationships, sexual coercion, and gender-based violence,[11] it is nonetheless striking that a comparison of gender equality[12] and HIV prevalence across African countries shows a strong positive, not negative, association. Participatory approaches that emphasize putative, largely unproven underlying structural or other social, economic, or political factors (although vital for other non-HIV reasons) can deflect emphasis from the major immediate cause of HIV infection: multiple sexual (and injecting) partnerships.[2–9,13–18]

Fourth, in southern Africa's epidemics of exceptionally high prevalence, the greatest challenge is not knowing your epidemic—but knowing how to bring about profound social and normative changes to reduce multiple, and especially concurrent, sexual partnerships.[5–8,11,14–18]

Once we better understand our epidemics, can we respond with proven approaches? Experience to date is sobering. If we face concentrated epidemics fuelled by sex work, we know what to do. Targeted interventions that promote education, condoms, sexual health, solidarity, empowerment, and rights for sex workers do work and have contained HIV in Asia's three main sexually ignited epidemics in Thailand, Cambodia, and south India.[2–9,13–16] Targeted interventions have also worked in several other developing-country epidemics where sex work contributes significantly to HIV transmission, such as the Dominican Republic.[19]

Where transmission in men who have sex with men fuels HIV epidemics, the real-world picture is less encouraging. However, there is greater room for optimism in contexts that are increasingly open to homosexuality, such as India, where the national AIDS authority recently petitioned the high court to legalise same-sex practices[20] or in Nepal, where the third gender—transgender—is a legal classification. Effective action is much more difficult in coercive contexts; in Egypt, a recent ground-breaking serosurvey hastened the imprisonment of homosexual men.[21]

And for injecting drug users, can we keep saying that harm reduction works in, for example, the former Soviet Union or Asia, when we still cannot convince the authorities that this is preferable to coercive approaches? We have only made limited progress towards the vital goal of large-scale harm-reduction programmes in Asia, with the partial exception of substitution therapy in China.

Turning to generalised epidemics, we face three overarching challenges. First, our most trusted prevention interventions—testing and counselling, condom promotion, school and youth (including abstinence) programmes, and treatment of other sexually transmitted infections (each of which may have other important public-health benefits)—are at best unproven, and at worst disproven, for reducing HIV incidence.[6–8,11,14,16,22–28]

Second, the most solidly proven preventive intervention to date, male circumcision, is barely advancing.[6,29,30] Since three randomised trials were terminated early nearly 2 years ago, due to highly preventive effect, lamentably few additional men have received this remarkable protective intervention. Yet the potential is immense. Seven of the eight countries with the highest HIV prevalence (with less than 2% of global population yet over a third of HIV infections) have male circumcision rates below 20%, and expansion of safe circumcision services in these countries could ultimately prevent many deaths.[6,29–31] In countries such as Zambia, with 15% adult HIV prevalence and nearly US $1 billion in aid annually for AIDS, much less than 1% of this funding goes for male circumcision services, and waiting lists for the procedure continue, as in other parts of Africa,[6,8,29,30] to grow at public facilities.[32] Even more disappointing is the fact that the countries where the trials were done (South Africa, Uganda, and Kenya) have yet to implement large-scale programmes. Under the Belmont principles of distributive justice, there is an ethical obligation to provide beneficial interventions to the populations in which studies were done.

Third, the major contributor to reduced HIV transmission in generalised epidemics has been reduction in multiple sexual partnerships.[5–9,11,14–18] Compelling evidence of this association has emerged in a growing number of African countries, such as Kenya,[6,7,33] Zimbabwe,[34] and Ethiopia.[6,35] Additionally, partner reduction seems to have contributed to HIV declines in Haiti and the Dominican Republic.[19] Yet, except for Uganda in the late 1980s, and more recently in Swaziland,[8] reductions in multiple partnerships seem to have mainly occurred despite, not because of, formal programmes.[5,6,9,14] Consequently, we know too little about how to effectively promote partner reduction. But this is no excuse not to immediately increase our commitment to well-evaluated programmes aimed at reducing multiple and concurrent sexual partnerships.

Lessons learned from the successes in reducing population-level HIV prevalence in countries such as Uganda may prove useful for prevention programming. It seems that the Ugandan response stimulated personalisation of risk in a way that fostered community mobilisation for behaviour change, without increasing stigma.[5,8,11,13,17,18,37,38] Second, the intensive use of a coordinated multilevel approach, involving clear and consistent risk-avoidance messaging at all levels, assisted in changing societal norms of behaviour.[14,17,18] And third, it seems that focusing such efforts for risk avoidance and partner reduction on adult men was key to reducing the sexual networks that fuel HIV transmission in high prevalence countries.[5,8,11,13,15,17,18,37,38]

Turning to the less clearly defined epidemics of parts of the Caribbean, central and west Africa, and the Pacific, we must resolve whether they are concentrated, low-intensity generalised, or mixed. If concentrated, we face the achievable goal of making sex work safe, and the more demanding task of reducing risk in men who have sex with men[39–41] (as well as addressing anal sex among heterosexuals, which also constitutes an under-recognised source of HIV transmission in Latin America and elsewhere[42]). If we determine that these are low-grade generalised epidemics, we face a perhaps greater challenge: how to convince countries with 1–3% adult HIV prevalence and numerous other competing health and social priorities, such as the Democratic Republic of the Congo or Sierra Leone, to invest in the fundamental normative and social change required for partner reduction.

Turning to a related question, what is a proportionate AIDS response? Global AIDS resources, while increasingly vast, are mainly concentrated in some 15–20 countries, mostly in southern and eastern Africa. In some of the eight most affected countries (all in southern Africa), where adult

HIV prevalence is above 15%, the question may not be whether we are distorting efforts too much, but whether we are prioritising enough? In Francistown, Botswana, where 70% of pregnant women aged 30–34 years have HIV, how can we possibly overemphasise AIDS? Yet, in much of east and west Africa, where HIV is lower than previously estimated, AIDS receives considerably more funding than much greater sources of disease burden, which highlights the need to reposition and integrate AIDS in support of other health challenges.[43,44] Conversely, in Thailand, AIDS accounts for over 10% of disease burden yet receives only 2% of recurrent health spending. In Indonesia, which faces Asia's fastest growing epidemic, fuelled by sexual transmission in the predominately non-circumcising island of Papua and by injecting drug use outside of Papua, HIV funding may fall, compromising vital programmes.

Furthermore, emerging research from around the world indicates that the growing availability of antiretroviral treatment—while a humanitarian godsend for millions of people—might also make behaviour change even more challenging, as AIDS is increasingly perceived as a chronic manageable disease.[39–41,45] Prevention efforts can backslide for other reasons. In Uganda, the intensive focus on zero grazing (ie, partner reduction) two decades ago, which helped lead to a dramatic reduction in multiple partnerships and a historically unprecedented decline in HIV prevalence, has in recent years been replaced by emphasis on other approaches, including social marketing of condoms and abstinence, and HIV incidence may now be increasing again, as are multiple partnerships.[8,17,18,46,47]

To conclude: first, the move to "know your epidemic, know your response" is welcome, but must not become overcomplicated—broad brushstrokes are sufficient for decisive, intelligent action. Second, concentrated epidemics driven by sex work are preventable, but protecting men who have sex with men and injecting drug users requires new and creative strategies and allies.[41,48] Third, in generalised epidemics, the core challenge is to begin reallocating resources from unproven or disproven approaches toward the two proven but admittedly sensitive approaches already at hand: male circumcision and partner reduction. Fourth, in the relatively few mixed epidemic settings, where there is significant transmission both from sex work and multiple partnerships in the general population (such as in Côte d'Ivoire and Haiti[19]) prevention must balance targeted and general population interventions according to transmission sources.

The challenge is clear. For too long, AIDS activists, academics, and national and international institutions have given insufficient emphasis to aligning prevention priorities with epidemic transmission dynamics, compromising effective prevention with mismatched or unfocused responses. And the AIDS community in its entirety has been slow to implement genuinely proven approaches at adequate scale. With the knowledge we already have, far more should have been, and can still be, done to curb HIV transmission globally.

References

1. UNAIDS. Practical guidelines for intensifying HIV prevention: towards universal access. 2007. http://data.unaids.org/pub/Manual/2007/20070306_Prevention_Guidelines_Towards_Universal_Access_en.pdf (accessed June 13, 2008).
2. Pisani E. *The wisdom of whores: bureaucrats, brothels, and the business of AIDS*. New York: W W Norton, 2008.

3. Chin J. *The AIDS pandemic: the collision of epidemiology with political correctness.* Oxford: Radcliffe Publishing, 2007.
4. Cohen J. Asia and Africa: on different trajectories? *Science* 2004; 304: 1932–38.
5. Wilson D. Partner reduction and the prevention of HIV/AIDS. *BMJ* 2004; 328: 848–49.
6. Potts M., Halperin D.T., Kirby D., et al. Reassessing HIV prevention. *Science* 2008; 320: 749–50.
7. Shelton D. Ten myths and one truth about generalised HIV epidemics. *Lancet* 2007; 370: 1809–11.
8. Halperin D.T., Epstein H. Why is HIV prevalence so severe in southern Africa? The role of multiple concurrent partnerships and lack of male circumcision: Implications for AIDS prevention. *South African J HIV Med* 2007; 26: 19–25.
9. Shelton J.D., Halperin D.T., Wilson D. Has global HIV incidence peaked? *Lancet* 2006; 367: 1120–22.
10. Mishra V., Bignami-Van Asscheb S., Greener R., et al. HIV infection does not disproportionately affect the poorer in sub-Saharan Africa. *AIDS* 2007; 21 (suppl 7): S17–28.
11. Southern African Development Community. Expert think tank meeting on HIV prevention in high-prevalence countries in southern Africa: report. May 10–12, 2006. http://www.sadc.int/downloads/news/SADCPrevReport.pdf (accessed June 13, 2008).
12. World Economic Forum. Global gender gap report 2007. http://www.weforum.org/pdf/gendergap/rankings2007.pdf (accessed June 19, 2008).
13. Pisani E. We can't wait for equality: the focus on female empowerment has made us forget the key role of men in Aids prevention. *Guardian* Dec 1, 2007. http://www.guardian.co.uk/commentisfree/2007/dec/01/comment.gender (accessed June 13, 2008).
14. Stoneburner RL, Low-Beer D. Population-level HIV declines and behavioral risk avoidance in Uganda. *Science* 2004; 304: 714–18.
15. Shelton JD, Halperin D.T., Nantulya V, Potts M, Gayle HD, Holmes KK. Partner reduction is crucial for balanced 'ABC' approach to HIV prevention. *BMJ* 2004; 328: 891–93.
16. Hearst N, Chen S. Condom promotion for AIDS prevention in the developing world: is it working? *Stud Fam Plann* 2004; 35: 39–47.
17. Green EC, Halperin D.T., Nantulya V, Hogle JA. Uganda's HIV prevention success: the role of sexual behavior change and the national response. *AIDS Behav* 2006; 10: 335–46.
18. Epstein H. *The invisible cure: Africa, the West and the fight against AIDS.* New York: Farrar Straus and Giroux, 2007.
19. Halperin D.T., de Moya A, Perez-Then E, Pappas G, Garcia Calleja JM. Understanding the HIV epidemic in the Dominican Republic: a prevention success story in the Caribbean? *J Acquir Immune Defic SynDr.* (in press).
20. Anonymous. Government's AIDS cell pushes to legalise homosexuality. *Times India* July 20, 2006. http://timesofindia.indiatimes.com/articleshow/1779097.cms (accessed June 13, 2008).
21. Human Rights Watch. Egypt: Court upholds HIV sentences, reinforces intolerance. May 29, 2008. http://hrw.org/english/docs/2008/05/29/egypt18959.htm (accessed June 13, 2008).
22. Shelton J. Counselling and testing for wide-scale HIV prevention. *Lancet* (in press).
23. Corbett EL, Makamure B, Cheung YB, et al. HIV incidence during a cluster-randomized trial of two strategies providing voluntary counselling and testing at the workplace, Zimbabwe. *AIDS* 2007; 21: 483–89.
24. Matovu JK, Gray R, Kiwanuka, et al. Repeat HIV counseling and testing (VCT), sexual risk behavior and HIV incidence in Rakai, Uganda. *AIDS Behav* 2007; 11: 71–81.

25. Kajubi P, Kamya MR, Kamya S, ChenS, McFarland W, Hearst N. Increasing condom use without reducing HIV risk: results of a controlled community trial in Uganda. *J Acquir Immune Defic SynDr.* 2005; 40: 77–82.
26. Gray RH, Wawer JM. Reassessing the hypothesis on STI control for HIV prevention. *Lancet* 2008; 371: 2064–65.
27. Gregson S, Adamson S, Papaya S, et al. Impact and process evaluation of integrated community and clinic-based HIV-1 control: a cluster-randomised trial in eastern Zimbabwe. *PLoS Med* 2007; 4: 547–55.
28. Hanley M. A realistic strategy for fighting African AIDS. *Mercatornet* Feb 29, 2008. http://www.mercatornet.com/articles/a_realistic_strategy_for_fighting_african_aids (accessed June 13, 2008).
29. Weiss HA, Halperin D.T., Bailey RC, Hayes R, Schmid G, Hankins C. Male circumcision for HIV prevention: from evidence to action? *AIDS* 2008; 22: 567–74.
30. Klausner JD, Wamai R, Bowa K, Agot K, Kagimba J, Halperin D.T.. Is male circumcision as good as the HIV vaccine we've been waiting for? *Future HIV Ther* 2008; 2: 1–7.
31. Auvert B, Marseille E, Korenromp EL. Estimating the resources needed and savings anticipated from roll-out of adult male circumcision in sub-Saharan Africa. *PLoS One* (in press).
32. *USA Today.* Zambian reporter gets circumcised to fight AIDS. Dec 1, 2007. www.usatoday.com/community/utils/idmap/30362328.story (accessed June 13, 2008).
33. Cheluget B, Baltazar G, Orege P, Ibrahim M, Marum LH, Stover J. Evidence for population level declines in adult HIV prevalence in Kenya. *Sex Transm Infect* 2006; 82 (suppl 1): i21–26.
34. Gregson S, Garnett GP, Nyamukapa CA, et al. HIV decline associated with behavior change in Eastern Zimbabwe. *Science* 2006; 311: 664–66.
35. Mekonnen Y, Sanders E, Aklilu M, et al. Evidence of changes in sexual behaviours among male factory workers in Ethiopia. *AIDS* 2003; 17: 223–31.
36. Halperin D.T.. The controversy over fear arousal in AIDS prevention and lessons from Uganda. *J Health Commun* 2006; 11: 266–67.
37. Helleringer S, Kohler HP. Sexual network structure and the spread of HIV in Africa: evidence from Likoma Island, Malawi. *AIDS* 2007; 21: 2323–32.
38. Kirby D. The changes in sexual behavior leading to the decline of HIV prevalence in Uganda—confirmation from multiple sources of evidence. *Sex Transm Infect* (in press).
39. Williamson LM, Dodds JP, Mercey DE, Hart GJ, Johnson AM. Sexual risk behaviour and knowledge of HIV status among community samples of gay men in the UK. *AIDS* 2008; 22: 1063–1070.
40. Bezemer D, de Wolf F, Boerlijst MC, et al. A resurgent HIV-1 epidemic among men who have sex with men in the era of potent antiretroviral therapy. *AIDS* 2008; 22: 1071–77.
41. Coates TJ. What is to be done? *AIDS* 2008; 22: 1079–80.
42. Halperin D.T.. Heterosexual anal intercourse: prevalence, cultural factors, and HIV infection and other health risks. *AIDS Patient Care* 1999; 13: 717–30.
43. England R. The writing is on the wall for UNAIDS. *BMJ* 2008; 336: 1072.
44. Halperin D.T.. Putting a plague in perspective. *New York Times* Jan 1, 2008: A19.
45. Cassell MM, Halperin D.T., Shelton JD, Stanton D. Risk compensation: the Achilles' heel of innovations in HIV prevention? *BMJ* 2006; 332: 605–07.
46. Timberg C. Uganda's early gains against HIV eroding: message of fear, fidelity diluted by array of other remedies. *Washington Post* March 29, 2007: A1.

47. Shafer LA, Biraro S, Kamali A, et al. HIV prevalence and incidence are no longer falling in Uganda—a case for renewed prevention efforts: evidence from a rural population cohort 1989–2005 and from ANC surveillance. XVI International AIDS Conference; Toronto, Canada; Aug 13–18, 2006: THLB0108 (abstr). http://www.aegis.com/conferences/iac/2006/ThLB0108.html (accessed June 19, 2008).
48. Coates TJ, Richter L, Caceres C. Behavioural strategies to reduce HIV transmission: how to make them work better. *Lancet* 2008; published online Aug 6. DOI:10.1016/S0140-6736(08)60886-7.

13.6

HIV Prevention Approach Reduces New Infections in Ugandan District

National Institutes of Health

At a Glance

- A combination of HIV prevention measures substantially reduced new HIV infections in a district of Uganda during a seven-year period.
- The results prove the approach can reduce new HIV infections in a population.

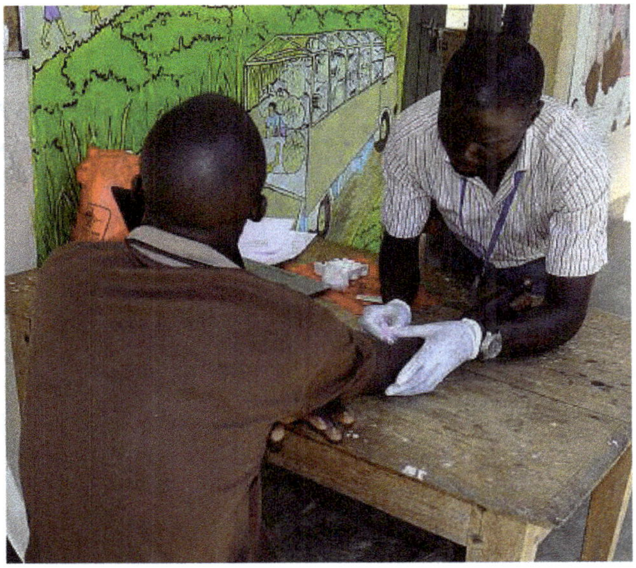

A RESEARCH assistant draws blood for HIV testing from a participant in the Rakai Community Cohort Study. Rakai Health Sciences Program

Researchers have found several strategies that can help stop the spread of HIV, the virus that causes AIDS. Voluntary, medically performed male circumcision, for example, significantly reduces a man's risk of acquiring HIV from his HIV-positive female partner. HIV-suppressing antiretroviral therapy (ART) prevents transmission of the virus to uninfected partners. Changes in sexual behavior, such as having only one sexual partner, can also help prevent HIV infection.

Source: https://www.nih.gov/news-events/nih-research-matters/hiv-prevention-approach-reduces-new-infections-ugandan-district.

The Rakai Health Sciences Program has been working to prevent the spread of HIV in the Rakai district of Uganda. The program promotes HIV testing, counseling, use of ART, and voluntary medical male circumcision to participants in the Rakai Community Cohort Study. In a new analysis, a team led by Dr. M. Kate Grabowski at Johns Hopkins University and the Rakai Health Sciences Program assessed the success of the program. The study, as well as the new analysis, were funded in part by NIH's National Institute of Allergy and Infectious Diseases (NIAID), Eunice Kennedy Shriver National Institute of Child Health and Human Development (NICHD), and National Institute of Mental Health (NIMH). Results were published on November 30, 2017, in the *New England Journal of Medicine.*

The analysis involved nearly 34,000 people, ages 15 to 49 years, from 30 communities. Every one or two years from April 1999 until September 2016, participants were tested for HIV and surveyed about their sexual behavior, use of ART, and male circumcision status.

The proportion of participants living with HIV who reported taking ART climbed from zero in 2003 to 69% in 2016. The proportion of males who were voluntarily circumcised grew from 15% in 1999 to 59% in 2016. The proportion of adolescents (ages 15 to 19) who reported never having sex rose from 30% in 1999 to 55% in 2016. Levels of condom use with casual partners and people reporting multiple sexual partners remained largely unchanged.

The researchers estimated that the annual number of new HIV infections fell 42%—from about 1.17 per 100 people in 2009 to about 0.66 per 100 in 2016. In addition, the proportion of participants living with HIV whose treatment suppressed the virus increased from 42% in 2009 to 75% in 2016.

HIV incidence dropped the most among circumcised men, by 57%. HIV incidence declined by 54% among all men but by only 32% among all women. The researchers anticipate that this gender imbalance will be addressed in the future. For example, pre-exposure prophylaxis (PrEP) could be added to the program's HIV prevention package.

"We expect that this multifaceted approach to HIV prevention will work as well in other populations as it has in rural Uganda," Grabowski says.

"Before this study, we knew that these HIV prevention measures worked at an individual level, yet it was not clear that they would substantially reduce HIV incidence in a population—or even if it would be possible to get large numbers of people to adopt them," says NIAID Director Dr. Anthony S. Fauci. "This new analysis demonstrates that scaling up combination HIV prevention is possible and can turn the tide of the epidemic."

References

HIV Prevention Efforts and Incidence of HIV in Uganda. Grabowski MK, Serwadda DM, Gray RH, Nakigozi G, Kigozi G, Kagaayi J, Ssekubugu R, Nalugoda F, Lessler J, Lutalo T, Galiwango RM, Makumbi F, Kong X, Kabatesi D, Alamo ST, Wiersma S, Sewankambo NK, Tobian AAR, Laeyendecker O, Quinn TC, Reynolds SJ, Wawer MJ, Chang LW; Rakai Health Sciences Program. N Engl J Med. 2017 Nov 30;377(22):2154-2166. doi: 10.1056/NEJMoa1702150. PMID: 29171817.

https://www.nih.gov/news-events/nih-research-matters/hiv-prevention-approach-reducesnew-infections-ugandan-district

13.7

Speeding HIV's Deadly Spread

Multiple, Concurrent Partners Drive Disease in Southern Africa

Craig Timberg

FRANCISTOWN, BOTSWANA—THE YOUNG AND HIP at ground zero of the AIDS epidemic meet, drink and pair off under the knowing gaze of bartender Brian Khumalo. Sometimes they first buy a three-pack of condoms from the box he keeps by the liquor, sometimes not.

Night after night they return for the carefree, beery vibe, with the same partners or new ones, creating a web of sexual interaction. A growing number of studies single out such behavior—in which men and women maintain two or more ongoing relationships—as the most powerful force propelling a killer disease through a vulnerable continent.

This new understanding of how the AIDS virus attacks individuals and their societies helps explain why the disease has devastated southern Africa while sparing other places. It also suggests how the region's AIDS programs, which have struggled to prevent new infections even as treatment for the disease has become more widely available, might save far more lives: by discouraging sexual networks.

"The problem of multiple partners who do not practice safe sex is obviously the biggest driver of HIV in the world," said Ndwapi Ndwapi, a top government AIDS official in Botswana, speaking in Gaborone, the capital. "What I need to know from the scientific community is, what do you do? ... How do you change that for a society that happens to have higher rates of multiple sexual partners?"

Khumalo, 25, tall and lanky with a crooked-toothed smile, described the problem succinctly as he pointed to a spiky-haired woman in a corner booth of the bar. "She's new around here, so every guy is going to talk to her," he said. "She will be with me today. Tomorrow she will be with my best friend. And I will be with somebody else."

Khumalo moved from Gaborone to Francistown last March, finding a city of 85,000 with a red-brick downtown, modest concrete homes and an accommodating sexual culture. The first night, he slept with a woman he had just met, he said. He did the same the second night, the third, the fourth.

Though he used condoms each time, he said, an alarmed friend soon drove him to the white, low-slung buildings of Francistown's biggest AIDS clinic. "I saw thousands of beautiful women going to get pills," Khumalo recalled.

It scared him, but not enough. By the end of the year, Khumalo had slept with more than 100 women, he said.

But the number of sexual partners is not the only factor that increases the risk of AIDS. The most potentially dangerous relationships, researchers say, involve men and women who maintain more than one regular partner for months or years. In these relationships, more intimate, trusting and long-lasting than casual sex, most couples eventually stop using condoms, studies show, allowing easy infiltration by HIV.

Researchers increasingly agree that curbing such behavior is key to slowing the spread of AIDS in Africa. In a July report, southern African AIDS experts and officials listed "reducing multiple and concurrent partnerships" as their first priority for preventing the spread of HIV in a region where nearly 15 million people are estimated to carry the virus—38 percent of the world's total.

But for many Batswana, as citizens of this landlocked desert country of 1.6 million call themselves, it is a strategy that has rarely been taught.

"There has never been equal emphasis on 'Don't have many partners,'" said Serara Selelo-Mogwe, a public health expert and retired nursing professor at the University of Botswana, who recalled stepping past broken bottles and used condoms as she arrived on campus each Monday morning. "If you just say, 'Use the condom' ... we will never see the daylight of the virus leaving us."

A Lethal Mix of Causes

International experts long regarded Botswana as a case study in how to combat AIDS. It had few of the intractable social problems thought to predispose a country to the disease, such as conflict, abject poverty and poor medical care. And for the past decade, the country has rigorously followed strategies that Western experts said would slow AIDS.

With its diamond wealth and the largess of international donors, Botswana aggressively promoted condom use while building Africa's best network of HIV testing centers and its most extensive system for distributing the antiretroviral drugs that dramatically prolong and improve the lives of those with AIDS.

But even though the relentless pace of funerals began to ease in recent years, the disease was far from under control. The national death rate fell from the highest in the world, but only to second-highest, behind AIDS-ravaged Swaziland. Men and women in Botswana continued to contract HIV faster than almost anywhere else on Earth.

Twenty-five percent of Batswana adults carry the virus, according to a 2004 national study, and among women in their early 30s living in Francistown, the rate is 69 percent.

Researchers increasingly attribute the resilience of HIV in Botswana—and in southern Africa generally—to the high incidence of multiple sexual relationships. Europeans and Americans often have more partners over their lives, studies show, but sub-Saharan Africans average more at the same time.

Nearly one in three sexually active men in Botswana reported having multiple, concurrent sex partners, as did 14 percent of women, in a 2003 survey paid for by the U.S. government. Among men younger than 25, the rate was 44 percent.

The distinction between having several partners in a year and several in a month is crucial because those newly infected with HIV experience an initial surge in viral loads that makes them far more contagious than they will be for years. During the three-week spike—which ends before standard tests can even detect HIV—the virus explodes through networks of unprotected sex.

This insight explained what studies were documenting: Africans with multiple, concurrent sex partners were more likely to contract HIV, and countries where such partnerships were common had wider and more lethal epidemics.

A model of multiple sexual relationships presented at a Princeton University conference in May showed that a small increase in the average number of concurrent sexual partners—from 1.68 to 1.86—had profound effects, connecting sexual networks into a single, massive tangle that, when plotted out, resembles the transportation system of a major city.

A second key factor helping the virus spread through southern Africa is low rates of circumcision. Before European colonialists arrived, most tribes in the region removed the foreskins of teenage boys during manhood rituals. Those rites, which were discouraged by missionaries and other Westerners who regarded them as primitive, have gradually declined as the region rapidly modernized.

Dozens of studies, including three experimental trials conducted in Africa in recent years, show that circumcised men are much less likely to contract HIV because the most easily infected cells have been removed.

These factors, researchers say, explain how North Africa, where Muslim societies require circumcision and strongly discourage sex outside monogamous and polygamous marriages, has largely avoided AIDS. They also explain why the epidemic is far more severe south of the Sahara, where webs of multiple sex partners are more common, researchers say.

West Africa has been partially protected by its high rates of circumcision, but in southern and eastern Africa—which have both low rates of circumcision and high rates of multiple sex partners—the AIDS epidemic became the most deadly in the world.

"That's the lethal cocktail," said Harvard University epidemiologist Daniel Halperin, a former AIDS prevention adviser in Africa for the U.S. government, speaking from suburban Boston. "There's no place in the world where you have very high HIV and you don't have those two factors."

No Word for 'Fidelity'

From under the broad thatched roof of Francistown's Customary Court, which handles minor crimes and misconduct, Chief Judge Ludo Margaret Mosojane had long suspected that the city's torrent of AIDS deaths flowed from its sexual culture. Each year brought more cases resulting from elaborate, overlapping relationships, she said.

"It explains why Africa is hardest hit by AIDS," Mosojane said. "The way we contract for sex is different from how others do it."

Polygamy once was common in the region, and in some parts still is; Swaziland's king has 13 wives. In generations past, even Batswana with just one spouse rarely expected monogamy. Husbands spent months herding cattle while their wives, staying elsewhere, tended crops, Mosojane said. On his return, a husband was not to be quizzed about his activities while he was away. He also was supposed to spend his first night back in an uncle's house, giving his wife time to send off boyfriends.

In Setswana, the national language, "the word 'fidelity' does not even exist," Mosojane said.

The few checks that traditional villages had on sexual behavior dwindled during the development frenzy after 1967, when diamonds were discovered. Batswana increasingly moved to cities for school or work.

Plentiful television sets delivered a flood of Western images, including racy soap operas and music videos featuring lightly clad women vying for the attention of wealthy, bejeweled men.

Francistown, with nearby mines, military camps and border posts overflowing with desperate refugees, changed faster than most cities. Amid the bustling malls, there was soon an unsettling concentration of young adults because so many people ages 35 to 50 had already died of AIDS complications, residents say.

Faruk Maunge, 36, a high school counselor whose dreadlocks, goatee and rectangular glasses give him a cosmopolitan air, noticed the changes when he returned from stays abroad. "They are just a lost bunch," he said. "They are very, very reckless."

Maunge said that rent, clothing, even cellphone airtime became part of implicit sexual exchanges. Men and women maintained two, three, even four regular partners. The toll was clear from the snapshots he kept in a green plastic first-aid box.

"This one is gone," Maunge said, pointing to a faded picture of a woman in a red top who was nibbling her fingernails. Moving deeper into the pile, he continued: "This one is gone, Mooketsi. And this one is gone, Themba. This one is gone, too, this one on the far left. This one is positive."

With a hint of frustration, Maunge said of one man, "He's sleeping around again." Maunge also grew irritated at a picture showing a friend with AIDS who seemed to father a child—he was awaiting his fourth—with every girlfriend.

Maunge said he once was reckless, too, having sex with three women in a week, sometimes without condoms. But after watching the disease kill more than 20 of his friends, he settled down with a new girlfriend and stayed faithful, he said.

"Praise God, I've been lucky," Maunge said. "It's like you have 10 bullets going through you and none hits you."

The Missing Message

On a hospital wall here, not far from the AIDS clinic that Khumalo visited with his friend, the painted image of a condom shimmers like a comic-book superhero. Giant, colorful block letters declare, "CONDOMISE AND STAY ALIVE!!"

In cramped black script below, it adds, "Abstain first."

Yet rarely seen among Botswana's AIDS prevention messages is one that has worked in other African countries: Multiple sex partners kill. Dubbed "Zero Grazing" by Ugandan President Yoweri Museveni, this approach dominated in East Africa, where several countries curbed HIV rates.

Fidelity campaigns never caught on in Botswana. Instead, the country focused on remedies favored by Western AIDS experts schooled in the epidemics of America's gay community or Thailand's brothels, where condom use became so routine it slowed the spread of HIV.

These experts brought not just ideas but money, and soon billboards in Botswana touted condoms. Schoolchildren sang about them. Cadres of young women demonstrated how to roll them on. The anti-AIDS partnership between the Bill & Melinda Gates Foundation and drugmaker Merck budgeted $13.5 million for condom promotion—25 times the amount dedicated to curbing dangerous sexual behavior.

But soaring rates of condom use have not brought down high HIV rates. Instead, they rose together, until both were among the highest in Africa.

The focus on condoms endured even after the arrival of internationally heralded "ABC" programs, named for their prescription of "Abstain, Be Faithful and Condomize." The middle concept—fidelity—often got lost.

The few posters advocating it in Francistown are old and torn; ads for condoms and abstinence are far more prominent. A 2004 government study measured the result: Three-quarters of Batswana surveyed knew that condoms could stop the spread of HIV. Half knew that abstinence would. Yet only one in five knew that fidelity to a single, uninfected partner prevented spreading the disease.

13.8

Pre-Exposure Prophylaxis (PrEP) for HIV Prevention

U.S. Center for Disease Control and Prevention

PRE-EXPOSURE PROPHYLAXIS (OR PREP) IS WHEN people at risk for HIV take daily medicine to prevent HIV. PrEP can stop HIV from taking hold and spreading throughout your body. When taken daily, PrEP is highly effective for preventing HIV from sex or injection drug use. PrEP is much less effective when it is not taken consistently.

Studies have shown that PrEP reduces the risk of getting HIV from sex by about 99% when taken daily. Among people who inject drugs, PrEP reduces the risk of getting HIV by at least 74% when taken daily.

[...]

What is PrEP?

Pre-exposure prophylaxis (or PrEP) is when people at risk for HIV take daily medicine to lower their chances of getting HIV. Two medications, sold under the brand names Truvada® and Descovy® are approved for daily use as PrEP to help prevent a person without HIV from getting the virus from sex or injection drug use. Studies have shown that PrEP is highly effective for preventing HIV if it is used as prescribed. PrEP is much less effective when it is not taken consistently.

Note: Truvada® for PrEP is recommended to prevent HIV for all people at risk through sex or injection drug use. Descovy® for PrEP is recommended to prevent HIV for people at risk through sex, ***excluding people at risk through receptive vaginal sex***. Descovy has not yet been studied for HIV prevention for receptive vaginal sex, so it may not be appropriate for some people.

[...]

Why take PrEP?

For those at risk for HIV, daily PrEP is highly effective for preventing HIV from sex or injection drug use. PrEP is much less effective when it is not taken consistently. [...]

U.S. Center for Disease Control and Prevention, "Pre-exposure Prophylaxis (PrEP) for HIV Prevention," pp. 1–2, 2014.

Is PrEP a vaccine?

No. PrEP does not work the same way as a vaccine. A vaccine teaches your body to fight off infection for several years. For PrEP, you take a pill every day by mouth. If you take PrEP daily, the presence of the medicine in your bloodstream can often stop HIV from taking hold and spreading in your body. If you do not take PrEP every day, there may not be enough medicine in your bloodstream to block the virus.

[...]

Should I consider taking PrEP?

PrEP is for people without HIV who are at risk for getting the virus from sex or injection drug use. The federal guidelines recommend that PrEP be considered for people who are HIV-negative who:

Have **had anal or vaginal sex in the past 6 months and**:

- Have a sexual partner with HIV (especially if the partner has an unknown or detectable viral load) or
- Have not consistently used a condom or
- Have been diagnosed with an STD in the past 6 months

PrEP is also recommended for **people who inject drugs and**

- have an injection partner with HIV or
- share needles, syringes, or other equipment to inject drugs (for example, cookers).

PrEP should also be considered for **people who have been prescribed non-occupational post-exposure prophylaxis (PEP) and**

- report continued risk behavior, or
- have used multiple courses of PEP.

If you have a partner with HIV and **are considering getting pregnant**, talk to your doctor about PrEP if you're not already taking it. PrEP may be an option to help protect you and your baby from getting HIV while you try to get pregnant, during pregnancy, or while breastfeeding.

Because PrEP involves daily medication and regular visits to a health care provider, it may not be right for everyone. And PrEP may cause side effects like nausea in some people, but these generally subside over time. These side effects aren't life threatening. [...]

How well does PrEP work?

Studies have shown that PrEP reduces the risk of getting HIV from sex by about 99% when taken consistently. Among people who inject drugs, PrEP reduces the risk of getting HIV by at least 74% when taken consistently. Since PrEP does not protect against other STDs, use condoms the right way every time you have sex.

[...]

Is PrEP safe?

PrEP can cause side effects like nausea in some people, but these generally subside over time. No serious side effects have been observed, and these side effects aren't life threatening. If you are taking PrEP, tell your health care provider about any side effects that are severe or do not go away.

[...]

I'm transgender, will PrEP interfere with my hormone therapy?

More studies are needed on this topic. But there are no known drug conflicts or interactions between the medicines used in PrEP and hormone therapy. There is no known scientific reason why the drugs cannot be taken at the same time. If you are worried that PrEP will affect your hormone therapy, ask your health care provider to check your hormone levels. People who use PrEP should see their health care provider every 3 months for follow up, HIV tests, and to have their prescriptions refilled. This visit could be combined with your hormone therapy appointments.

[...]

If I take PrEP, can I stop using condoms when I have sex?

No, you should not stop using condoms because you are taking PrEP. PrEP doesn't give you any protection against other STDs, like gonorrhea and chlamydia.

If used the right way every time you have sex, condoms are highly effective in preventing HIV and some STDs you can get through body fluids, like gonorrhea and chlamydia. However, they provide less protection against STDs spread through skin-to-skin contact, like human papillomavirus or HPV (genital warts), genital herpes, and syphilis.

[...]

How long do I need to take PrEP?

You must take PrEP daily for it to work. But there are several reasons people stop taking PrEP. For example,

- If your risk of getting HIV infection becomes low because of changes in your life, you may want to stop taking PrEP.
- If you find you don't want to take a pill every day or often forget to take your pills, other ways of protecting yourself from HIV infection may work better for you.

- If you have side effects from the medicine that are interfering with your life, or if blood tests show that your body is reacting to PrEP in unsafe ways, your provider may stop prescribing PrEP for you.

[...]

How long do I have to take PrEP before it is effective?

When taken every day, PrEP is safe and highly effective in preventing HIV. PrEP reaches maximum protection from HIV for **receptive anal sex** at about **7 days** of daily use. For **receptive vaginal sex** and **injection drug use**, PrEP reaches maximum protection at about **21 days** of daily use. No data are yet available about how long it takes to reach maximum protection for **insertive anal or insertive vaginal sex**.

[...]

Does taking PrEP long-term have harmful health effects?

In people without HIV and have taken PrEP for up to 5 years, no significant health effects have been seen.

[...]

Can you start PrEP after you have been exposed to HIV?

PrEP (pre-exposure prophylaxis) is only for people who are at risk of getting HIV. But **PEP (post-exposure prophylaxis)** is an option for someone who thinks they've recently been exposed to HIV during sex or through injection drug use.

PEP means taking antiretroviral medicines after a potential exposure to HIV to prevent getting the virus. PEP must be started within 72 hours of possible exposure to HIV. If you're prescribed PEP, you'll need to take it once or twice daily for 28 days. [...]

[...]

13.9

PEP 101

U.S. Center for Disease Control and Prevention

PEP (POST-EXPOSURE PROPHYLAXIS) MEANS TAKING ANTIRETROVIRAL medicines (ART) after being potentially exposed to HIV to prevent becoming infected.

PEP should be used only in emergency situations and must be started within 72 hours after a recent possible exposure to HIV. If you think you've recently been exposed to HIV during sex or through sharing needles and works to prepare drugs or if you've been sexually assaulted, talk to your health care provider or an emergency room doctor about PEP right away.

[...]

What is PEP?

PEP stands for post-exposure prophylaxis. It means taking antiretroviral medicines (ART) after being potentially exposed to HIV to prevent becoming infected.

PEP must be started within 72 hours after a recent possible exposure to HIV, but the sooner you start PEP, the better. Every hour counts. If you're prescribed PEP, you'll need to take it once or twice daily for 28 days. PEP is effective in preventing HIV when administered correctly, but not 100%.

[...]

Is PEP right for me?

If you're HIV-negative or don't know your HIV status, and in the last 72 hours you

1. think you may have been exposed to HIV during sex (for example, if the condom broke),
2. shared needles and works to prepare drugs (for example, cotton, cookers, water), or
3. were sexually assaulted,

talk to your health care provider or an emergency room doctor about PEP right away.

U.S. Center for Disease Control and Prevention, "PEP 101," https://www.cdc.gov/hiv/pdf/programresources/cdc-hiv-npep-guidelines.pdf, 2018.

PEP should be used only in emergency situations and must be started within 72 hours after a recent possible exposure to HIV. It is not a substitute for regular use of other proven HIV prevention methods, such as pre-exposure prophylaxis (PrEP), which means taking HIV medicines daily to lower your chance of getting infected; using condoms the right way every time you have sex; and using only your own new, sterile needles and works every time you inject.

PEP is effective, but not 100%, so you should continue to use condoms with sex partners and safe injection practices while taking PEP. These strategies can protect you from being exposed to HIV again and reduce the chances of transmitting HIV to others if you do become infected while you're on PEP.

If you're a health care worker and think you've had a possible HIV exposure at work, see the following question.

[...]

I'm a health care worker, and I think I've been exposed to HIV at work. Should I take PEP?

PEP should be considered if you've had a recent possible exposure to HIV at work. Report your exposure to your supervisor, and seek medical attention immediately.

Occupational transmission of HIV to health care workers is extremely rare, and the proper use of safety devices and barriers can help minimize the risk of exposure while caring for patients with HIV.

A health care worker who has a possible exposure should see a doctor or visit an emergency room immediately. PEP must be started within 72 hours after a recent possible exposure to HIV. The sooner, the better; every hour counts.

CDC issued updated guidelines in 2013 for the management of health care worker exposures to HIV and recommendations for PEP.

Clinicians caring for health care workers who've had a possible exposure can call the PEPline (1-888-448-4911), which offers around-the-clock advice on managing occupational exposures to HIV, as well as hepatitis B and C. Exposed health care workers may also call the PEPline, but they should seek local medical attention first.

[...]

When should I take PEP?

PEP must be started within 72 hours after a possible exposure. The sooner you start PEP, the better; every hour counts.

Starting PEP as soon as possible after a potential HIV exposure is important. Research has shown that PEP has little or no effect in preventing HIV infection if it is started later than 72 hours after HIV exposure. If you're prescribed PEP, you'll need to take it once or twice daily for 28 days.

[...]

Does PEP have any side effects?

PEP is safe but may cause side effects like nausea in some people. These side effects can be treated and aren't life-threatening.

[...]

Where can I get PEP?

Your health care provider or an emergency room doctor can prescribe PEP. Talk to them right away if you think you've recently been exposed to HIV.

[...]

How can I pay for PEP?

If you're prescribed PEP after a sexual assault, you may qualify for partial or total reimbursement for medicines and clinical care costs through the Office for Victims of Crime, funded by the US Department of Justice (see the contact information for each state).

If you're prescribed PEP for another reason and you cannot get insurance coverage (Medicaid, Medicare, private, or employer-based), your health care provider can apply for free PEP medicines through the medication assistance programs run by the manufacturers. Online applications can be faxed to the company, or some companies have special phone lines. These can be handled urgently in many cases to avoid a delay in getting medicine.

If you're a health care worker who was exposed to HIV on the job, your workplace health insurance or workers' compensation will usually pay for PEP.

[...]

Can I take a round of PEP every time I have unprotected sex?

PEP should be used only in emergency situations.

PEP is not the right choice for people who may be exposed to HIV frequently—for example, if you often have sex without a condom with a partner who is HIV-positive. Because PEP is given after a potential exposure to HIV, more drugs and higher doses are needed to block infection than with PrEP, or *pre-exposure* prophylaxis. PrEP is when people at high risk for HIV take HIV medicines (sold under the brand name Truvada) daily to lower their chances of getting HIV. [...]

Algorithm for evaluation and treatment of possible nonoccupational HIV exposures

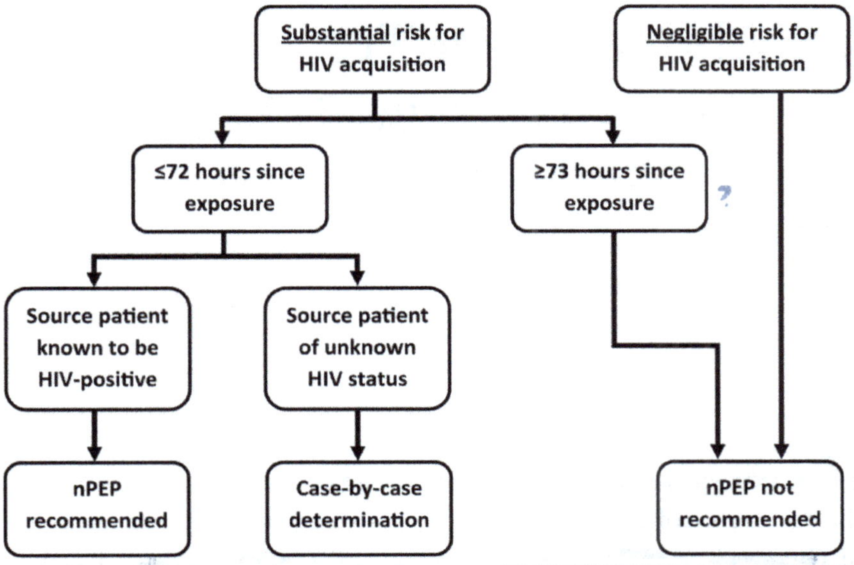

Substantial Risk for HIV Acquisition

Exposure of:
Vagina, rectum, eye, mouth, or other mucous membrane, nonintact skin, or percutaneous contact

With:
Blood, semen, vaginal secretions, rectal secretions, breast milk, or any body fluid that is visibly contaminated with blood

When:
The source is known to be HIV-positive

Negligible Risk for HIV Acquisition

Exposure of:
Vagina, rectum, eye, mouth, or other mucous membrane, intact or nonintact skin, or percutaneous contact

With:
Urine, nasal secretions, saliva, sweat, or tears if not visibly contaminated with blood

Regardless:
Of the known or suspected HIV status of the source

nPEP = non-occupational post-exposure prophylaxis

Reference:

Updated Guidelines for Antiretroviral Postexposure Prophylaxis After Sexual, Injection Drug Use, or Other Nonoccupational Exposure to HIV— United States, 2016
from the Centers for Disease Control and Prevention
https://www.cdc.gov/hiv/pdf/programresources/cdc-hiv-npep-guidelines.pdf

13.10

Beliefs About Better Treatment for HIV Leads Gay Men to Engage in Riskier Sex

Condomless Intercourse Among Men Who have Sex with Men Again on the Rise

Springer

A SURVEY SPANNING 19 YEARS OF PARTICIPANTS at a gay pride event in the US notes a consistent increase in the occurrence of condomless anal sex among men, as well as a rise in how many sex partners they have. Condomless receptive anal sex among HIV uninfected men has doubled, while insertive condomless anal sex has more than tripled among HIV-positive men. The findings show that, although antiretroviral therapies (ART) have revolutionized the treatment and prevention of HIV infections, knowing that they have ART as a protective back-up against contracting or transmitting the disease makes people complacent. This complacency can lead to increased risks when it comes to sex and their health, says study leader Seth Kalichman of the University of Connecticut in an article in Springer's journal *Archives of Sexual Behavior.*

Trials have shown that early treatment with ART prevents HIV transmission. This shifted the focus of HIV prevention campaigns away from condom use as a form of protection toward detecting and treating those already infected. Despite these efforts there have not yet been significant reductions in new HIV infections in major cities, for instance. In addition, HIV infections remain stable or are rising among gay men in countries that have scaled-up HIV testing programs and access to ART.

Kalichman and his team analyzed surveys conducted in 1997, 2005, 2006, and 2015 at the Atlanta Gay Pride Festival. Through self-administered surveys 1,831 gay men provided anonymous information about their substance use, sexual behavior, beliefs about HIV treatment, and how they perceive sexual risks in relation to the HIV treatment status of potential sex partners.

Among uninfected men and those who did not know their HIV status, condomless anal sex increased from 43 percent in 1997 to 61 percent in 2015. The number of those having multiple sex partners also rose from 9 percent in 1997 to 33 percent in 2015. This pattern is also reflected among HIV-positive men. Condomless anal sex increased from 25 percent in 1997 to 67 percent in 2015. In 1997 only 9 percent of men in this group reported having had unprotected intercourse with two or more partners in the six months before the survey. By 2015 this figure rose to 52 percent. In 1997 condoms were used about eight out of ten times (82 percent) when HIV-positive men had intercourse, but it dropped by 2015 to less than one in two (47 percent) instances. These shifts in behavior create increased risks for sexually transmitted infections, which in turn can increase risks for HIV transmission.

HIV-positive men as well as those who had not tested positive held increased beliefs reflecting public health messages that ART prevents HIV and therefore make condomless anal sex safe. Also consistent with public health messaging, they believed their risk of contracting HIV to be much lower when their partner had an undetectable blood plasma viral load.

"Treatment-related behavioral beliefs in this study paralleled a resurgence in condomless anal sex among men who have sex with men measured over nearly two decades," explains Kalichman. "The current study adds to the mounting evidence that substantial changes have occurred in community-held beliefs that condomless anal sex is safer in the era of HIV treatment as prevention."

Journal Reference

Seth C. Kalichman, Devon Price, Lisa A. Eaton, Kaylee Burnham, Matthew Sullivan, Stephanie Finneran, Talea Cornelius, Aerielle Allen. Diminishing Perceived Threat of AIDS and Increasing Sexual Risks of HIV Among Men Who Have Sex with Men, 1997–2015. *Archives of Sexual Behavior*, 2017; DOI: 10.1007/s10508-016-0934-9

13.11

HIV and Disclosure

A Doctor's Moral Dilemma

Lisa Fitzpatrick

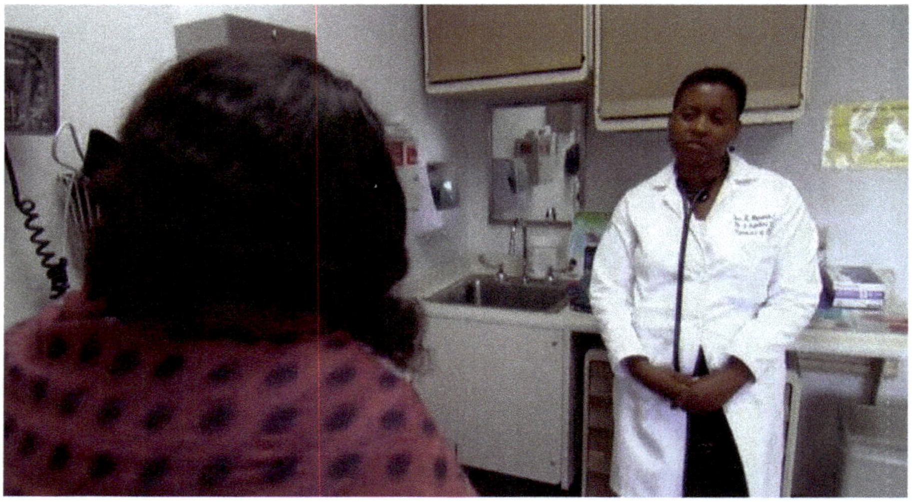

Dr. Lisa Fitzpatrick is a CDC-trained epidemiologist and practicing infectious diseases physician in Washington D.C. At the CDC, she led teams that produced landmark studies on HIV transmission among black college students, black women and in the Georgia prison system. From 2005 to 2007, she served as a U.S. diplomat, and was director of the CDC's Global AIDS Program in the Caribbean, responsible for implementing the President's Emergency Plan for AIDS Relief (PEPFAR). Fitzpatrick is an associate professor of medicine at Howard University and the director of infectious diseases services at United Medical Center.

RECENTLY I HAD AN UNUSUALLY DISTRESSING day at my clinic. I work in an impoverished neighborhood with some of the city's most indigent patients. Each one faces a social challenge—unemployment, chronic hunger with no access to food, lack of transportation, homelessness. But the challenge I faced with my new patient made these issues seem like a walk in the park.

The patient was a newly diagnosed woman with a single-digit CD4 count, which means her immune system had been destroyed by HIV. In the previous months she had been evaluated by four internists, none of whom thought to test her for HIV. This information bothered me, but wasn't the source of my distress. Experiencing no physical relief from these providers, she had decided to "lay down and die."

However, upon what she describes as "fierce" insistence by her partner of 10 years, she agreed to go to a hospital ER, and after a rapid test, learned she was HIV positive.

As she sat in front of me and told me her story, her partner, who had accompanied her—the one she credits with saving her life—sat quietly in the corner. This partner was the source of my distress. She told me he was also HIV positive. I turned my attention to him and asked if he was in care. He said no and indicated he wanted to establish care with us. Then I asked if he had previously been on medication. Angst and frustration grew inside me as I listened to his answer.

He gazed at the medication chart and pointed out his previous regimen. The cocktail contained indinavir. Based on this information I knew immediately that he had been withholding his secret from her for over a decade. I couldn't remember the last time I prescribed indinavir. An awkward moment passed as I reflected on their scenario.

The silence is perpetuating disease.

His secret led to her infection. I then wondered if this was the reason he "fiercely" insisted she seek help despite her resolve to lay down and die.

For the remainder of the visit I maintained objectivity externally, but inside I was wrestling with endless questions and my own moral dilemma. As a physician, I am not allowed to reveal any medical information about my patients or their circumstances without their written permission. The confidentiality between a patient and provider is sacred. Therefore, it is not my duty or my right to disclose or report such blatant injustice. But now this constraint feels inappropriate and morally irresponsible.

Unfortunately this is not an isolated case. A personal urgency is building for me to seek answers, incite a conversation or influence our murky policies that provide no guidance about or latitude for wandering outside the lines of confidentiality even if for the health benefit of another. The urgency is building because I have witnessed countless scenarios many of which are variations on this theme.

A few months ago, a patient arrived at her visit urgently wanting to know her viral load—which would tell her the amount of HIV floating in her bloodstream. She had a new boyfriend and had decided if the amount of virus in her blood remained low enough and was controlled by her HIV medication she would not have to disclose her HIV status. She has since decided to wait until they are married to disclose her status to him.

I encouraged her to tell him by asking how she would feel if she were in his place. She then asked if she could bring him for a visit; they could both be tested and she could feign shock, awe and distress when I revealed her diagnosis. It is a clever response that painfully demonstrates why support must accompany disclosure. She did not feel strong enough to divulge her secret on her own and thought she could draw strength from my presence as I diffused what might become a tense and awkward situation. However, as I played the scenario out with her, she realized this would create additional ethical dilemmas and a series of untruths and dishonesty from which neither of us could recover.

These issues around disclosure, personal responsibility and the need for clarity around my role as a health care provider give me heartburn. Am I complicit in these behaviors? Why doesn't the law speak clearly and guide me about how to address these issues? Whose responsibility is it to inform unknowing, uninfected partners when their infected partner refuses to disclose? What should be the ramifications for failure to disclose? What should our response be? What should the community expectations be? How do we balance personal responsibility while minimizing HIV-associated stigma and shame?

As a public health practitioner whose goals in life include fostering community wellness and halting the spread of disease, these questions around the failure to disclose HIV status and our response to it have become the moral dilemma of my career. Most of my patients are so comfortable with me they know they can tell me anything without shame, embarrassment or fear of judgment. The trust between us is sacred and this deepens my conflict all the more.

But the secrecy is not OK. The silence is perpetuating disease. If we expect to end the epidemic, we cannot continue to ignore these questions, which are blatantly staring us in the face. They are pervasive and until we develop the moral courage to craft a balanced response and discuss these issues aloud and in the open, any notions of ending the epidemic is merely lip service and a pipe dream.

13.12

Knowingly Exposing Others to HIV Will No Longer Be a Felony in California

Patrick Mcgreevy

GOV. JERRY BROWN SIGNED A BILL Friday that lowers from a felony to a misdemeanor the crime of knowingly exposing a sexual partner to HIV without disclosing the infection.

The measure also applies to those who give blood without telling the blood bank that they are HIV-positive.

Modern medicine allows those with HIV to live longer lives and nearly eliminates the possibility of transmission, according to state Sen. Scott Wiener (D-San Francisco) and Assemblyman Todd Gloria (D-San Diego), authors of the bill.

"Today California took a major step toward treating HIV as a public health issue, instead of treating people living with HIV as criminals," Wiener said in a statement. "HIV should be treated like all other serious infectious diseases, and that's what SB 239 does."

Supporters of the change said the current law requires an intent to transmit HIV to justify a felony, but others noted cases have been prosecuted where there was no physical contact, so there was an argument intent was lacking.

Brown declined to comment on his action.

HIV has been the only communicable disease for which exposure is a felony under California law. The current law, Wiener argued, may convince people not to be tested for HIV, because without a test they cannot be charged with a felony if they expose a partner to the infection.

"We are going to end new HIV infections, and we will do so not by threatening people with state prison time, but rather by getting people to test and providing them access to care," Wiener said.

Supporters of the bill said women engaging in prostitution are disproportionately targeted with criminal charges, even in cases where the infection is not transmitted.

Republican lawmakers including Sen. Joel Anderson of Alpine voted against the bill, arguing it puts the public at risk.

"I'm of the mind that if you purposefully inflict another with a disease that alters their lifestyle the rest of their life, puts them on a regimen of medications to maintain any kind of normalcy, it should be a felony," Anderson said during the floor debate. "It's absolutely crazy to me that we should go light on this."

Anderson said the answer could be to extend tougher penalties to those who expose others to other infectious diseases.

13.13

Healthcare Worker Safety

World Health Organization

Aide-Mémoire

For a Strategy to Protect Health Workers from Infection with Bloodborne Viruses

Health workers are exposed to blood and other body fluids in the course of their work. Consequently, they are at risk of infection with bloodborne viruses including human immunodeficiency virus (HIV), hepatitis B virus (HBV) and hepatitis C virus (HCV). The risk of infection for health workers depends on the prevalence of disease in the patient population and the nature and frequency of exposures. Occupational exposure to blood can result from percutaneous injury (needle-stick or other sharps injury), mucocutaneous injury (splash of blood or other body fluids into the eyes, nose or mouth) or bold contact with non-intact skin. The most common form of occupational exposure to blood and the most likely to result in infection, is needle-stick injury. The most common causes of needle-stick injury are two-handed recapping and the unsafe collection and disposal of sharps waste. Health workers in areas such as operating, delivery and emergency rooms and laboratories have a higher risk of exposure. Cleaners, waste collectors and others whose duties involve handling blood-contaminated items are also at risk.

Among the 35 million health workers worldwide, about 3 million experience percutaneous exposures to bloodborne pathogens each year; two million of those to HBV, 0.9 million to HCV and 170,000 to HIV. These injuries may result in 15,000 HCV, 70,000 HBV and 1,000 HIV infections. More than 90% of these infections occur in developing countries.

Most blood exposures in health settings are preventable. Strategies to protect health workers include implementation of Universal Precautions, immunization against hepatitis B, provision of personal protection and the management of exposures. Elimination of unnecessary sharps and injections also minimizes the potential for exposure. Successful implementation of these strategies requires an effective infection control committee with support from the health setting management team.

Words of Advice

- Set up and empower an Infection Control Committee
- Use surveillance to identify risk situations and procedures and modify them wherever possible

- Achieve compliance with Universal Precautions through ongoing commitment, training of all staff members and provision of supplies
- Immunize health workers against hepatitis B early in their career
- Ensure availability of personal protective equipment
- Manage cases of exposure to blood and body fluids
- Enforce safe practices through monitoring and supervision

Checklist

Universal Precautions

- Hand washing after any direct contact with patients
- No needle recapping
- Safe collection and disposal of sharps
- Gloves for contact with body fluids, non-intact skin and mucous membranes
- Wearing a mask, eye protection and a gown if blood or other body fluids might splash
- Covering cuts and abrasions
- Cleaning up spills of blood and other body fluids
- Safe system for hospital waste management and disposal

Personal Protection

- Where possible, use needle-stick prevention devices
- Ensure adequate supplies
- Involve staff in the selection of personal protective equipment
- Train staff in correct use
- Use influential senior staff as role models
- Monitor compliance and inappropriate use
- Dispose safely

Post-exposure Management

- Guidelines outlining all procedures
- Dissemination of guidelines
- Information, education and communication
- Support and counseling
- Where possible, provision of post-exposure prophylactic medication for high-risk exposures
- Analysis of surveillance data

Key Elements

Universal Precautions

Universal Precautions are a simple set of effective practices designed to protect health workers and patients from infection with a range of pathogens including bloodborne viruses. These practices are used when caring for all patients regardless of diagnosis. They are applied universally. It is not feasible, effective or cost-effective to test all patients for all pathogens prior to giving care in order to identify those who are infected and take precautions only with them. Knowing a patient is infected does not prevent occupational exposure to blood. Thus, decisions regarding the level of precautions to use are based on the nature of the procedure and not on the actual or assumed serological status of the patient. It is not safe to take precautions only with those from so-called risk groups for infection with bloodborne pathogens as many people belonging to risk groups are not infected and many infected people do not belong to risk groups. In practice, the implementation of Universal Precautions includes the following interventions:

- Hand washing after any direct contact with patients
- Preventing two-handed recapping of needles
- Safe collection and disposal of needles (hypodermic and suture) and sharps (scalpels, blades, Lancets, razors, scissors), with required puncture- and liquid-proof safety boxes in each patient care area
- Wearing gloves for contact with body fluids, non-intact skin and mucous membranes
- Wearing a mask, eye protection and a gown (and sometimes a plastic apron) if blood or other body fluids might splash
- Covering all cuts and abrasions with a waterproof dressing
- Promptly and carefully cleaning up spills of blood and other body fluids
- Using a safe system for health care waste management and disposal

Personal Protection

Personal protective equipment includes gloves, goggles or glasses, masks, gowns and plastic aprons.

- Where possible, use needle-stick prevention devices (i.e., devices where the sharp is sheathed or retracted after use)
- Ensure adequate supplies of personal protective equipment in all areas
- Involve staff in the selection of personal protective equipment, as equipment that is of poor quality or uncomfortable to wear will not be used
- Train staff in the correct use of personal protective equipment
- Use influential senior staff as role models to promote personal protective equipment
- Monitor compliance and inappropriate use. Inappropriate glove use wastes resources. Compliance with eye protection often requires additional efforts
- Dispose of used personal protective equipment safely

Post-Exposure Management

The risk of infection following a needle-stick injury with needle from an infected source patient is ~0.3% for HIV, 3% for hepatitis C and 6–30% for hepatitis B. An effective response to occupational exposure to blood or other body fluids involves the following:

- Development of guidelines outlining the first aid required, reporting mechanism and procedure to be followed for post-exposure prophylaxis and follow-up testing
- Dissemination of guidelines
- Information, education and communication
- Provision of support and counseling
- Where possible and indicated, provision of post-exposure prophylactic medication
- Analyze reported cases of exposure to improve practices

13.14

HIV and the Opioid Epidemic

5 Key Points

Lindsey Dawson and Jennifer Kates

Background

The opioid epidemic represents a significant and worsening public health crisis in the United States. In 2016, 2.1 million Americans were estimated to have an opioid use disorder and nearly 12 million to have misused opioids at some point during the preceding year.[1] Death rates from opioid overdoses nearly doubled between 2012 and 2016, rising from 7.4 to 13.3 per 100,000, and in 2016, an estimated 115 people per day died of an opioid overdose.[2]

As the opioid epidemic has worsened, there has been growing concern about how injection drug use might fuel transmission of infectious disease. Those misusing opioids commonly move from oral use to insufflation to injection use.[3] In fact, an estimated 10–20% of people who abuse prescription opioids move on to inject either opioids or heroin.[4] Injection drug use increases the risk of blood-borne infections including HIV, hepatitis, and bacterial endocarditis, which spread efficiently through needle sharing.

In 2015, opioid use resulted in an HIV outbreak in Scott County, Indiana, with 181 individuals diagnosed with HIV by year-end, most of whom were co-infected with hepatitis C (HCV).[5,6] In response to this outbreak and the threat posed by the opioid epidemic more broadly, the Centers for Disease Control and Prevention (CDC) identified 220 jurisdictions particularly vulnerable to a similar type of outbreak in an effort to detect and prevent additional events.[7] Indeed, recent reports suggest new outbreaks may in fact be occurring. In the context of HIV, this has raised particular concerns given that, prior to the opioid epidemic, HIV infections due to injecting drug use had fallen dramatically.

This graphic series highlights key things to know about the intersection of the nation's HIV and opioid epidemics.

Lindsey Dawson and Jennifer Kates, "HIV and the Opioid Epidemic: 5 Key Points," *The Kaiser Family Foundation*, pp. 1–6.

1. **The decline in HIV infections associated with injection drug use has been a major success in the fight against HIV in the U.S.,** with the share of new HIV infections attributed to injection drug use falling from an estimated 40% in 1990 to just 6% in 2015.

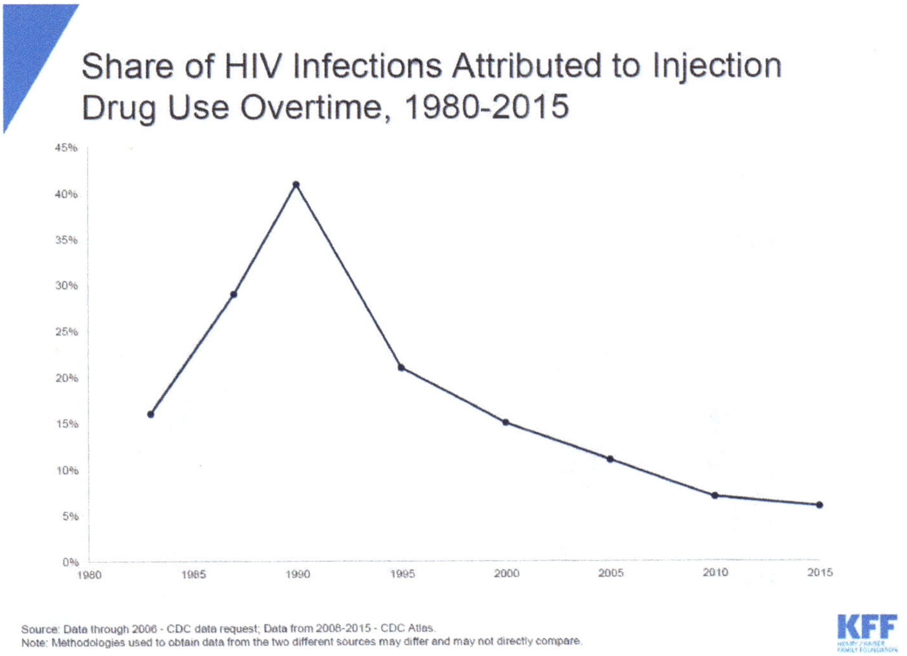

2. **However, 2015 marked the first time in two decades where the number of HIV diagnoses attributed to IDU increased,** largely associated with the opioid epidemic and subsequent HIV outbreak in Scott County, Indiana. (Early data suggests a decline in 2016, back to 2014 levels, after the peak of this localized outbreak.)[8]

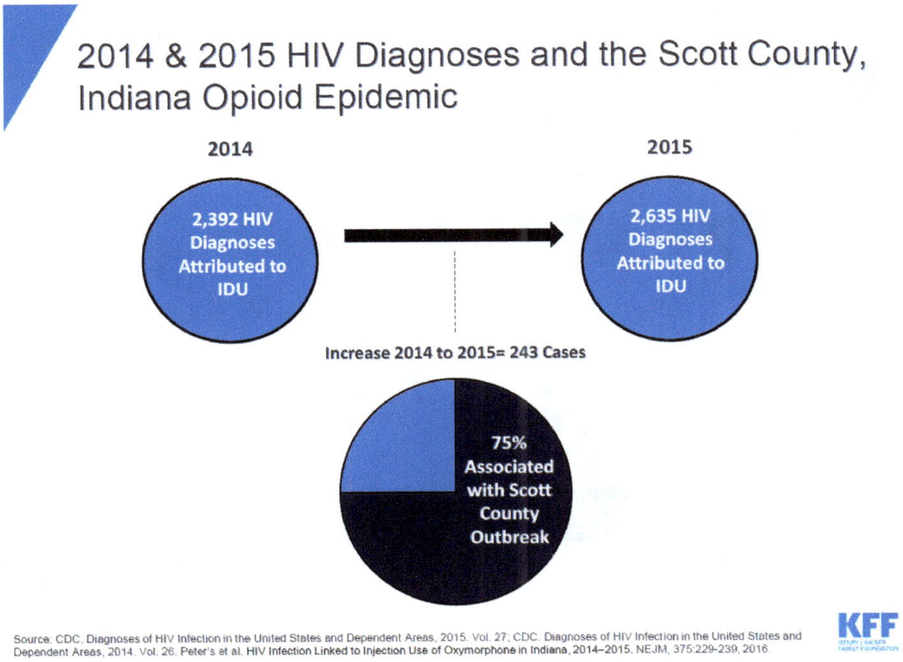

3. **The demographics of people with HIV attributed to injection drug are increasingly similar to those most at risk for opioid use and addiction**, with greater shares of those newly diagnosed being white and younger, relative to earlier years in the epidemic.

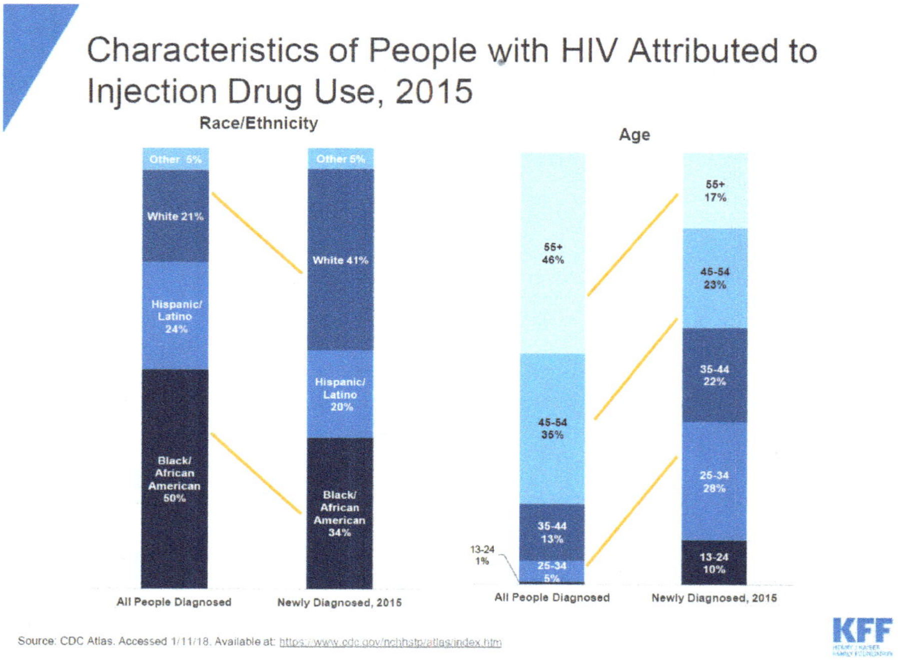

4. While there are several proven strategies available to reduce risk of infectious disease associated with injection drug use, including the provision of Syringe Exchange Programs (SEPs), access varies significantly across the country and does not always align with opioid epidemic epicenters.[9] Of the 220, mostly rural, counties CDC determined were potentially vulnerable to an HIV or HCV outbreak among people who inject drugs, just 8% have an SEP in place.[10,11]

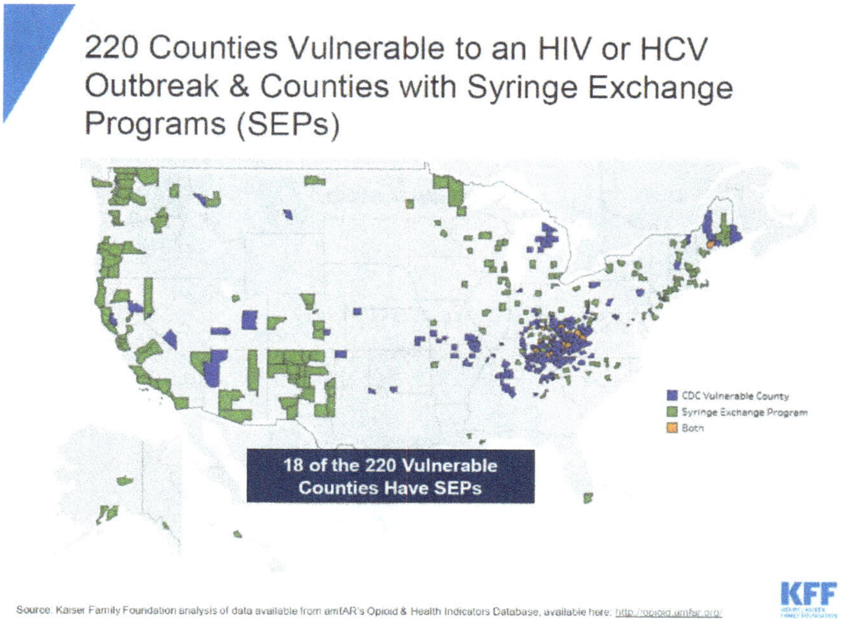

5. **While all Medicaid programs and some private plans cover Medication-Assisted Treatments (MATs) to address substance use problems, the AIDS Drug Assistance Program (ADAP) of the federal Ryan White HIV/AIDS Program offers an additional source of support for people with HIV with limited or no insurance coverage.**[12,13] However, access varies across the country with just half (26) of state ADAPs covering at least one of the three commonly prescribed MATs for opioid addiction.[14,15]

ADAPs with Medication-Assisted Treatment for Opioid Addiction on Formulary, 2018

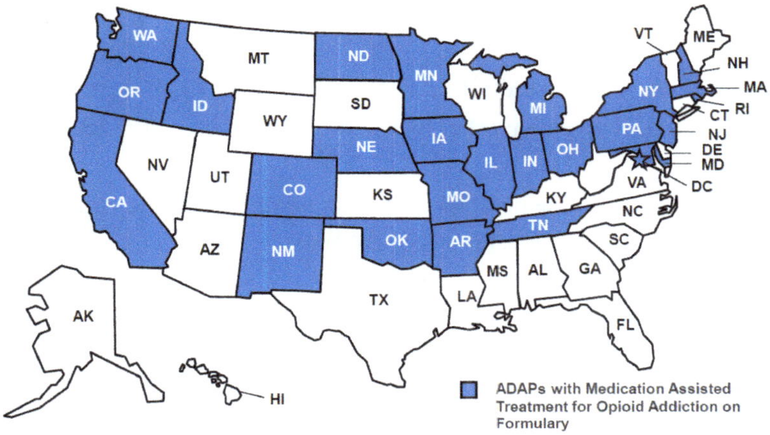

Source: Kaiser Family Foundation Analysis of NASTAD's 2018 ADAP formulary database: https://www.nastad.org/adap-formulary-database.

Endnotes

1. SAMHSA. 2016 National Survey on Drug Use and Health. https://www.samhsa.gov/data/sites/default/files/NSDUH-FFR1-2016/NSDUH-FFR1-2016.pdf
2. Kaiser Family Foundation. State Health Facts. Opioid Overdose Deaths. https://www.kff.org/other/state-indicator/opioid-overdose-deaths-by-gender/
3. Peters, P., et al. (2016.) "HIV Infection Linked to Injection Use of Oxymorphone in Indiana, 2014–2015." New England Journal of Medicine. 375:229–239.
4. Van Handle, M., et al. (2016). "County-level Vulnerability Assessment for Rapid Dissemination of HIV or HCV Infections among Persons who Inject Drugs, United States." Journal of AIDS. 73:3, 323–331
5. Peters, P., et al. (2016.) "HIV Infection Linked to Injection Use of Oxymorphone in Indiana, 2014–2015." New England Journal of Medicine. 375:229–239.
6. See for example, Zibell, J., et al. (2018). "Increases in Acute Hepatitis C Virus Infection Related to a Growing Opioid Epidemic and Associated Injection Drug Use, United States, 2004 to 2014. AJPH: Hepatitis C and Opioids. 108:2,175–181 and Van Handle, M., et al. (2016). "County-level Vulnerability Assessment for Rapid Dissemination of HIV or HCV Infections among Persons who Inject Drugs, United States." Journal of AIDS. 73:3, 323–331.

7. Van Handle, M., et al. (2016). "County-level Vulnerability Assessment for Rapid Dissemination of HIV or HCV Infections among Persons who Inject Drugs, United States." Journal of AIDS. 73:3, 323–331.
8. Centers for Disease Control and Prevention. NCHHSTP AtlasPlus. Updated 2017. https://www.cdc.gov/nchhstp/atlas/index.htm. Accessed February 2018.
9. Wejnert, et al. (2016). MMWR. "Vital signs: Trends in HIV Diagnoses, Risk Behaviors. And Prevention Among Persons Who Inject Drugs–United States." 65:47,1336–1342.
10. Kaiser Family Foundation analysis of data available from amfAR's Opioid & Health Indicators Database. Maps from amfAR database, available here: http://opioid.amfar.org/. 220 Vulnerable Counties originally identified in Van Handle, M., et al. (2016). "County-level Vulnerability Assessment for Rapid Dissemination of HIV or HCV Infections among Persons who Inject Drugs, United States." Journal of AIDS. 73:3, 323–331.
11. The original article identifying these counties also notes that 43% of the counties did not have a buprenorphine-waivered physician (another indicator of limited capacity to respond to an emerging opioid epidemic).
12. Kaiser Family Foundation. 2018. Medicaid's Role in Addressing Opioid Addiction. https://www.kff.org/infographic/medicaids-role-in-addressing-opioid-epidemic/
13. Peters, R. Wengle, E. 2016. The Urban Institute. Coverage of Substance-Use Disorder Treatments in Marketplace Plans in Six Cities. https://www.urban.org/sites/default/files/publication/81856/2000838-Coverage-of-Substance-Use-Disorder-Treatments-in-Marketplace-Plans-in-Six-Cities.pdf
14. The three common MATs are buprenorphine; Methadone, and Naltrexone.
15. 23 ADAP formularies include buprenorphine, 16 include Methadone, and 20 cover Naltrexone. NASTAD's 2018 ADAP formulary database: https://www.nastad.org/adap-formulary-database.

13.15

Syringe Exchange Programs in California

An Overview

California Department of Public Health

SYRINGE EXCHANGE PROGRAMS (SEPS) HAVE BEEN operating in California since the late 1980s, providing sterile syringes, collecting used ones, and acting as a point of access to health education and help for people who inject drugs.

Currently

- There are more than 40 SEPs operating in California.
- California SEPs provide a wide range of services in addition to syringe exchange and disposal. These services may include HIV and hepatitis C testing, overdose prevention training, and referrals to drug treatment, housing, and mental health services. Most SEPs also provide first aid and basic supplies, such as clean socks and bottled water, to meet the needs of homeless clients.
- California SEPs operate in a variety of settings, including in health clinics, mobile vans, storefronts and churches. Some offer street-based services in multiple locations; others offer services daily during standard business hours; still others provide home delivery services.
- Since 1999 the California State Legislature has acted several times to expand access to sterile syringes through SEPs authorized by local government. Most syringe exchange programs currently operating in California have been authorized by their county boards of supervisors or city councils.
- In 2012, Assembly Bill (AB) 604, (Skinner, Chapter 744, Statutes of 2011) also granted authority to the California Department of Public Health, Office of AIDS to permit organizations to apply directly to the Department for authorization to provide syringe exchange services. Existing SEPs are not required to apply for state certification, and local governments may continue to authorize local programs.

"Syringe Exchange Programs in California: An Overview," pp. 1–4, 2018.

Research in California: The CalSEP Study[1]

- The California Syringe Exchange Program (CalSEP) study fund by the Centers for Disease Control and Prevention examined the impact of syringe exchange legislation over several years in sixteen counties. Researchers found that for most SEP clients, contact with SEPs was the only contact they had with health care or social services of any kind. Of 10 recommended preventive services received by SEP clients, 76 percent were received exclusively from SEPs.
- In addition to syringe exchange, eighty-three percent of SEPs participating in the study offered HIV counseling and testing on site and 63 percent offered screening for hepatitis C virus. All SEPs offered safer sex materials, first aid, and referrals to drug treatment.
- In a survey of 75 clients recruited from 25 California SEPs, more than 90 percent would recommend SEPs to friends with similar needs.

Additional Research Findings

- A study of 81 cities around the world compared HIV infection rates among IDUs in cities that had SEPs to cities that did not. In the 29 cities with SEPs, HIV infection rates decreased by an average of 5.8 percent per year. By contrast, in the 52 cities without SEPs, HIV infection rates increased by 5.9 percent per year.[2]
- Researchers studying a San Francisco SEP found that the program did not encourage drug use, either by recruiting young or new IDUs, or by increasing drug use among current IDUs. In fact, during the five-year study period, injection frequency among IDUs decreased from 1.9 injections per day to 0.7, and the percentage of new IDUs in the community decreased from 3 percent to 1 percent.[3]
- Economic studies have predicted that SEPs could prevent HIV infections among clients, their sex partners, and offspring at a cost of about $13,000 per infection averted.[4] This is significantly less than the lifetime cost of treating an HIV-infected person, which is estimated to be $385,200.
- Hundreds of studies of SEPs have been conducted and have been summarized in a series of federally funded reports beginning in 1991. Each of the eight reports has concluded that SEPs do not appear to lead to increased drug use, increased neighborhood crime, or increased syringe litter in the communities that are home to these programs.[5]

---

1 Bluthenthal, R. Syringe Exchange Program Diversity and Correlates of HIV Risk: Preliminary results from the California Syringe Exchange Program Study. Presentation to the California Department of Health Services, Office of AIDS, April 22, 2003. Sacramento, CA.

2 Hurley, S.F., Jolley, D.J., Kaldor, J.M. Effectiveness of needle-exchange programmes for prevention of HIV infection. Lancet 1997; 349:1797–1800.

3 Watters, J.K., Estilo, M.J., Clark, G.L., et al. Syringe and needle exchange as HIV/AIDS prevention for injection drug users. Journal of the American Medical Association 1994; 271:115–120.

4 Cohen, D.A., Wu, S-Y., Farley, T.A. Cost-effective allocation of government funds to prevent HIV infection. Health Affairs 2005; 24:915–926.

5 Report from the NIH Consensus Development Conference. February 1997.

- A comprehensive review of international studies on syringe access programs, including both syringe exchange and nonprescription pharmacy sale concluded, "There is compelling evidence that increasing the availability, accessibility, and both the awareness of the imperative to avoid HIV and utilization of sterile injecting equipment by IDUs reduces HIV infection substantially."[6]
- The National Institutes of Health Consensus Panel on HIV Prevention stated, "An impressive body of evidence suggests powerful effects from needle exchange programs. ... Studies show reduction in risk behavior as high as 80 percent, with estimates of a 30 percent or greater reduction of HIV in IDUs."[7]

Related California Legislation

- AB 1743 (Ting, Statutes of 2014) allows licensed pharmacies throughout California to sell syringes to adults without a prescription and removes prior limits on the number of syringes that may be sold. It allows adults 18 years of age and older to purchase and possess an unlimited number of syringes for personal use when acquired from a pharmacy, physician or authorized SEP.
- AB 604 (Skinner, Statutes of 2011) added CDPH/OA to the list of government entities that may authorize SEPs. As of January 1, 2012 OA has authority to establish a program that allows entities to provide syringe exchange services anywhere in the state where OA determines that the conditions exist for rapid spread of HIV, viral hepatitis, or other blood-borne diseases.

---

6 Wodak A, Cooney A. Do needle syringe programs reduce HIV infection among injecting drug users: a comprehensive review of the international evidence. Subst Use Misuse. 2006;41(6–7):777–813.

7 National Institutes of Health. Consensus development statement. Interventions to prevent HIV risk behaviors, February 11–13, 1997; 7–8.

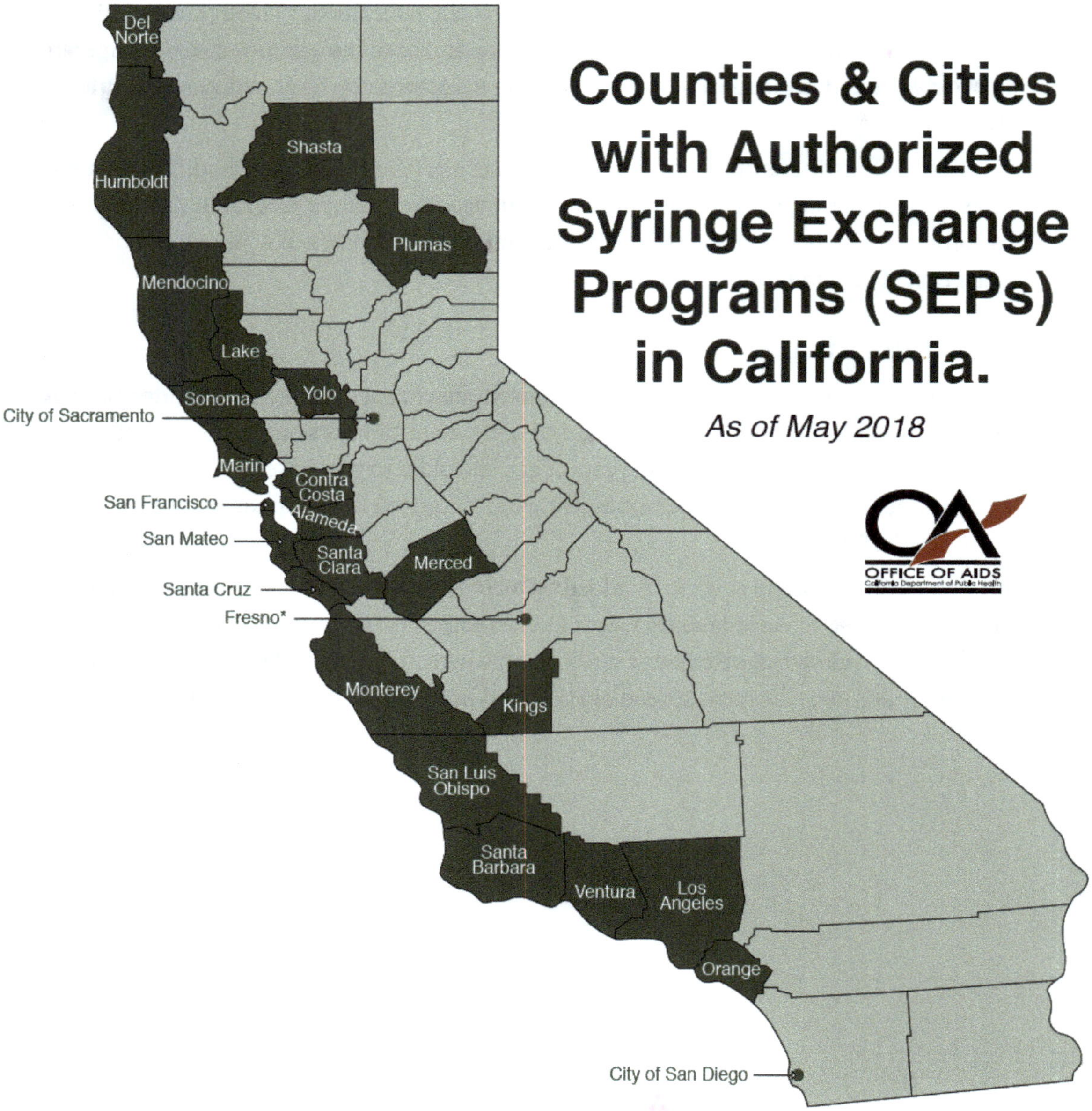
Counties & Cities with Authorized Syringe Exchange Programs (SEPs) in California.
As of May 2018
OFFICE OF AIDS
Del Norte
Humboldt
Shasta
Plumas
Mendocino
Lake
Yolo
Sonoma
City of Sacramento
Marin
Contra Costa
Alameda
San Francisco
San Mateo
Santa Clara
Merced
Santa Cruz
Fresno*
Monterey
Kings
San Luis Obispo
Santa Barbara
Ventura
Los Angeles
Orange
City of San Diego

13.16

Editorial

Reassessing Blood Donation by Men Who Have Sex with Men

Y. Tony Yang, Elizabeth Wiley, Robbert J. Duvivier

FOLLOWING THE PULSE NIGHTCLUB SHOOTINGS in Orlando, FL, USA, on June 12, 2016, many gay men were barred from donating blood in aid of the surviving victims because of the deferral policy of the US Food and Drug Administration (FDA). The policy is aimed at reducing the risk of HIV transmission through blood products, but in the wake of the shooting was criticised by lawmakers and activists as antiquated and discriminatory. Now, as the USA faces a severe blood shortage, the FDA is reconsidering its stance.

On Dec 21, 2015, the FDA replaced the lifetime ban on men who have sex with men (MSM) donating blood with a deferral for those who reported having sexual contact with another man in the past 12 months, in line with the UK, Canada, and Australia. But critics such as Paul Volberding, director of the AIDS Research Institute at the University of California at San Francisco, contend that the current policy is "based on fear and stigma" and should change.

The unfortunate reality, however, is that rates of new, and hence acute, HIV infection are extremely high among MSM. Although they represent approximately 2% of the US population, gay and bisexual men accounted for an estimated 65% of new HIV diagnoses in 2013. New infections are particularly problematic for blood screening, as even the most sensitive tests can miss early infections.

Of course, not all MSM partake in high-risk behaviour. In 2001, Italy lifted its ban on MSM donating blood, replacing it with an individual risk assessment, and has not reported any cases of transfusion-related HIV transmission since the shift. This kind of screening, however, relies on accurate self-reporting of sexual behaviours—something that might prove challenging in the context of communities where MSM still face stigma and marginalisation.

Ultimately, any change in policy must be based on rigorous evidence-based risk analysis. Whatever the outcome of the review, the reasoning behind the decision must be communicated effectively to show that science, not discrimination, has prevailed. Marginalisation has no place in public health.

Response: US Policy on Blood Donation by Men Who Have Sex with Men

by Y. Tony Yang, Elizabeth Wiley, Robbert .J Duvivier

A recent *Lancet* Editorial (Aug 6, p 534) reassessed the US Food and Drug Administration (FDA) policy on blood donations from men who have sex with men (MSM) after the Orlando terrorist attack.[1] MSM donor policies vary throughout the world, but in the past 20 years many countries have relaxed their outright bans (eg, Australia, Canada, and the UK) or have eliminated deferrals and implemented individualised risk assessment screening for all donors, regardless of their gender and that of their partners (eg, Chile, Mexico, Russia, and Spain).[2] Although we agree that any policy change must be based on evidence-based risk analysis, it should be emphasised that certain sexual practices, not sexual orientation, put individuals at risk for HIV.

The US 12-month deferral is inconsistent with current science. With up-to-date tests, the window between the time of HIV infection and the time when diagnostic tests can detect HIV is shorter, with an average duration of 12 days.[3] Fourth generation combination HIV tests are conclusive at 3 months.[4] Moreover, there have been no reported cases of transfusion- related HIV transmission in countries that have changed deferral policy.[5]

The USA is experiencing a severe blood shortage. The 12-month deferral prevents 4·2 million MSM from donating blood: lifting this deferral would lead to 360 600 potential new donors and 615 300 more pints of blood available per year (2–4% increase in supply). It is time to move the US debate from precautionary to risk management policies, using available evidence from other countries, toward a national blood system that is safe, caring, and inclusive.

1. Reassessing blood donation by men who have sex with men. *Lancet* 2016; **388:** 534.
2. Wilson K, Atkinson K, Keelan J. Three decades of MSM donor deferral policies. What have we learned? *Int J Infect Dis* 2014; **18:** 1–3.
3. Food and Drug Administration. FDA approves first nucleic acid test (NAT) system to screen whole blood donors for infections with human immunodeficiency virus (HIV) and hepatitis C virus (HCV). Feb 28, 2002. https://aidsinfo.nih. gov/news/593/fda-approves-first-nucleic-acid-test-(nat)-system-to-screen-whole-blood-donors-for-infections-with-human-immuno-deficiency-virus-(hiv)-and-hepatitis-c-virus-(hcv) (accessed Aug 9, 2016).
4. Centres for Disease Control and Prevention. Laboratory testing for the diagnosis of HIV infection. June 27, 2014. http://www.cdc.gov/ hiv/pdf/hivtestingalgorithmrecommendation-final.pdf (accessed Aug 9, 2016).
5. Suligoi B., Pupella S., Regine V, Raimondo M., Velati C., Grazzini G. Changing blood donor screening criteria from permanent deferral for men who have sex with men to individual sexual risk assessment: no evidence of a significant impact on the human immunodeficiency virus epidemic in Italy. *Blood Transfusion*

Section XIV

Disease Progression

14.1

Symptoms of HIV Infection

National Institute of Allergy and Infectious Diseases, U.S. National Institutes of Health

What Are the Early Symptoms of HIV Infection?

Many people do not have any symptoms when they first become infected with HIV. Some people, however, have a flu-like illness within a month or two after exposure to the virus.
This illness may include:

- Fever
- Headache
- Tiredness
- Enlarged lymph nodes (glands of the immune system easily felt in the neck and groin)

These symptoms usually disappear within a week to a month and are often mistaken for those of another viral infection. During this period, people are very infectious, and HIV is present in large quantities in genital fluids.

More persistent or severe symptoms may not appear for 10 years or more after HIV first enters the body in adults, or within two years in children born with HIV infection. This period of **"asymptomatic" infection** is highly individual. Some people may begin to have symptoms within a few months, while others may be symptom-free for more than 10 years.

Even during the asymptomatic period, the virus is actively multiplying, infecting, and killing cells of the immune system. HIV's effect is seen most obviously in a decline in the blood levels of CD4 positive T cells (also called T4 cells)—the immune system's key infection fighters. At the beginning of its life in the human body, the virus disables or destroys these cells without causing symptoms.

As the immune system worsens, a variety of complications start to take over. For many people, their first sign of infection is large lymph nodes or "swollen glands" that may be enlarged for more than three months. Other symptoms often experienced months to years before the onset of AIDS include:

- Extreme and unexplained tiredness
- Rapid weight loss
- Recurring fever or profuse night sweats

NIAID (NIH), "Symptoms of HIV infection," HIV Infection and AIDS: An Overview, 2002.

- Persistent or frequent yeast infections (oral or vaginal)
- Persistent skin rashes or flaky skin
- Prolonged swelling of the lymph glands in the armpits, groin, or neck
- Pelvic inflammatory disease in women that does not respond to treatment
- Short-term memory loss

Some people develop frequent and severe herpes infections that cause mouth, genital, or anal sores, or a painful nerve disease called shingles. Children may grow slowly or be sick a lot.

What Is AIDS?

The term AIDS applies to the most advanced stage of HIV infection. CDC developed official criteria for the definition of AIDS and is responsible for tracking the spread of AIDS in the United States.

CDC's definition of AIDS includes all HIV-infected people who have fewer than 200 CD4 positive T cells per cubic millimeter of blood. (Healthy adults usually have CD4 positive T-cell counts of 1,000 or more.) In addition, the definition includes 26 clinical conditions that affect people with advanced HIV disease. Most of these conditions are opportunistic infections that generally do not affect healthy people. In people with AIDS, these infections are often severe and sometimes fatal because the immune system is so ravaged by HIV that the body cannot fight off certain bacteria, viruses, fungi, parasites, and other microbes.

Symptoms of opportunistic infections common in people with AIDS include:

- Coughing and shortness of breath
- Seizures and lack of coordination
- Difficult or painful swallowing
- Severe and persistent diarrhea
- Sores of the mouth, anus, or genitals
- Fever
- Pneumonia
- Vision loss
- Nausea, abdominal cramps, and vomiting
- Weight loss and extreme fatigue
- Severe headaches
- Mental symptoms such as confusion, forgetfulness, depression, and other neurologic disorders
- Coma

Children with AIDS may get the same opportunistic infections as do adults with the disease. In addition, they also have severe forms of the bacterial infections all children may get, such as conjunctivitis (pink eye), ear infections, and tonsillitis.

People with AIDS are particularly prone to developing various cancers, especially those caused by viruses such as Kaposi's sarcoma and cervical cancer, or cancers of the immune system known as lymphomas. These cancers are usually more aggressive and difficult to treat in people with AIDS. Signs of Kaposi's sarcoma in light-skinned people are round brown, reddish, or purple spots that develop in the skin or in the mouth. In dark-skinned people, the spots are more pigmented.

During the course of HIV infection, most people experience a gradual decline in the number of $CD4^+$ T-cells, although some may have abrupt and dramatic drops in their $CD4^+$ T-cell counts. A person with $CD4^+$ T-cells above 200 may experience some of the early symptoms of HIV disease. Others may have no symptoms even though their $CD4^+$ T-cell count is below 200.

Many people are so debilitated by the symptoms of AIDS that they cannot hold steady employment or do household chores. Other people with AIDS may experience phases of intense life-threatening illness followed by phases in which they function normally.

A small number of people first infected with HIV 10 or more years ago have not developed symptoms of AIDS. Scientists are trying to determine what factors may account for their lack of progression to AIDS, such as particular characteristics of their immune systems or whether they were infected with a less aggressive strain of the virus, or if their genes may protect them from the effects of HIV. Scientists hope that understanding the body's natural method of control may lead to ideas for protective HIV vaccines and use of vaccines to prevent the disease from progressing.

14.2

2014 CDC Definition of HIV Infection Stages

U.S. Center for Disease Control and Prevention

TREATMENT CAN SLOW OR PREVENT PROGRESSION from one stage to the next. If a person does not receive treatment, they will progress through the following stages:

Stage 1: Acute HIV Infection

Within *2 to 4 weeks* after infection with HIV, people may experience a flu-like illness. Flu-like symptoms include fever, chills, rash, night sweats, muscle aches, sore throat, fatigue, swollen lymph nodes, or mouth ulcers. This is the body's natural response to infection. These symptoms can last anywhere from a few days to several weeks. But some people may not feel sick during this stage.

During this time, HIV infection may not show up on an HIV test, but people who have it are highly infectious and can spread the infection to others. When people have acute HIV infection, they have a large amount of virus in their blood and are very contagious. But people with acute infection are often unaware that they're infected because they may not feel sick right away or at all. To know whether someone has acute infection, either a fourth-generation antibody/antigen test or a nucleic acid (NAT) test is necessary.

Stage 2: Clinical Latency (HIV Inactivity or Dormancy)

This period is sometimes called *asymptomatic HIV infection* or *chronic HIV infection*. During this phase, HIV is still active but reproduces at very low levels. People may not have any symptoms or get sick during this time. For people who aren't taking medicine to treat HIV, this period can last a decade or longer, but some may progress through this phase faster. People who are taking medicine to treat HIV (ART) the right way, every day may be in this stage for several decades. It's important to remember that people can still transmit HIV to others during this phase, although people who are on ART and stay virally suppressed (having a very low level of virus in their blood) are much less likely to transmit HIV than those who are not virally suppressed. At the end of this phase, a person's viral load starts to go up and the CD4 cell count begins to go down. As this happens, the person may begin to have symptoms as the virus levels increase in the body, and the person moves into Stage 3.

U.S. Center for Disease Control and Prevention, "2014 CDC Definition of HIV Infection Stages," *Morbidity and Mortality Weekly Report*.

Stage 3: Acquired Immunodeficiency Syndrome (AIDS)

AIDS is the most severe phase of HIV infection. People with AIDS have such badly damaged immune systems that they get an increasing number of severe illnesses, called opportunistic illnesses.

Without treatment, people with AIDS typically survive about 3 years. Common symptoms of AIDS include chills, fever, sweats, swollen lymph glands, weakness, and weight loss. People are diagnosed with AIDS when their CD4 cell count drops below 200 cells/μL or if they develop certain opportunistic illnesses. People with AIDS can have a high viral load and be very infectious.

HIV INFECTION stage based on age-specific $CD4^+$ T-lymphocyte count or $CD4^+$ T-lymphocyte percentage of total lymphocytes

	Age on date of CD4+ T-lymphocyte test					
	<1 yr		1–5 yrs		≥6 yrs	
Stage	**Cells/μL**	**%**	**Cells/μL**	**%**	**Cells/μL**	**%**
1	≥1,500	≥34	≥1,000	≥30	≥500	≥26
2	750–1,499	26–33	500–999	22–29	200–499	14–25
3	<750	<26	<500	<22	<200	<14

The stage is based primarily on the $CD4^+$ T-lymphocyte count; the $CD4^+$ T-lymphocyte count takes precedence over the CD4 T-lymphocyte percentage, and the percentage is considered only if the count is missing.

If a stage-3-defining opportunistic illness has been diagnosed (below), then the stage is 3 (AIDS) regardless of CD4 T-lymphocyte test results.

An adult has AIDS (stage 3) if:

1. They are HIV positive
   AND
2. One of the following is true:
   a. Their $CD4^+$ T cell count is below 200 cells/μl blood.
   b. Their $CD4^+$ T cells/total lymphocytes is less than 14%.
   c. They have a Stage-3- (AIDS-) defining illness.

Stage-3- (AIDS-) Defining Opportunistic Illnesses in HIV Infection:

1. Bacterial infections, multiple or recurrent*
2. Candidiasis of bronchi, trachea, or lungs
3. Candidiasis of esophagus
4. Cervical cancer, invasive†
5. Coccidioidomycosis, disseminated or extrapulmonary
6. Cryptococcosis, extrapulmonary
7. Cryptosporidiosis, chronic intestinal (>1 month's duration)
8. Cytomegalovirus disease (other than liver, spleen, or nodes), onset at age >1 month
9. Cytomegalovirus retinitis (with loss of vision)

10. Encephalopathy attributed to HIV[§]
11. Herpes simplex: chronic ulcers (>1 month's duration) or bronchitis, pneumonitis, or esophagitis (onset at age >1 month)
12. Histoplasmosis, disseminated or extrapulmonary
13. Isosporiasis, chronic intestinal (>1 month's duration)
14. Kaposi sarcoma
15. Lymphoma, Burkitt (or equivalent term)
16. Lymphoma, immunoblastic (or equivalent term)
17. Lymphoma, primary, of brain
18. *Mycobacterium avium* complex or *Mycobacterium kansasii*, disseminated or extrapulmonary
19. *Mycobacterium tuberculosis* of any site, pulmonary[†], disseminated, or extrapulmonary
20. Mycobacterium, other species or unidentified species, disseminated or extrapulmonary
21. *Pneumocystis jirovecii* (previously known as "*Pneumocystis carinii*") pneumonia
22. Pneumonia, recurrent[†]
23. Progressive multifocal leukoencephalopathy
24. *Salmonella* septicemia, recurrent
25. Toxoplasmosis of brain, onset at age >1 month
26. Wasting syndrome attributed to HIV

---

[*] Only among children aged <6 years.
[†] Only among adults, adolescents, and children aged ≥6 years.

References

Morbidity and Mortality Weekly Report
Revised Surveillance Case Definition for HIV Infection—United States, 2014
April 11, 2014/63(RR03);1-10
https://www.cdc.gov/mmwr/preview/mmwrhtml/rr6303a1.htm?s_cid=rr6303a1_e
What are the stages of HIV?
updated March 2018, accessed May 22, 2018
https://www.cdc.gov/hiv/basics/whatishiv.html

14.3

How HIV Causes AIDS

National Institute of Allergy and Infectious Diseases, U.S. National Institutes of Health

Overview

Untreated HIV disease is characterized by a gradual deterioration of immune function. Most notably, crucial immune cells called **CD4 positive ($CD4^+$) T cells** are disabled and killed during the typical course of infection. These cells, sometimes called "T-helper cells," play a central role in the immune response, signaling other cells in the immune system to perform their special functions.

A healthy, uninfected person usually has 800 to 1,200 $CD4^+$ T cells per cubic millimeter (mm^3) of blood. During untreated HIV infection, the number of these cells in a person's blood progressively declines. When the $CD4^+$ T cell count falls below 200/mm^3, a person becomes particularly vulnerable to the **opportunistic infections** and cancers that typify AIDS, the end stage of HIV disease. People with AIDS often suffer infections of the lungs, intestinal tract, brain, eyes, and other organs, as well as debilitating weight loss, diarrhea, neurologic conditions, and cancers such as **Kaposi's sarcoma** and certain types of lymphomas.

Most scientists think that HIV causes AIDS by directly inducing the death of $CD4^+$ T cells or interfering with their normal function, and by triggering other events that weaken a person's immune function. For example, the network of signaling molecules that normally regulates a person's immune response is disrupted during HIV disease, impairing a person's ability to fight other infections. The HIV-mediated destruction of the lymph nodes and related immunologic organs also plays a major role in causing the **immunosuppression** seen in people with AIDS. Immunosuppression by HIV is confirmed by the fact that medicines, which interfere with the HIV lifecycle, preserve $CD4^+$ T cells and immune function as well as delay clinical illness.

[...]

Early Events in HIV Infection

Research suggests that immune system cells of the dendritic cell type, which live in the mucosa, may begin the infection process after sexual exposure by binding to and carrying the virus from the site of

NIAID (NIH), "How HIV Causes AIDS."

infection to the lymph nodes where other immune system cells become infected. A molecule on the surface of dendritic cells, DC-SIGN, may be critical for this transmission process.

Once it enters the body, HIV infects a large number of $CD4^+$ T cells and replicates rapidly. During this **acute** or **primary phase** of infection, the blood contains many viral particles that spread throughout the body, seeding various organs, particularly the **lymphoid organs.**

Two to 4 weeks after exposure to the virus, up to 70 percent of HIV-infected people suffer flu-like symptoms related to the acute infection. Their immune system fights back with **killer T cells** (**$CD8^+$ T cells**) and **B-cell**-produced **antibodies**, which dramatically reduce HIV levels. A person's $CD4^+$ T cell count may rebound somewhat and even approach its original level. A person may then remain free of HIV-related symptoms for years despite continuous replication of HIV in the lymphoid organs that had been seeded during the acute phase of infection.

One reason that HIV is unique is the fact that despite the body's aggressive immune responses, which are sufficient to clear most viral infections, some HIV invariably escapes. This is due in large part to the high rate of mutations that occur during the process of HIV replication. Even when the virus does not avoid the immune system by mutating, the body's best soldiers in the fight against HIV—certain subsets of killer T cells that recognize HIV—may be depleted or become dysfunctional.

In addition, early in the course of HIV infection, people may lose HIV-specific $CD4^+$ T cell responses that normally slow the replication of viruses. Such responses include the secretion of interferons and other antiviral factors, and the orchestration of $CD8^+$ T cells.

Finally, the virus may hide within the chromosomes of an infected cell and be shielded from surveillance by the immune system. Such cells can be considered as a **latent reservoir** of the virus. Because the antiviral agents currently in our therapeutic arsenal attack actively replicating virus, they are not effective against hidden, inactive viral DNA (so-called provirus). New strategies to purge this latent reservoir of HIV have become one of the major goals for current research efforts.

Course of HIV Infection

Among people enrolled in large epidemiologic studies in Western countries, the median time from infection with HIV to the development of AIDS-related symptoms has been approximately 10 to 12 years in the absence of antiretroviral therapy. Researchers, however, have observed a wide variation in disease progression. Approximately 10 percent of HIV-infected people in these studies have progressed to AIDS within the first 2 to 3 years following infection, while up to 5 percent of individuals in the studies have stable $CD4^+$ T cell counts and no symptoms even after 12 or more years.

Factors such as age or genetic differences among individuals, the level of virulence of an individual strain of virus, and co-infection with other **microbes** may influence the rate and severity of disease progression. Drugs that fight the infections associated with AIDS have improved and prolonged the lives of HIV-infected people by preventing or treating conditions such as *Pneumocystis carinii* pneumonia, cytomegalovirus disease, and diseases caused by a number of fungi.

HIV Co-receptors and Disease Progression

Recent research has shown that most infecting strains of HIV use a co-receptor molecule called CCR5, in addition to the CD4 molecule, to enter certain of its target cells. HIV-infected people with a specific mutation in one of their two copies of the gene for this receptor may have a slower disease course than people with two normal copies of the gene. Rare individuals with two mutant copies of the CCR5 gene appear, in most cases, to be completely protected from HIV infection. Mutations in the gene for other HIV co-receptors also may influence the rate of disease progression.

Viral Burden and Disease Progression

Numerous studies show that people with high levels of HIV in their bloodstream are more likely to develop new AIDS-related symptoms or die than those with lower levels of virus. For instance, in the Multicenter AIDS Cohort Study (MACS), investigators showed that the level of HIV in an untreated person's plasma 6 months to a year after infection—the so-called viral "set point"—is highly predictive of the rate of disease progression; that is, patients with high levels of virus are much more likely to get sicker faster than those with low levels of virus. The MACS and other studies have provided the rationale for providing aggressive antiretroviral therapy to HIV-infected people, as well as for routinely using newly available blood tests to measure viral load when initiating, monitoring, and modifying anti-HIV therapy.

Potent combinations of three or more anti-HIV drugs known as highly active antiretroviral therapy, or HAART, can reduce a person's "viral burden" (amount of virus in the circulating blood) to very low levels and in many cases delay the progression of HIV disease for prolonged periods. Before the introduction of HAART therapy, 85 percent of patients survived an average of 3 years following AIDS diagnosis. Today, 95 percent of patients who start therapy before they get AIDS survive on average 3 years following their first AIDS diagnosis. For those who start HAART after their first AIDS event, survival is still very high at 85 percent, averaging 3 years after AIDS diagnosis.

Antiretroviral regimens, however, have yet to completely and permanently suppress the virus in HIV-infected people. Recent studies have shown that, in addition to the latent HIV reservoir discussed above, HIV persists in a replication-competent form in resting $CD4^+$ T cells even in people receiving aggressive antiretroviral therapy who have no readily detectable HIV in their blood. Investigators around the world are working to develop the next generation of anti-HIV drugs that can stop HIV, even in these biological scenarios.

A treatment goal, along with reduction of viral burden, is the reconstitution of the person's immune system, which may have become sufficiently damaged that it cannot replenish itself. Various strategies for assisting the immune system in this regard are being tested in clinical trials in tandem with HAART, such as the Evaluation of Subcutaneous Proleukin in a Randomized International Trial (ESPRIT) exploring the effects of the T cell growth factor, IL2.

HIV Is Active in the Lymph Nodes

Although HIV-infected people often show an extended period of **clinical latency** with little evidence of disease, the virus is never truly completely latent, although individual cells may be latently infected. Researchers have shown that even early in disease, HIV actively replicates within the lymph nodes and related organs, where large amounts of virus become trapped in networks of specialized cells with long, tentacle-like extensions. These cells are called **follicular dendritic cells (FDCs)**. FDCs are located in hot spots of immune activity in lymphoid tissue called **germinal centers**. They act like flypaper, trapping invading **pathogens** (including HIV) and holding them until B cells come along to start an immune response.

Over a period of years, even when little virus is readily detectable in the blood, significant amounts of virus accumulate in the lymphoid tissue, both within infected cells and bound to FDCs. In and around the germinal centers, numerous $CD4^+$ T cells are probably activated by the increased production of cytokines such as TNF-alpha and IL-6 by immune system cells within the lymphoid tissue. Activation allows uninfected cells to be more easily infected and increases replication of HIV in already infected cells.

While greater quantities of certain cytokines such as TNF-alpha and IL-6 are secreted during HIV infection, other cytokines with key roles in the regulation of normal immune function may be secreted in decreased amounts. For example, $CD4^+$ T cells may lose their capacity to produce IL-2, a cytokine that enhances the growth of other T cells and helps to stimulate other cells' response to invaders. Infected cells also have low levels of receptors for IL-2, which may reduce their ability to respond to signals from other cells.

Breakdown of Lymph Node Architecture

Ultimately, with chronic cell activation and secretion of inflammatory cytokines, the fine and complex inner structure of the lymph node breaks down and is replaced by scar tissue. Without this structure, cells in the lymph node cannot communicate and the immune system cannot function properly. Investigators also have reported recently that this scarring reduces the ability of the immune system to replenish itself following antiretroviral therapy that reduces the viral burden.

Role of $CD8^+$ T Cells

$CD8^+$ T cells are critically important in the immune response to HIV. These cells attack and kill infected cells that are producing virus. Thus, vaccine efforts are directed toward eliciting or enhancing these killer T cells, as well as eliciting antibodies that will neutralize the infectivity of HIV.

$CD8^+$ T cells also appear to secrete soluble factors that suppress HIV replication. Several molecules, including RANTES, MIP-1alpha, MIP-1beta, and M.D.C appear to block HIV replication by occupying the coreceptors necessary for many strains of HIV to enter their target cells. There may be other immune system molecules—including the so-called CD8 antiviral factor (CAF), the defensins (type of antimicrobials), and others yet undiscovered—that can suppress HIV replication to some degree.

Rapid Replication and Mutation of HIV

HIV replicates rapidly; several billion new virus particles may be produced every day. In addition, the HIV reverse transcriptase enzyme makes many mistakes while making DNA copies from HIV RNA. As a consequence, many variants or strains of HIV develop in a person, some of which may escape destruction by antibodies or killer T cells. Additionally, different strains of HIV can recombine to produce a wide range of variants.

During the course of HIV disease, viral strains emerge in an infected person that differ widely in their ability to infect and kill different cell types, as well as in their rate of replication. Scientists are investigating why strains of HIV from people with advanced disease appear to be more virulent and infect more cell types than strains obtained earlier from the same person. Part of the explanation may be the expanded ability of the virus to use other co-receptors, such as CXCR4.

Central Nervous System Damage

Although monocytes and macrophages can be infected by HIV, they appear to be relatively resistant to being killed by the virus. These cells, however, travel throughout the body and carry HIV to various organs, including the brain, which may serve as a hiding place or "reservoir" for the virus that may be relatively resistant to most anti-HIV drugs.

Neurologic manifestations of HIV disease are seen in up to 50 percent of HIV-infected people, to varying degrees of severity. People infected with HIV often experience

- Cognitive symptoms, including impaired short-term memory, reduced concentration, and mental slowing
- Motor symptoms such as fine motor clumsiness or slowness, tremor, and leg weakness
- Behavioral symptoms including apathy, social withdrawal, irritability, depression, and personality change

More serious neurologic manifestations in HIV disease typically occur in patients with high viral loads, generally when a person has advanced HIV disease or AIDS.

Neurologic manifestations of HIV disease are the subject of many research projects. Current evidence suggests that although nerve cells do not become infected with HIV, supportive cells within the brain, such as astrocytes and microglia (as well as monocytes/macrophages that have migrated to the brain) can be infected with the virus. Researchers postulate that infection of these cells can cause a disruption of normal neurologic functions by altering cytokine levels, by delivering aberrant signals, and by causing the release of toxic products in the brain. The use of anti-HIV drugs frequently reduces the severity of neurologic symptoms, but in many cases does not, for reasons that are unclear. The impact of long-term therapy and long-term HIV disease on neurologic function is also unknown and under intensive study.

Role of Immune Activation in HIV Disease

During a normal immune response, many parts of the immune system are mobilized to fight an invader. $CD4^+$ T cells, for instance, may quickly multiply and increase their cytokine secretion, thereby signaling other cells to perform their special functions. Scavenger cells called macrophages may double in size and develop numerous **organelles**, including lysosomes that contain digestive enzymes used to process ingested pathogens. Once the immune system clears the foreign antigen, it returns to a relative state of quiescence.

Paradoxically, although it ultimately causes immune deficiency, HIV disease for most of its course is characterized by immune system hyperactivation, which has negative consequences. As noted above, HIV replication and spread are much more efficient in activated $CD4^+$ T cells. Chronic immune system activation during HIV disease also may result in a massive stimulation of B cells, impairing the ability of these cells to make antibodies against other pathogens.

Chronic immune activation also can result in apoptosis, and an increased production of cytokines that not only may increase HIV replication but also have other deleterious effects. Increased levels of TNF-alpha, for example, may be at least partly responsible for the severe weight loss or wasting syndrome seen in many HIV-infected people.

The persistence of HIV and HIV replication plays an important role in the chronic state of immune activation seen in HIV-infected people. In addition, researchers have shown that infections with other organisms activate immune system cells and increase production of the virus in HIV-infected people. Chronic immune activation due to persistent infections, or the cumulative effects of multiple episodes of immune activation and bursts of virus production, likely contributes to the progression of HIV disease.

New Clinical Signs of HIV in the Era of HAART Therapy

The clinical spectrum of disease among people with HIV has changed dramatically in the era of HAART. NIAID and its grantees are actively studying the new clinical syndrome of disease among persons on long term-therapy. Research is concentrating on the impact of HIV over the long term, the toxicity of the medicines used to control HIV, and the effects of aging on HIV disease progression. People with HIV have a variety of conditions including diabetes, heart disease, neurocognitive decline, and cancers that may, or may not, be directly due to HIV or its treatment. Long-term studies of people with HIV in the United States and abroad are underway.

14.4

Selections from How We Die

Sherwin B. Nuland

Note: This poignant description of AIDS was published in 1994, after AZT was available, but before the potent antiretroviral cocktails. It provides a glimpse into how the epidemic impacted patients prior to effective treatments for AIDS. Even today, the picture is not so different for some HIV-positive people who are not receiving treatment.

The Story of AIDS

"Call me Ishmael." She smiled at the recollection of that irony, and looked beyond me with wistful eyes into the room where the father of a young family lay dying.

"It was only four months ago, but it's a lifetime, really. I walked into the clinic that day, and there he was, sitting in a cubicle waiting for the great miracle-doctor who was coming to help him. The doctor was me. 'Good morning, Mr. Garcia,' I said, just as bright and breezy as a new interne is supposed to be. And he jumped up, this little Hispanic guy with a great big smile on his face. 'Call me Ishmael' was what he said—imagine it! I guess he never read the book. Melville's Ishmael survived, and mine never had a chance. He'll be dead in a few days, but I'll remember him the rest of my life." ...

One crisis after another had taken place since that summertime afternoon when Ishmael[1] Garcia leaped up from the chair and stuck out his open palm to shake hands with Dr. Mary Defoe, and both of them had vastly changed from what they had been. Though she had seen plenty of AIDS patients while in medical school, Mary never quite realized the full magnitude of individual catastrophe until she actually took on the intimidating responsibilities of a newly graduated doctor.

From the sunny July afternoon when he first presented himself to the AIDS clinic until the chilly gray November morning when she was destined to pronounce him dead, Mary Defoe and Ishmael Garcia would be doctor and patient. Whether hospitalized or being followed in the outpatient clinic, he thought of her as his personal physician. From time to time, other interns assumed his care for brief periods when

---

1 His name was officially Ismail, which is the Spanish form. But since he and others used the English form Ishmael more or less interchangeably with the Spanish, I will refer to him as Ishmael.

Mary rotated to a different service, but they always found each other again and resumed their journey toward the grim conclusion they both knew lay ahead.

Early in training, most doctors develop relationships with patients that become models on which they will base their responses to sickness and death for the rest of their careers. For Mary Defoe, Ishmael Garcia will surely represent a reawakening of an old image long lost to modern generations of healers—impotence in the face of a plague of death upon the young.

In the calculus of death, no one before 1981 could have factored in HIV, the human immunodeficiency virus. The first hints of its gathering fury struck just at the instant when biomedical science was beginning to offer cautious congratulations to itself on having achieved a state of advancement where the final conquest of infectious disease seemed at last within sight. AIDS not only confounded the microbe hunters; it shook the confidence held by all of us that technology and science can keep humanity safe from the whims of nature. In a very few explosive years, virtually every young doctor in training was treating his or her share of those dying who were meant to live.

Dr. Defoe and I stepped into Ishmael's room—noiselessly, though he was far beyond hearing any sound we might have made. It was more out of respect than necessity that we were so quiet. When a man is dying, the walls of his room enclose a chapel, and it *is* right to enter it in hushed reverence.

How different this scene from the frenzied drama so often played out during a patient's last moments, as desperate attempts are made to revive him to yet another few weeks or months of waiting for death—and sometimes only hours or days. After the incalculable miseries of Ishmael Garcia's descent into the valley of fever and incoherence, this oblivion was earned; it was fitting that the end, at least, should be undisturbed.

The room's overhead illumination had been turned off and the blinds were closed against the glare of midday autumn sunshine, bathing the entire space in a uniformity of subdued daylight. The unconscious man in the bed had a high fever—the yellowish skin of his forehead glistened against the stark whiteness of his freshly changed pillowcase. Ravaged as he was by the wasting effects of his disease, it could be seen that he had once been very handsome.

I had read Ishmael's chart, and I knew that with his very last breath, the tranquillity would be shattered by a full-scale attempt at resuscitation. In a moment of terror months earlier, he had begged his wife to see to it that the doctors did everything possible to preserve his life—that she not allow them to give up. And now, Carmen could not make herself believe what the AIDS team was telling her: that the possible had become impossible. She clung to that part of her pledge which would destroy the easy exit of an essence in which she devoutly believed—the immortal soul of her husband.

Though Ishmael had been separated from his wife for three years prior to his illness, she was nevertheless his legal next-of-kin, and she spoke for his family. In reality, she spoke only for herself, because Carmen and her husband had together made the unyielding decision to keep the diagnosis to themselves. Neither Ishmael's parents nor his two sisters knew the name of his disease. If they did, they never spoke of it.

When she realized just how sick Ishmael was, Carmen had let him return home. Somehow, she found the strength to put aside his years of unfaithfulness and drug dependence, and even the near-poverty into which his irresponsibility had thrown her and their three daughters. He came back so that she could be his nurse and the only one of his family or friends to share his knowledge of the ultimate end. In spite of everything, he had been a good father, she said, and she owed him this much. For the sake of their three girls and for the recollections of a life that once had been, she permitted her dying husband to return.

In refusing to let him die when his time came, Carmen insisted that she was doing one last kindness for Ishmael—it was, after all, what she believed she had promised him. She refused to discuss with the doctors why she would not listen to their reasoned arguments, and none of them had the heart to press her. They supposed, they told me, that somewhere in the depths of her awareness, Ishmael's obvious devotion to their girls made Carmen feel some unjustified element of guilt about her rejection of her prodigal husband and her obdurate refusal to respond to his sputtering intervals of good behavior and promises of reform. The staff had gone so far as to seek a consultation with the chairman of our hospital's Bioethics Committee, but when they told him that a successful resuscitation might be possible, he would not overrule the dictates of Carmen's heart. In circumstances like this, who knows where wisdom lies?

Ishmael was never alone in that room. The three girls were always with him, a constant presence watching over their adored father through the plastic facing of a three-by-two-foot blown-up photograph standing on the wide windowsill. There they were, three beautiful curly-haired kids in party dresses, smiling out at the world and their father on a day much happier than this. I gestured toward the picture, wordlessly asking Mary a question.

"Yes," she replied, "the two older ones come here almost every day, but Carmen doesn't bring the littlest one. The six-year-old just plays by herself around the foot of the bed—she doesn't really understand. The ten-year-old cries; she stands by her father's bedside every minute she's here, wiping his face and stroking it, and she can't stop crying. I try not to come into the room when they're here—it's more than I can bear." ...

There is a good deal more to AIDS than its bare clinical facts disclose. Although such a statement may be made about any disease, how much more so may it be said of this specific plague? But no matter the cultural and societal implications of AIDS, certain of its clinical and scientific manifestations must be understood before the full tragedy unfolds of how it kills its victims. The case of Ishmael Garcia is archetypical.

In February 1990, Garcia had his first positive blood test for HIV. The test was done as part of the evaluation of a nonhealing open sore on his left forearm, which brought him to the medical clinic of the Yale–New Haven Hospital. The infection was almost certainly caused by his intravenous drug habit. Because he felt quite well otherwise, especially when the sore cleared rapidly with a short outpatient course of antibiotics, he never kept any follow-up appointment beyond the one at which he was told his diagnosis. In January 1991, he developed a dry cough that gradually worsened over a period of several weeks. As the cough progressed, a feeling of tightness appeared in Ishmael's chest, aggravated by coughing or a deep inspiration. After more than a month during which things gradually worsened, he began to be frightened by the appearance of two new symptoms: a fever, and shortness of breath brought on by even minor activity. When his breathing difficulty reached the point where it increased with no greater movement than walking around his small furnished room in New Haven's barrio, he knew the time had come to go to the hospital. In the emergency room, a chest X-ray demonstrated that Ishmael's lung fields were diffusely infiltrated with a thin whitish haze, representing the large areas in which an infection of some sort was preventing proper aeration. Analysis of arterial blood revealed an abnormally low level of oxygen, reflecting inefficient uptake by the infected lung tissue. When the admitting resident looked into his feverish patient's mouth, he saw the familiar clue exhibited by virtually every new case of AIDS—Ishmael's tongue was coated with the telltale milky white fungus of thrush.

The chest findings were consistent with the form of pneumonia most common in AIDS, caused by a parasite called *Pneumocystis carinii*. Ishmael was admitted to the hospital and the doctors passed a snakelike viewing device called a bronchoscope down into the depths of his windpipe, from where a small sample was taken for culture and the microscopic study that revealed the tightly packed globular structures of *Pneumocystis*. He was given antifungal medication for the thrush and started on a course of a highly specific antibiotic for the pneumonia (called pentamidine), and he gradually recovered. During the hospitalization, Ishmael was found to be anemic and to have a low white blood cell count. Although he insisted that he had been eating well, he was sufficiently malnourished that the protein level in his blood was decreased. On being weighed, he was surprised to find that he had lost 4 of his accustomed 140 pounds. The worst news he was given, however, was something he was not yet able to understand: The marker cell of HIV infection, the T4, or CD4, lymphocyte was found to be at a level of 120 per cubic millimeter of blood, very far below normal.

It is not known whether Ishmael complied with discharge instructions to take his prescribed medications, whose function was to prevent further episodes of the lung infection he had by then learned to call PCP, *Pneumocystis carinii* pneumonia. Most likely he did not, because he returned eleven months later, in January 1992, with similar but even worse symptoms. This time, he complained in addition of severe headache and nausea and seemed somewhat confused. An evaluation of his spinal fluid demonstrated the presence of meningitis caused by a yeastlike organism called *Cryptococcus neoformans*. He was also found to have a bacterial infection of the right ear, but he was too mentally befuddled to be aware of it. His CD4 count was down to 50—HIV's destruction of the immune system was progressing rapidly. Although Ishmael almost succumbed to the combination of three separate forms of infection, skillful management by the Yale–New Haven AIDS team got him through. After three weeks in the hospital, he was able to go back to Carmen and the girls, having amassed a bill of some twelve thousand dollars. Because he had long since lost his health insurance after being fired from his factory job as the result of the drug habit, the costs were assumed by the state of Connecticut.

In early July of 1992, Ishmael, who by that time was scrupulously keeping his appointments at the clinic, developed a large painful abscess in his left armpit, requiring surgical drainage. It was on this visit that he first met Mary Defoe. Over the next few weeks, she supervised his outpatient treatment for sinusitis and another ear infection, while the abscess healed as well.

As Ishmael was recovering from his bacterial illnesses, he once again noted that he was often light-headed and dizzy and sometimes had trouble maintaining his balance. Shortly after the onset of these disturbing symptoms, his memory began increasingly to fail him. Carmen became aware that he did not always comprehend even simple sentences. The symptoms progressed over the next month, to the point where he was confused and lethargic most of the time. In spite of Carmen's gratitude to the physicians, she gave in to his entreaties not to be taken to the emergency room. Both she and Ishmael were afraid of what another hospitalization might mean. He was now losing weight more rapidly, and they knew that, once admitted, he might never come home.

Carmen finally called an ambulance when she awoke one morning and found her husband too far gone to resist. By then, Ishmael was almost in a coma, his left arm was twitching uncontrollably, and he barely responded to commands shouted into his ear. From time to time, his entire left side would go into a brief convulsion. A CT scan showed findings most consistent with the type of brain infection caused by a protozoan called *Toxoplasma gondii*, although the blood tests did not confirm that diagnosis. The pictures were striking and consisted of multiple small masses on both sides of the brain. Similar lesions are often found in AIDS patients who have a malignancy called lymphoma, but Ishmael's looked more like those of toxoplasmosis.

At this point, the medical staff decided that even though the diagnosis was not firmly established, it would be safest to begin treatment for *Toxoplasma*, in view of its greater frequency than lymphoma in AIDS patients. When only slight improvement could be discerned after two weeks of drug therapy, Ishmael was taken to the operating room, where the neurosurgeons drilled a small hole in his skull and took a tiny bit of brain for biopsy. Microscopic study of the tissue did not identify the protozoa in the brain, but it did show changes the pathologist believed to be caused by healing of the *Toxoplasma*-induced disease. This encouraged the AIDS team to continue their treatment even in the face of residual uncertainty about the diagnosis. Within a week, however, it became clear that Ishmael's condition was worsening. Because no definite *Toxoplasma* had been identified, those members of the team who had argued against that diagnosis now recommended radiation therapy for a presumed lymphoma of the brain. Before the advent of HIV, brain lymphoma was exceedingly rare, but it is now seen with frequency in AIDS patients.

At first, Ishmael responded to the X-ray treatments by a partial awakening from what had become a profound coma. He even reached the point where he was able to swallow small amounts of custard and pureed foods spooned into his mouth by a nurse or Carmen. But the gains were short-lived. The coma returned, his low-grade fever rose to levels of 102°–103° each day, and he developed a bacterial pneumonia in addition to some other generalized infection whose nature was obscure and, in any case, resistant to treatment. This is how things stood on that November noon when Mary Defoe and I stood at Ishmael's bedside.

Although he was deeply unconscious, Ishmael's face was troubled. Perhaps there was some flickering comprehension of his struggles to move air in and out of those infected lungs, or of the decreasing amounts of oxygen being carried to his gasping tissues. He had become septic, and the entire mechanism of his life was failing. Or maybe his troubled expression had nothing to do with the physical distress of breathless tissues. Possibly, something within him was trying to communicate that he was too exhausted to continue—that he was trying to die but couldn't. And yet, is it really possible that he longed for death? Would not any struggle be worth the anguish, for the chance to see his girls one more time? No one knows why the faces of dying men and women look the way they do—an appearance of discomfort may be as meaningless as an appearance of serenity.

Ishmael's travail ended the next morning. Carmen, feeling the closeness of death, had taken the day off from her job in a New Haven cardboard box factory and sat at his bedside as the seconds grew slowly longer between his respirations, until they stopped altogether. Without being approached again, she had told Mary the night before that there was to be no resuscitation—she could see that her promise to her husband had been kept; everything possible had been done. When Ishmael stopped breathing, she simply stepped outside to inform the nurse who had been sitting with her most of the morning. And then, Carmen did something she had refused over and over again while Ishmael was still alive—she asked to be tested for HIV. ...

It is no easy matter to explain or understand the mechanism by which the many opportunistic invaders lay waste the body of an adult or child with AIDS. Such a baffling array of problems is faced by the HIV-infected and their caregivers that one cannot but contemplate with a sense of awestruck gratitude that so much has already been accomplished. When a doctor of my generation makes hospital rounds with an AIDS team of physicians and nurses, all he can do is figuratively gasp at how much these skilled clinicians know and what a large proportion of it has been learned in so short a time. Every patient on the unit carries a multitude of infections and sometimes one or two cancers; each *is* receiving four to ten or even more medications, without any certainty of predictable response or toxicity—Ishmael Garcia was on fourteen. Daily, and sometimes more often, new decisions must be made about everyone being treated (my hospital's relatively small AIDS area has forty beds, and they are always full).

As if the immensity of the clinical challenges were not enough, distraught families wait nearby for answers, and for consolation as well; there are reports for the staff to fill out, charts to review, tests to order, students to teach, conferences to attend, and an ever-burgeoning new literature to read and often to contribute to. And always, the most important charge is to care for those dreadfully stricken brothers and sisters of all of us, the sickest of whom are wasted, feverish, swollen, and anemic, their eyes seeking some reassurance and the unspoken promise of relief from their torment, which too often will come only with death. No matter the perseverance and moral strength so many patients muster in the face of lethal certainty, the pitiless process by which they die is dispiriting anew with every reenactment.

The Life of a Virus and the Death of a Man

... [T]he immune system is gradually laid waste by HIV. Although some have protested the use of military analogies to portray the pathophysiology of disease, AIDS lends itself particularly well to such descriptive comparisons. The process, in fact, is not unlike a gradual buildup of forces, during the later stages of which a prolonged artillery and air bombardment destroys a country's defenses in preparation for a massive land invasion carried out by a large coalition of belligerents, allied together to accomplish total annihilation. The army of microbes that kills the victim of AIDS after HIV has knocked off his CD4 cells includes many different kinds of divisions, and every one of them has its own target and its own lethal mechanism of attack. ...

The virus often shows its hand very soon after entering a new host. Within a month or less, rapid replication causes its concentration in the blood to become extremely high, and it stays that way for about two to four weeks. Although many newly infected people remain without symptoms, others during this period develop low-grade fevers, swollen glands, muscle aches, a rash, and sometimes central nervous system symptoms such as headaches. Because these symptoms are not specific and may also be accompanied by a general sense of fatigue, they are often erroneously attributed to flu or mononucleosis. As this brief syndrome is ending, the first antibodies against HIV begin to appear in the blood; a blood test will detect them, and the patient is henceforth seropositive. Although the short symptomatic period ends, the virus continues to replicate.

Very likely, the brief mononucleosis-like syndrome is caused by the first response of the body's immune system to the alarm set off by the massive number of new virus particles that have by then been produced. The body is initially successful, and the number of virus-particles in the blood drops dramatically to low levels. What seems to have happened at this point is a retreat by the remaining microbes into CD4 lymphocytes, lymph nodes, bone marrow, the central nervous system, and spleen, where they lie dormant for years or replicate so slowly that the total low concentration in the blood remains stable. Actually, only 2 to 4 percent of the body's CD4 cells are in the blood. Most likely, those in the lymph nodes, spleen, and marrow are being gradually destroyed during the long dormant period, but the destruction is not reflected in the blood until the end of this time, when the CD4 counts, having remained constant till then, begin to drop dramatically, allowing the multiple secondary infections that characterize AIDS to ensue. At that point, the amount of virus in the blood rises again. The reason for the prolonged period of relative inactivity is unknown, but it does suggest that the body's immune system may be playing some role in mitigating the infection, at least that part of it which is restricted to the blood itself. When the immune system has sufficiently deteriorated, the amount of virus in the lymphocytes and free in the blood increases markedly.

This sequence of events may explain why most HIV-positive people develop swollen lymph glands in the neck and armpits during the early two-to-four-week period of symptoms, which do not recede at the end of it. When that period is over, patients continue to feel well for an average of three to five years or even ten years, by the end of which time examination of the blood will usually reveal that the number of CD4 cells has declined considerably, from a normal count of 800 to 1,200 per cubic millimeter to below 400. This means that 80 to 90 percent of these lymphocytes have been destroyed. On an average of eighteen months later, standard skin tests for allergy begin to show that the immune system is becoming impaired. The CD4 cell count continues to drop, but patients at this stage of disease still may not have begun to show evidence of clinical illness. In the meantime, the level of virus in the blood is rising and the swollen lymph nodes are slowly being destroyed.

When the CD4 cell count falls below 300, the majority of patients will develop the fungal infections of the tongue or oral cavity called thrush, which presents itself as white patches in those areas. Other infections that may begin to appear when the count is below 200 are herpes around the mouth, anus, and genitals, as well as a severe vaginal infection with the same fungus that caused the thrush. A characteristic finding is a condition called oral hairy leukoplakia (from the Greek *leukos*—meaning "white," and *plakoeis*—meaning "flat") a group of fuzzy-looking vertical white patches standing upright like corrugations along the lateral margins of the tongue. These lesions are due to a virus-induced thickening of the surface layers.

Within a year or two of this time, many patients are beginning to develop opportunistic infections in areas beyond the skin and body openings. By then, the CD4 cell count has usually fallen well below 200 and is dropping rapidly. The entire syndrome of immune deficiency begins to make itself evident as diseases appear that are caused by microbes ordinarily living in perfectly healthy people whose normal physiological defenses prevent trouble. The stage has now been reached at which serious pathology can be caused by any organism that requires intact immunity to combat it. Although people with AIDS are highly susceptible to well-known diseases such as tuberculosis and bacterial pneumonia, they are also set upon by a group of otherwise-unusual sicknesses due to a variety of parasites, fungi, yeasts, viruses, and even bacteria that physicians rarely encountered before the advent of HIV. For some of these organisms, there was no effective treatment until the late 1980s, when the efforts of university laboratories and the pharmaceutical industry were finally rewarded with the development of a group of drugs that have shown varying degrees of clinical success.

Every variety of microbial invader attacking the shattered defenses of the immune-compromised person with AIDS is equipped with its own unique assault weapons and directs its onslaughts against specific objectives. With little remaining CD4 cell resistance to bar their way, the individual divisions and regiments of opportunistic killers devastate the territory that comprises the patient's tissues. Sometimes by exhausting a person's energy and small supply of reserve firepower, and sometimes by knocking out a central structure like the brain, the heart, or the lungs, the swarming bits of infection will have their way. Though the pestilential offensives may be slowed or halted for a while by one or another of the newer pharmaceutical agents, they will always in time resume, if not in one form, then in another. A skirmish may be won here and there, or a battle prevented by timely use of prophylactic drugs, and some months of stability thereby achieved—but the eventual outcome of the struggle is preordained. The determined microbial aggressors will accept nothing less than the unconditional surrender that comes only with the death of their involuntary host.

Although AIDS patients may die of any of a number of pathological processes, a relatively small group of microbes is involved in the vast majority of deaths. Foremost among these is *Pneumocystis carinii,* the first one to be identified at the very outset of the worldwide pestilence. The figures are now declining because of prophylactic medication, but until fairly recently, more than 80 percent of patients had at least one experience of PCP, and many died during an episode, either from the respiratory insufficiency itself or from problems associated with it. Depending on the severity of the onslaught, an individual episode used to kill between 10 and 50 percent of its victims before effective means had been found to combat it. It remains a significant factor in the death of nearly half of all AIDS sufferers, but the percentage continues to decrease.

The symptoms of PCP are essentially those experienced by Ishmael Garcia as his breathing became progressively compromised until he sought treatment. Occasionally, the organism may be found in other parts of the body than the lungs, and in autopsies of patients who die of this infection it is sometimes disseminated throughout virtually every major organ, most particularly the brain, heart, and kidneys.

Like patients with other types of pneumonia, those who die with PCP are asphyxiated by the infected lung's inability to be aerated. As wider areas of tissue become involved, more and more alveoli are destroyed, and a point is reached where arterial oxygen levels cannot be raised in spite of every available means of forcing the gas into the soggy and plugged tissues. The lack of oxygen and the buildup of carbon dioxide damage the brain and finally stop the heart. Sometimes destruction of tissue has been so severe that cavities have been created in the areas of disintegration, very much as in tuberculosis.

The lung is the organ most commonly assaulted by AIDS. Virtually every one of the opportunists, as well as the tumors, looks to the lung as a target. On hospital rounds I have attended, tuberculosis, pus-forming bacteria, the herpes-like cytomegalic virus (CMV), and toxoplasmosis are among the most common problems discussed. Except for the last, they all seek out a home in the respiratory tissue. The incidence of tuberculosis in AIDS patients is some five hundred times what it is in the general population.

Toxoplasmosis is a disease that was at one time so rare that I had difficulty remembering just what it was when I first encountered it in an early AIDS patient. In little more than a decade, it has become a major belligerent in the HIV invasion, and I will never again have to search my memory about its details, so devastating are the things I have seen it do to defenseless people. The organism itself is a protozoan commonly found infecting birds, as well as cats and other small mammals. Most commonly, it is transmitted to humans in inadequately cooked meat or is ingested when food is contaminated with animal feces. *Toxoplasma* lives harmlessly in anywhere from 20 to 70 percent of Americans, its frequency depending on the social and economic group tested. In an immunodeficient patient, however, it manifests itself by fever, pneumonia, enlargement of the liver or spleen, rash, meningitis, encephalitis, and sometimes involvement of the heart or other muscles. Its most common focus of attack in AIDS is the central nervous system, where it can cause fever, headache, neurological deficits, seizures, and mental changes ranging from confusion to deep coma. On CT scans, the infected areas of the brain sometimes so much resemble the lesions of lymphoma that they are differentiated only with difficulty. This was the diagnostic dilemma that caused so much uncertainty in the care of Ishmael Garcia.

It is a rare AIDS patient whose nervous system escapes the pillaging of the disease. Even in the early period of HIV infection, some few people go through a transient period of neurological disabilities, which may sometimes appear even before AIDS itself has supervened; fortunately, this particularly distressing complication is far less common in early than in late stages of HIV disease, when it is more severe and called the AIDS dementia complex. Its eventual effects on cognition, motor function, and behavior can be devastating, but most frequently present initially as simple forgetfulness and loss of concentration. After a while, apathy and withdrawal become common symptoms, while some smaller number of patients complain of headaches or develop seizures. Should these findings not pass off when they occur early in HIV infection, they slowly worsen. In that case or in those far more common patients whose symptoms appear in the AIDS period, intellectual function often declines and difficulty with balance or muscular coordination appears. In the most advanced stages of the complex, patients are severely demented and show little response to their surroundings; they may be paraplegic and suffer tremors or occasional convulsions. These complications exist without any relationship to those processes caused by cerebral toxoplasmosis, lymphoma of the brain, or other opportunistic neurological disabilities such as meningitis caused by the yeastlike fungus cryptococcus. AIDS dementia complex is thought to be due to the virus itself, but its exact cause is unknown, and the cerebral atrophy seen on CT scan and biopsy is unrelated to any other factor. Of the many neurological problems associated with AIDS, this one and toxoplasmosis are the most common. Fortunately, the beneficial effects of AZT have resulted in some decline in its frequency.

Two cousins of the tuberculosis germ share the distinction of being the bacteria most frequently disseminated throughout the body of people with AIDS. *Mycobacterium avium* and *Mycobacterium intracellulare* (MAI), jointly called the *Mycobacterium avium* complex (MAC), are present in about half of AIDS patients when they die, having caused a wide variety of symptoms during life. MAI is now a more frequent cause of death than PCP. Fever, night sweats, weight loss, fatigue, diarrhea, anemia, pain, and jaundice are often attributable to these marauding twins. Although the complex rarely causes death on its own, its wasting effects are major contributors to the general debilitation and malnourishment that further weaken defenses against other invaders.

These are just a few of the manifestations of AIDS. Lengthening the list serves only to name some of the other common problems that beset patients, but it cannot even approach the complete inventory of suffering: the blindness of the retinitis resulting from CMV or *Toxoplasma* infection; the massive diarrhea that can have any of five or six causes, or sometimes none that are identifiable; the meningitis or occasional pneumonia of cryptococcosis; the thrush or swallowing difficulties of candidiasis, and perhaps the slimy wet ooze of its skin lesions; the discomfort of herpes around the anus; the fungal pneumonia or bloodstream seeding of histoplasma; the bacteria typical and atypical; the more than a score of creeping, crawling things with names like *Aspergillus, Strongyloides, Cryptosporidium, Coccidioides, Nocardia*—their time has come and they act like looters after a natural disaster, which is exactly what they are. Though they pose no danger to people with normal immunity, every one of them is a bane to those with a depleted store of CD4 lymphocytes. ...

When bacterial infection is no longer controllable, the familiar picture of sepsis supervenes. All the while, malnutrition and anemia are further weakening the body's ability to slow down the processes of destruction. The malnutrition is often aggravated by huge protein losses through the damaged kidneys, resulting from a rapidly progressive condition of uncertain cause, called HIV-associated nephropathy (kidney disease). The nephropathy may go on to terminal uremia within three to four months of onset.

Even without direct involvement by infection, the heart in AIDS patients occasionally becomes enlarged and may fail, or it may develop a rhythm irregularity leading to sudden death. The liver, too, is susceptible to attack, not only because of AIDS itself but because so many patients are concomitantly infected with the hepatitis B virus. CMV, MAI, tuberculosis, and several of the fungi have a predilection for the liver. The hapless organ is not only battered by the disease but by attempts to treat it, as drug toxicity affects its performance in many ways. The liver is found to be abnormal in some way or other in 85 percent of autopsied patients.

The entire length of the gastrointestinal tract is a vast twisting tunnel of opportunity for the various predators of AIDS. From the herpes and that wide assortment of ulcerations and infections around and in the mouth to the running sores and problems of continence at the anus, the torment of the final months may be magnified by the involvement of so many structures that it inhibits eating, interferes with digestion, and produces uncontrollable watery diarrhea that not only is a source of constantly recurring distress but also makes it difficult to maintain proper hygiene of the raw areas around the anus and rectum. To imagine extracting a scrap of dignity from this kind of death is beyond the comprehension of most of us. And yet the indignity itself sometimes brings out moments of nobility that overcome for a while the reality of anguish—arising from sources so deep, they can only be marveled at, for they surpass understanding.

An intact immune system is needed not only to resist infection but to inhibit growth of tumors as well. In the absence of an effective defense, certain kinds of malignant processes find a favorable environment in which to make their appearance. HIV has been particularly conducive to one form of cancer previously so rare that I had seen exactly one case, in an elderly Russian immigrant, since my graduation from medical school almost forty years ago. The incidence of this malignancy, Kaposi's sarcoma, has been magnified by a factor of well over a thousand—from 0.2 percent of the general population to more than 20 percent of Americans with AIDS. It is by far the most common tumor seen with this disease, and for as-yet-uncertain reasons, it afflicts a greater percentage of homosexual men (40 to 45 percent) than IV drug abusers (2 to 3 percent) or hemophiliacs (1 percent). These figures reflect only the people in whom the diagnosis is made during life. When autopsies are done, the frequency of KS triples or quadruples, making its presence somewhere in the bodies of gay men even more common.

In 1879, Moritz Kaposi, a professor of dermatology at the University of Vienna Medical School, described an entity he called "multiple pigment sarcoma," consisting of a group of reddish brown or bluish red nodules that originates on the hands and feet and advances along the extremities until reaching the trunk and head. In time, stated his report, the lesions enlarge, ulcerate, and spread to the internal organs. "Fever, bloody diarrhea, haemoptysis [coughing of blood] and marasmus set in at this stage, and are followed by death. At the autopsy, similar nodules are found in large numbers in the lungs, liver, spleen, heart and intestinal tract."

Sarcoma is derived from the Greek *sark,* meaning "flesh," and *oma,* meaning "tumor." These growths originate in the same kinds of cells that give rise to connective tissue, muscle, and bone. In spite of Kaposi's admonition about his disease that "the prognosis is unfavorable ... and fatal termination could not be prevented by extirpation, local or general, or the administration of arsenic [a favored treatment for cancer at the time]," physicians for a century underestimated the danger of this unusual malignancy.

Because the progression of KS was known to be slow, requiring "three to eight years or more," subsequent textbooks most commonly employed the word *indolent* to describe its course. Thus was conveyed an erroneous message about the basically lethal nature of the malignancy, even though some authorities continued to write of its deadly manifestations, such as massive intestinal bleeding. The word *indolent,* in fact, appears in the original 1981 reports in British and American medical journals of outbreaks of Kaposi's sarcoma among gay men. So alarmed, however, were the authors of those reports by the sudden raging aggressiveness of a disease traditionally regarded as lethargic that the American article saw fit to remind its readers that the course had sometimes been known to be "fulminant, with extensive visceral involvement"; the paper published in England made the same case and gave it immediacy by pointing out that "half our patients were dead within 20 months of diagnosis." Clearly, this was a new form of KS, suddenly far more worrisome than even Kaposi had warned.

Decades before KS became associated in physicians' minds with HIV infection, it was being recognized too often for coincidence as an accompaniment of various forms of the lymphatic cancer called lymphoma. Today, KS and lymphoma, not necessarily concomitant, are the two leading malignancies that prey on people with AIDS. Except for reasons of immunodeficiency, the relationship between the two has not yet been clarified. AIDS-related lymphoma, which most often involves the central nervous system, gastrointestinal tract, liver, and bone marrow, is no less aggressive than KS. ...

Respiratory failure, sepsis, destruction of brain tissue by tumor or infection—these are the more common immediate causes of death; some patients bleed into the brain, or the lung, or even the gastrointestinal tract, and some succumb to widespread tuberculosis or sarcoma; organs fail, tissues bleed, infection is everywhere. And invariably, there is malnutrition. No matter the magnitude of methods activated to fight it, starvation cannot be prevented. A care unit for terminal AIDS patients is peopled by emaciated, wraithlike men and women whose shrunken eyes look dully out from cavernous sockets, their faces often without expression, their bodies wizened with the shriveled frailty of prematurely advanced age. Most are beyond courage. The virus has robbed them of their youth, and it is about to rob them of the rest of their lives.

Autopsy pathologists distinguish between two separate designations for the cause of death: They refer to the proximate cause of death and the immediate cause of death (officially known by the acronyms PCOD and ICOD). For all of these young people, the PCOD will be AIDS—the specific ICOD seems hardly to matter. The quantity of suffering is the same for all, even though the quality varies. I talked about these matters not long ago with Dr. Peter Selwyn, one of the several Yale professors whose single-minded devotion to the care of AIDS patients has animated the efforts of many of the residents and students at our school. Despite his authoritative contributions to current understanding of HIV infection, he is a reticent man who expresses large concepts with few words. He said simply, “My patients die, I think, when their time comes.” It seemed an incongruous statement, floating there in the company of the biomedical complexities still hanging in the air from our long discussion of molecular biology and bedside management. And yet it made sense. At the end, he said, so many things go wrong that there comes a time when the depleted forces of gasping life just seem to give out. Death comes with sepsis and organ failure and starvation and with the final departure of the spirit, all at once. Selwyn has seen it many times, and he knows.

I am a hundred miles away from the hospital. This is one of those unexpected afternoons in mid-autumn when everything under nature’s cloudless blue sky has become exactly the way it should be, but almost never is. The summer just passed was rainy, and perhaps for that reason the hills surrounding my friend’s farm have taken on those heartbursting effusions of color that are almost more than my city-bred soul can comprehend or contain. Nature is being kind without knowing it, as nature can be cruel without knowing it. At such an instant, it seems as though no other day will ever attain the impossible splendor of this one. Already, I feel a nostalgia for today even as I live it. I am obsessed with an urge to memorize the image of every tree because I know its blazing flourish will begin to fade as soon as tomorrow, and never appear precisely like this again. When a thing is beautiful and good, it should be seen so clearly, and held so snugly, that no one will ever forget how it looks and how it feels.

I am sitting in the sunny kitchen of John Seidman’s farmhouse, built a century ago in the midst of twenty acres of fertile land, near the town of Lomontville in upper New York State. In an upstairs bedroom, ten years ago, John’s best friend, David Rounds, died in his arms at the end of a long and difficult illness. John and David were more than best friends; they shared a love that was meant to endure. But cancer determined otherwise. David was taken from John, and from those others of us who also loved him in our variety of ways, at a time when the future seemed secure and certain for both of them. David had won a Tony Award for Best Supporting Actor on Broadway only two years before, and John’s stage career was showing increasing promise. In that farmhouse, grief was a long time in passing before life resumed its proper rhythms.

I have known John Seidman for almost twenty years, and Sarah, my wife, shared a house with him and David long before that. He has been so close a friend to my family that my two youngest children call him Uncle. And yet there is a large part of his life that he and I have never discussed and about which I know almost nothing. On this splendorous day just before the fleeting grandeur of autumn disappears, the two of us are sitting together and we are talking about death—and AIDS.

Death has become much too familiar to John. It is as though the loss of David was the prelude to a succession of sorrows, during which friends, colleagues in the theater, and even mere acquaintances sickened, withered, and died. In the past decade, John has repeated with one after another the cycle of discovery of seropositivity, disease progression, watchful caregiving, descent to terminal illness, and death—again and again. In his early forties, he is one of tragedy's witnesses. There have been many others, and more than a few are now dead. The young men, and the few young women, who have companioned one another to the grave have been taken in the most productive years of their lives—what might have been and what should have been is lost. The vigor, the talent, and undoubtedly the genius of a generation are diminished, and so is our society.

We talk about John's friend Kent Griswold, who died in 1990 with toxoplasmosis and a trio of the common acronyms: CMV, MAI, and several bouts of PCP. Could there, I wanted to know, be any dignity in such a death? Can anything be salvaged of what once was, to bring a sense of himself to a man near his final hour, when he has been through so much? John thought a long time before answering, not because he had never considered the question before but because he wanted to be sure I would understand. The search for the elusive dignity, he said, may become irrelevant to the person who is dying—he has already carried out his struggle, and so often near the end, those around him can detect no recognizable conscious thought. Dignity is something, said John, that the survivors snatch—it is in their minds that it exists, if it exists at all:

> Those of us left behind search for dignity in order not to think ill of ourselves. We try to atone for our dying friend's inability to achieve a measure of dignity, perhaps by forcing it on him. It's our one possible victory over the awful process of this kind of death. With a disease like AIDS, we need to deal with the sadness that comes with seeing a beloved friend lose his particularity, his uniqueness. Toward the end, he becomes just like the last person you saw go through this. You feel the sadness of seeing someone lose his individuality and become a clinical model.
>
> How much of the "good death" is for the person dying and how much for the person helping him? They're obviously related to one another, but the question is how. To me, the concept of a good death is generally not something that can be managed very well for the one who is dying. A "good death" is only a relative thing, and what it really means is decreasing the mess. There isn't much you can manage beyond trying to keep things neat and keep things painless—keeping someone from being alone. But leading up to those final moments, I think even the importance of one's not being alone is something we infer.
>
> In retrospect, and in a way this sounds brutal, my own experience is that the only means we have of knowing if we have helped someone to a better death is whether or not we feel regret, or whether there is anything we feel sorry about or have left undone. If we can truly say that we missed no opportunity to do what we could, we've done the best job that's possible. But even that, as an absolute achievement, only has absolute

> value to oneself. What you're left with at the end is a situation that makes no one happy. The fact is that you've lost someone. There's no way to feel good about it.
>
> The one bond we do need to believe is absolutely unbreakable in death is love. If love is what we feel we're providing at those mysterious moments leading up to death, that, I suppose, is what makes a death "good," if anything really can. But it's such a subjective quality.

During his terminal weeks in the hospital, Kent was never alone. Whatever help they could or could not provide him at the final hours, there is no question that the constant presence of his friends eased him beyond what might have been achieved by the nursing staff, no matter the attentiveness of their care. It is impossible to observe homosexual AIDS patients without being struck by the way a circle of friends, not necessarily all gay, will almost predictably come together as a man's family and assume responsibility for what a wife or parents might otherwise do. Dr. Alvin Novick, one of the earliest of America's AIDS activists and among the most highly respected, has called this phenomenon of joined commitment "the caregiving surround." It is a communal act of love, but it is also something more. John describes it:

> AIDS is happening to people, especially in the case of gay men, who have created families by a conscious affinity—we have chosen the people who will be our family. Our sense of responsibility to each other isn't based on the usual social forms. In many cases, the traditional family has rejected us. So the affinitive family is much more important.
>
> A lot of the greater community really do feel that what is happening to us *should* happen to us—it's some kind of visitation on us for our sinful and abnormal ways. And so it's in our mutual interest not to leave someone alone with that judgment of society. Those of us who suffer from some kind of self-loathing may find it very easy to think of AIDS as a form of punishment, but even those of us who don't are aware that much of society does see it that way. To neglect our friends who have to deal with the disease themselves is somehow to abandon them to the judgment of the straight world.

Kent's last few weeks, John tells me, were like those of so many other people with AIDS, and of so many people with any of the diseases that slowly eat away at life's ebbing strength. Following the long months during which he had been forced to fight off one unanticipated problem after another, he seemed to undergo a suspension of any understanding that an incremental reduction of control was accompanying each new complication. As he stopped trying to comprehend, he also stopped struggling against the successive assaults, as though it seemed now less important to resist—there was no longer any point to it. Or perhaps the effort required to grasp the significance of events simply sapped too much of his limited energy.

The details of a latest onslaught lost their urgency. There are those who would call such exhausted indifference acceptance, but the very word implies a welcoming. Perhaps it is rather the recognition of defeat, the involuntary acknowledgment that the time has come to quit fighting. Most of the dying, not only of AIDS but of any prolonged sickness, seem unaware that they have reached this stage. For some few, mental faculties remain so intact that they are able to consciously decide, but much more often the decision is made for them by a lapse into a degree of lessened sensibility or even coma. This is the phase of dying in which William Osler and Lewis Thomas seldom saw aught but serenity. For most of us, it will come much too late to give consolation to those who watch at the bedside.

While Kent had been less sick, he had sometimes spoken of his concern about how much physical pain he would be able to withstand, how uncomfortable his last weeks might be. He expressed a wish to find that critical moment when he could knowingly make up his own mind whether to continue the struggle. No one around him could tell for sure whether that wish was granted.

An influential friend had somehow gotten Kent a commodious private room in the hospital, and in that large space he appeared daily to become smaller. He seemed almost hard to find. In John's words, "He dwindled further and further beneath the sheets." Even when he was at his strongest, Kent needed help to get to the bathroom, but the rest of the time he was completely bedridden. Never a large man, he seemed now to be disappearing. As John describes Kent's withering, I think again of Thomas Browne watching his dying friend go through the same process 350 years earlier: "He came to be almost half himself and left a great part behind him which he carried not to the grave."

Because of Kent's toxoplasmosis, he was losing cognition to the point where he was unable to comprehend what was going on around him. CMV retinitis blinded first one eye and then the other. He had by then wasted to such a degree that it was impossible to read his face or decipher his expressions—was he smiling, or was it a grimace that twisted the corners of his silent mouth? John says it so well: "A form of communication is lost when someone is so diminished." The dying man's whole body had grown very dark, especially his face.

Early on, Kent had made it clear that no aggressive treatment was to be used once it became evident that it would be futile. Guided by that, his "caregiving surround" consulted with the doctors, and together they tried to make correct decisions as each succeeding necessity arose. Finally, there were no longer any decisions to make. It had become so clear—there was nothing further to be done. It was just as Peter Selwyn says—Kent's time had come.

Kent was less and less conscious of any sort of discomfort. No longer was it important that he receive medical help of any kind. "It became our mission just to keep him surrounded, just to keep him connected, at least as much as he was capable of sensing any connection. The most important thing was that we didn't want him to be alone." At the end, Kent just slipped away. John now comes to the final part of the story.

> I wasn't in New York when he died—I was up here at the farm for a few days. I got off a bus at the Port Authority and called in to my machine. There was a message that Kent was gone, and it shocked me. When I'd last seen him, he wasn't recognizably living, certainly not recognizably Kent. Even though he was expected to die any minute, somehow the idea that he was actually gone—I suppose the shock had to do with the fact that after all the time I had spent with him I had to find out about it in that rotten way—standing there alone in a grimy phone booth, hearing it from my answering machine.

Kent died among companions who had helped sustain him in his last two years of life. He was not one of the many homosexuals and drug abusers who have been ostracized by their families—he was the only child of older parents and they had died years before. Without the devotion of his friends, his death, and his life as well, would have been soon forgotten.

Nothing that has been written here should be construed to imply that traditional families are only seldom involved in the care of their sons and daughters (or husbands and wives) dying of AIDS. Quite the opposite is true. Gerald Friedland describes the return, the reuniting of parents, mothers in particular, with the children whose lives and friends they had years before rejected. This is true not only of the families of gay men but of those of drug abusers as well. Of course, not all homosexuals and not all drug abusers have separated from their roots in the first place, and so it is not uncommon that the last months of a young man or woman with AIDS are spent in the nurturing care of siblings or parents, sometimes together with a small group of their child's friends or a lover. It is usually a great deal easier for a middle-class parent to leave employment or a distant home than it would be for members of a family from an inner-city ghetto or barrio, where even a day's absence from work means loss not only of income but possibly of the low-paying job itself. I have been told of mothers with as many as four children at once dying of AIDS—the cruelty of the virus reaches magnitudes beyond any imaginable reality.

At the bedsides of dying young people watch mothers and wives, husbands and lovers—sisters, brothers, and friends—doing what they can to buffer the onslaughts of messy death. As in ages past when a child is mortally ill, murmuring voices of parents are heard, sometimes barely audible in the hush that precedes a life's departure. They are soft words of encouragement and they are prayers. In English or in Spanish, and in other languages throughout the world, there has been repeated so many times one variant or another of the words spoken by the biblical King David as he wept over the body of his slain son, the rebellious Absalom, from whom he had been for so many years estranged:

> O my son Absalom,
> my son, my son Absalom!
> Would God I had died for thee,
> Oh Absalom, my son, my son.

Gerald Friedland speaks of the "inversion of the expected life cycle—parents are burying their children." An aberration has recurred from earlier centuries, just when we had complacently concluded that our science had conquered it. Not only the virus is turned back to front but so is the pattern of natural logic by which the young should bury the old. There is finally a metaphoric lesson here—in the therapy that is at present our best means of inhibiting the propagation of HIV: With AZT and other drugs, we try to stop the reverse transcriptase, and thereby stop the reversal, too, that turns the cycle of life on its head. Our scheme works, but not as well as we would like, and death continues to pursue the young and even the very young, while their elders can only stand by and mourn.

What dignity or meaning can be snatched from such a death will never be known, except by those whose lives have embraced the life just lost. The young people who provide the hospital care for the young people who die—and here I refer not only to doctors and nurses but to every one of those dedicated personnel—look on and wonder that such selflessness exists in a world they have been taught is cynical. Their own daily deeds belie the cynicism—they, too, are heroes of a sort. Their heroism is contemporary and unique to the path they have chosen as health workers who conquer their own fears and vanquish their feelings of vulnerability for the sake of those afflicted with AIDS. They make no moral judgments—they do not distinguish between social classes, manners of infection, or memberships in those categories called risk groups. Camus described it well: "What's true of all the evils in the world is true of plague as well. It helps men to rise above themselves."

In the midst of the stories that still come to us of unwilling physicians here or HIV-phobic surgeons there (and the more than 20 percent of surveyed American medical residents who would treat people with HIV but if given the opportunity would choose not to), it is heartening to know that the AIDS-affected are being watched over by people like these. For our children who care for our children stricken by HIV, the burden is made still greater with the sorrow of being stewards to the mortality of men and women their own age or perhaps only a decade older. In that injustice lies the source of the most outraged of those many reproaches we hurl at insensate nature, whose mindless tinkering created HIV—that it robs us of great pieces of the fabric from which we are entitled to fashion our future. Of the youthful legions lost to AIDS, it is proper to speak the words written seventy years ago by the neurosurgeon Harvey Gushing as he grieved over his companions martyred in World War I. They are, Gushing lamented, "doubly dead in that they died so young."

14.5

HIV-Infected People Are Living for Years, But Age-Related Diseases Set in Early

Marlene Cimons

DAVID HARDY HAS BEEN TREATING HIV-INFECTED patients since the early 1980s, when the epidemic began. In those days, people newly diagnosed with AIDS lived for only about six months. Hardy, an infectious-disease specialist and internist, was ecstatic when powerful new drug combinations came into widespread use in 1996, enabling HIV-infected people to measure their lives in decades rather than months. But in recent years, his euphoria has turned bittersweet.

"Most people assume that the medicines have worked and that everything has gone back to normal, and that's not really true," says Hardy, who directs research for Whitman-Walker Health in Washington and who still sees patients weekly. "While we have suppressed HIV very well, we've now discovered that the medicines only treat part of the problem."

Many HIV-infected people, now in their 50s and 60s, who have lived for years with HIV under control, are developing aging-related conditions—heart, liver and kidney disease, certain cancers and frailty, for example—at a rate significantly higher than uninfected people of the same age. "These are things that people develop all the time as they get old, but they are occurring at an earlier age in HIV-positive people," Hardy says.

"The first goal was to save someone from dying of HIV infection," agrees Anthony S. Fauci, director of the National Institute of Allergy and Infectious Diseases (NIAID) and a leading researcher involved in developing the AIDS drug combinations. "After we started successful therapy that suppressed the virus and extended lives, we began to notice that people were getting diseases associated with aging sooner than their chronological age would indicate they should be getting them."

An Aging HIV Population

In 2014, an estimated 45 percent of Americans living with HIV were older than 50, amounting to 428,724 people, according to the Centers for Disease Control and Prevention, while 27 percent were older than 55 and 6 percent were 65 and older. These include people diagnosed a decade or more before life-prolonging drugs became available, as well as older Americans diagnosed with late-stage AIDS who did not begin HIV drug therapy until then.

Experts believe this timing—the point at which someone starts therapy after infection—is key to understanding what is happening now. It involves how the body's immune system behaves following infection with HIV.

"If you are in your 50s today and you were infected when you were 20, you had about 10 years of living without therapy before the drugs came along and helped you survive," says Carl Dieffenbach, director of NIAID's AIDS division. In this group, and in older people diagnosed with late-stage AIDS, the period without treatment "led to a tremendous amount of damage to their immune system."

HIV not only damages the immune system, it also turns on that system indefinitely, meaning the immune response triggered by HIV never really shuts down, even once drugs have begun to quell the virus. "With most infectious invaders, the immune system responds and then is supposed to rest, like a fire engine waiting to come out when there is a fire to be fought," Dieffenbach says. "With HIV, those firetrucks keep driving around looking for fires, even when there are none."

Fauci agrees. "It isn't only the [initial] immune response against HIV," he says. "It's a global turning-on of the immune system—and the longer you wait to take drugs, the more robust the immune activation."

Many AIDS researchers believe that this "immune activation" is the primary mechanism underlying the accelerated rate of age-related diseases. HIV-infected patients must take multiple medications daily, some with side effects, but experts believe the AIDS drugs aren't a major contributor to these conditions. "It's much less the drugs; it's the immune activation," Fauci says.

Medications Don't Cure

HIV medications control HIV, but they don't cure it. The virus persists in numerous reservoirs in the body, including the lymph nodes, which prompt immune activation as well as chronic inflammation. "Inflammation and immune activation accelerate heart disease and stroke, and chronic HIV infection results in both," says Robert T. Schooley, a longtime AIDS researcher and professor of medicine in the infectious-diseases division at the University of California at San Diego. "One can calculate a given patient's risk for stroke or heart attack based on how elevated laboratory markers of inflammation are."

Several studies have shown the heightened risk of cardiovascular disease among those with HIV. They have a 50 percent higher risk of heart attack compared with noninfected controls, and a more than fourfold higher rate of sudden cardiac death compared with the general population. They also are in greater danger from complications associated with heart failure.

Certain cancers are increasing among them as well. Early in the epidemic, some cancers—Kaposi's sarcoma, non-Hodgkin's lymphoma and invasive cervical cancer, for example—often developed in HIV-infected individuals, signaling the onset of full-scale AIDS. These "AIDS-defining" cancers initially decreased with the introduction of anti-HIV drugs and have remained relatively steady during the past two decades. However, the burden of non-AIDS-defining cancers—anal cancer, lung cancer, Hodgkin's lymphoma, liver cancer and head and neck cancers, among others—has grown during that period. Many of these are caused by viruses other than HIV. (These include hepatitis B and C viruses and liver cancer; human papillomavirus and head, neck and anal cancers; and Epstein Barr virus and Hodgkin's lymphoma.)

Experts believe these arise in HIV-infected people predominantly because their impaired immune systems can't effectively fight the viruses responsible. Lung cancer is an exception because it is not caused by a virus. But many HIV-infected people smoke, and also suffer lung infections and other assaults.

These cancers account for a growing number of cancer-related deaths among the HIV population. "As people are dying less often of AIDS and opportunistic infections, cancer is becoming one of the most common causes of death in people with HIV," says Robert Yarchoan, chief of the National Cancer Institute's HIV and AIDS malignancy branch. "Also, the incidence of most cancers increases as people age, and HIV-infected people are becoming more susceptible, just like the rest of us."

One ongoing study has shown that patients who start AIDS antiretroviral drug therapy early generally fare better than those who wait, including significantly reducing their chances of developing full-scale AIDS. But even a brief period between infection and the onset of therapy can harm the immune system and cause problems, experts say.

Leaky Gut

"Very shortly after someone is infected, the lymphatic system in the gastrointestinal tract undergoes a major transformation" known as microbial translocation, often called "leaky gut," a condition where microbes from the GI tract escape and enter the bloodstream, according to Amy Justice, a professor of medicine at Yale University who studies HIV among veterans. "It happens quickly after infection, and we're not very good at preventing it. Even when we treat them [with anti-HIV drugs] early, they still have more microbial translocation than people who don't have HIV—and it feeds the chronic inflammation."

Moreover, drinking alcohol exacerbates leaky gut, "so drinking when you have HIV is not a good thing," she says.

In fact, drinking, smoking, recreational drug use and obesity—a common side effect of antiretroviral therapy—also probably contribute to the medical problems of HIV patients, experts say. "The challenge is to try to get them to change ingrained health behaviors at midlife," Justice says. "This is hard for anyone, with or without HIV, but probably more important if you've got HIV."

While the risk of developing age-related conditions "is substantially increased" for people with HIV, the situation isn't necessarily all grim, Justice says. "Not everyone is miserable and sick," Justice says. "Many are doing incredibly well. A lot is in their control, if they can change their health behaviors."

The NIAID's Dieffenbach agrees. "Everybody has his or her own set of risk factors, and what HIV infection tends to do is magnify your lifestyle choices, or your genetics," he says. "What we are grappling with now is defining this. Aging occurs, and with it the risk of getting one or more of these diseases. What is it about HIV that hastens the process? Can we do anything about it? Those are the things we are trying very hard to address."

what does leaky gut do

Section XV

Immunological Interventions

15.1

HIV Vaccine Approaches

Stephen J. Kent

Speed of Response: The Adaptive Immune System's Achilles Heel

The human immune system is a complex network of cells and molecules capable of mounting highly specific, potent protective responses against a broad range of invading pathogens. Nonetheless. infectious diseases are still a major problem, due in part to an inherent weakness of the immune system: the extended time taken to generate protective adaptive responses if innate immune mechanisms fail. This weakness is an unavoidable consequence of the principal dilemma that faces the immune system that infectious episodes cannot be predicted in advance. The adaptive immune system attempts to solve this problem by preparing for every eventuality: it generates billions of T and B lymphocytes, each with a unique antigen receptor, in the hope that a small fraction of these cells will recognise any particular infectious agent. However, the sheer number of receptors needed to provide the necessary breadth of antigen recognition dictates that each unique specificity can be represented on only very few lymphocytes, well below that needed for an effective immune response. Thus, pathogen-specific T and B cells must undergo massive expansion in the early days of infection before protective responses can be generated. This provides a window of opportunity for infection to take hold, generate symptoms and possibly lead to death. Vaccination attempts to limit this window of vulnerability by preparing the immune system in advance to respond faster and better when infection strikes. In the case of natural HIV infection, however, the virus establishes an effectively permanent infection by integrating successfully into the host genome. The long lag time for the development of adaptive immunity means that once HIV infection is established beyond the very first days of infection, it is very difficult to eliminate, described previously as 'too little too late' (Reynolds *et al.*, 2005).

Vaccines Induce Immunological Readiness

Vaccines are pathogen-specific antigenic preparations that attempt to stimulate protective immune responses and are one of the most powerful and cost-effective health interventions. Indeed, protective vaccines are a major success of modern medicine and were the driving force behind the birth of immunology as a scientific discipline. Since Edward Jenner's first attempts to protect against smallpox by the administration of cowpox in 1796, the goal of vaccination has been to prepare the immune system in advance to respond faster and better to infectious agents, minimising the time in which pathogens could cause death and disease. Vaccines aim to provide lifelong protection by inducing a prolonged state of immunological readiness. The precise mechanism by which this state is maintained is still the subject of debate (Ahmed and Gray, 1996: Zinkernagel and Hengartner. 2006), but it is fair to say that it capitalises on the ability of the immune system to preserve useful 'memory' lymphocytes; essentially, an increased frequency of protective pathogen-specific cells that will respond rapidly and efficiently to reinfection. [...] Normally, this heightened state of readiness can only be reached by engaging pathogen in a full-blown infectious setting. Vaccination attempts to mimic these interactions, selecting useful lymphocytes for use in later immune responses, but importantly doing so in the absence of the very great dangers of disease. For HIV, as the virus rapidly establishes a permanent infection, there is potentially a need to have a large number of effective immune responses constantly ready at the site of possible infection—this poses a significant challenge faced by few if any other pathogens (Masopust and Picker, 2012).

Vaccines Must Induce Appropriate Immune Responses

The goal of vaccination is to initiate long-term protective immune responses. The optimal control of infection commonly involves both the cell-mediated (T cell) and humoral (antibody) arms of the immune response. Protective immunity can be distilled into two main areas: the induction of protective CD4+ and CD8+ T cells and the induction of B cells capable of generating neutralising antibodies. These key elements combine to neutralise invading pathogens before they establish an infectious foothold and allow the rapid expansion and mobilisation to appropriate anatomical locations of large numbers of pathogen-specific lymphocytes that subsequently regulate all elements of a coordinated immune response. However, the vaccine-induced generation of an appropriate balance between these key elements is not always straightforward, as effective immunity against different pathogens commonly requires specific immune effectors. Thus, modern research into vaccination seeks to promote appropriate and specific combinations of immune responses targeted to particular pathogens, especially those against which the more basic approaches of vaccination have so far failed. An understanding of precise immune responses that 'correlate with protective immunity' allows the vaccine field to move forward in a rational direction. For HIV, despite decades of research, there is still a need to more precisely define protective immune responses (Corey *et al.*, 2015).

Vaccination Success and Failure: Lessons to Be Learned

Successful vaccines are now used to immunise children against a variety of diseases that include smallpox, polio, measles, mumps, rubella, influenza, chickenpox, diphtheria, tetanus, pertussis, hepatitis B and rabies. Nonetheless, despite concerted efforts, vaccines remain unavailable for tuberculosis, leprosy, malaria, hepatitis C, leishmania, dengue fever and, of course, HIV/AIDS. Key questions are as follows: What distinguishes or links these two sets of diseases? And what can we learn for future vaccine development?

Diseases against which successful vaccines are available are invariably acute, cytopathic and often lethal infections that generate an abundance of antigen. Protection in all cases is due to establishment of high titres of specific neutralising antibody that prevent significant infection. Interestingly, natural immunisation through passage of maternal neutralising antibodies across the placenta and via breast milk is thought to attenuate these acute childhood infections if exposed too early in early infancy, helping the child's immune system to establish protective responses of its own. These types of infection are relatively easily imitated by current vaccination protocols which are often over 90% effective.

By contrast, diseases such as HIV/AIDS against which vaccine development has been unsuccessful tend to be persistent infections that evade or subvert adaptive responses. In natural infection, these are usually better controlled by activated T cells, especially cytotoxic T cells (CTLs), although neutralising antibodies are also involved. However, prolonged CTL function can result in exhaustion of these cells, limiting their capacity to control infection. Persistent infections do not kill the host quickly and coexist with low-grade immune responses for years.

Chronic viral pathogens are often capable of rapid variation, evading any protective responses that are generated (Ha *et al.*, 2008). HIV-1, in particular, is extraordinarily diverse. Within a single infected individual, up to 10^9 variants are produced daily (Pang *et al.*, 1992). The plasticity of HIV means that virtually every type of immune response directed against HIV has been shown to be subject to mutational escape from recognition over time (Chung *et al.*, 2011: Ferrari *et al.*, 2011). Indeed, the difficulties of the immune system in dealing with HIV/AIDS and other chronic infections are reflected in our failure, so far, to devise successful vaccine strategies against them.

Through infecting CD4 T cells HIV also causes substantial immune dysfunction that limits the host immune response. HIV-specific CD4 T cells are even more highly susceptible to infection and dysfunction, rendering their central role in coordinating both cellular and humoral immunity weakened (Douek *et al.*, 2002). Successful vaccines for HIV will need to block the establishment of infection in CD4 T cells before these cells die and become dysfunctional.

Common Vaccine Strategies That Have Failed to Make an Impact of HIV Immunity

Critically important considerations directly impact on the success of a vaccine. These condense to several key issues. First the vaccine preparation must be immunogenic; it must induce pathogen-targeted protective immunity that avoids or breaks tolerogenic and inhibitory mechanisms. Unfortunately, the HIV envelope, a key target of humoral immunity, is relatively weakly immunogenic. Second, the vaccine should induce immunity at appropriate anatomical sites that ideally reflect the likely route of pathogen entry. Immunity at mucosal sites is particularly relevant for HIV as sexual contact is the major route of infection, and the gut-associated lymphoid tissue (GALT) is a major site of replication. Site-specific immunity can be achieved by administering the vaccine orally or through mucosal, intramuscular or intravenous inoculation. This allows distinct antigen-presenting cells to prime local T- and B-cell responses, influencing the subsequent compartmentalisation and nature of the induced immune response. There is a growing interest in the role that 'resident-memory T cells' may have in protective immunity at mucosal surfaces (Tan *et al.*, 2016b). Indeed, there is a relative paucity of studies effectively inducing mucosal immunity to HIV (Tan *et al.*, 2016a). Third, the vaccine must represent the global extent of expected pathogen diversity. For HIV/AIDS, vaccines for specific geographical regions may also be a consideration, but as yet there is no evidence to suggest that this might be a feasible strategy. The global diversity of HIV is strikingly large, and many strategies concentrate on subtypes of HIV that are especially common, such as subtype C in southern Africa. Finally, the vaccine must provide continuous and sufficient presentation of antigen in secondary lymphoid organs that allow long-term protective responses to become established. This may be particularly relevant for HIV/AIDS as highly exposed, persistently seronegative Kenyan sex workers displayed potent virus-specific CTL responses which waned when their constant exposure to HIV stopped, often resulting in the recurrence of susceptibility to HIV infection (Kaul *et al.*, 2001).

With the earlier considerations in mind, a myriad of vaccination strategies have been derived that range from passive transfer of antibodies through to the postgenomic vaccines based on modelling protein structure, many of which are being explored to combat HIV/AIDS. Early vaccines were pathogen derived; heat or chemically inactivated pathogens were used in the Salk polio vaccine and for cholera, influenza and plague. These are relatively safe but require adjuvants and stimulate poor cell-mediated responses owing to limited MHC (major histocompatibility complex) class-I presentation. Other vaccines, for example, against measles, mumps and rubella, and the Sabin polio vaccine, use live attenuated pathogens with greatly decreased virulence. These preparations have the advantage of entering both the class-I and class-II pathways of antigen presentation inducing both cell mediated and humoral immunity. However, reversion to more virulent forms is always a dangerous possibility, preventing the use of this strategy against rapidly mutating pathogens such as HIV. For HIV, reversion to virulence has been documented in both animal models and humans who have naturally acquired attenuated strains (Learmont *et al.*, 1999). As technology has progressed, subunit vaccines have become more prominent and are a more appropriate strategy for HIV. Examples have included toxoid-derived vaccines (e.g. against tetanus and diphtheria), vaccines derived from capsular polysaccharides, either alone or conjugated to a protein carrier (e.g. against bacteria, meningitis) and vaccines that use recombinant DNA (deoxyribonucleic acid) technology (e.g. against hepatitis B virus—HBV). These are generally low risk but invariably require the correct choice of adjuvant to ensure sufficient immunogenicity and often fail to stimulate a full range of immune responses because, like killed vaccines, they have limited access to appropriate pathways of antigen presentation. Envelope protein approaches alone have to date not induced neutralising antibodies and earlier approaches were not protective in human efficacy trials

15.2

A Step Forward for HIV Vaccines

Dan H. Barouch

Development of a safe and effective HIV vaccine will probably be essential to achieve a durable end to the HIV pandemic.[1,2] However, only four HIV vaccine regimens have been assessed for clinical efficacy in the 35-year history of the HIV epidemic.[2] The main challenges facing the development of an HIV vaccine are scientific and are unprecedented in the history of vaccinology, including the need to protect against globally diverse virus strains and unclear immune correlates of protection. In *The Lancet HIV*, Linda-Gail Bekker and colleagues report an important next chapter in the quest to develop an HIV vaccine.[3]

In 2009, the RV144 trial showed the first, and to date only, positive results from an HIV vaccine efficacy trial in human beings.[4] This vaccine included priming with canarypox ALVAC vectors and boosting with alum-adjuvanted envelope (env) gp120 proteins, and it provided 31% efficacy in a low-risk population in Thailand. Although not sufficient for licensure, these data catalysed a wave of enthusiasm to understand the immune correlates of protection and to try to improve this vaccine. Findings from an immune correlates analysis indicated that antibodies against env variable loops 1 and 2 (V1V2) correlated inversely with infection risk,[5] and a sieve analysis similarly showed vaccine-induced immune pressure on env V1V2.[6]

These data led to a hypothesis that vaccine-elicited binding antibodies against V1V2 might have accounted for the protection observed in RV144. Additional potential correlates of protection that emerged from RV144 included IgG3 responses and CD4+ T-cell responses. A validated and predictive immune correlate of protection would be a major advance for the HIV vaccine field. Thus, a key priority has been to test this potential V1V2 immune correlate prospectively in another study.

Bekker and colleagues aimed to adapt the RV144 vaccine regimen to the clade C epidemic in South Africa. New ALVAC vectors (vCP2438, expressing clade C *env gp120* and clade B *env gp41/gag/pro*) and bivalent clade C env gp120 proteins (TV1/1086) were manufactured, and instead of the alum adjuvant used in RV144, the more potent squalene-based adjuvant MF59 was used. Bekker and colleagues assessed the safety and immunogenicity of this new vaccine in the HIV Vaccine Trials Network (HVTN) 100 trial[3]—a placebo-controlled, randomised, double-blind, phase 1/2 trial in South Africa. A late boost was added to the RV144 vaccine schedule at 12 months, with vaccine administered at months 0, 1, 3, 6, and 12. Thus, the RV144 and HVTN 100 trials differed by many variables. Binding antibody responses were of a higher magnitude and cellular immune responses were of a higher frequency in HVTN 100 compared with RV144, but V1V2-specific antibody responses were lower in HVTN 100 than in RV144. The reasons for these differences are not entirely clear but could be related to the specific env strains selected for the vaccines and the more potent adjuvant used in HVTN 100.

The findings of HVTN 100 are important because prespecified immunological go/no-go criteria were achieved, including IgG antibody binding and CD4+ T-cell responses, which led to initiation of a phase 2b/3 efficacy trial (HVTN 702) to ascertain the capacity of this vaccine to protect against HIV acquisition in South Africa (NCT02968849). HVTN 702 will also test prospectively whether vaccine-elicited V1V2-binding antibodies correlate with protection. Validation of this immune correlate would be useful because it could then be used as a surrogate biomarker that would greatly accelerate HIV vaccine development moving forward.

As the area of HIV vaccine research awaits efficacy results from HVTN 702, additional HIV vaccine candidates are also being pursued. These include adenovirus vectors expressing mosaic immunogens with an env gp140 protein boost, cytomegalovirus vectors that induce persistent T-cell responses, native-like env trimers, and sequential env immunisation approaches that aim to induce broadly neutralising antibodies.[2] One lesson from the RV144, HVTN 100, and HVTN 702 trials is that the time and resources needed to bring a vaccine candidate into efficacy trials are substantial. However, only such clinical efficacy trials can establish if a vaccine candidate protects humans. Moreover, efficacy data in humans helps to refine preclinical models and immunological assays. Therefore, we need to increase the number of efficacy trials to test a broad range of ideas for vaccines if we are to achieve the ultimate objective of developing an HIV vaccine and ending the HIV pandemic.

I declare grants from the National Institutes of Health, the Gates Foundation, the Ragon Institute, the Henry Jackson Foundation, The Foundation for AIDS Research, the Defense Advanced Research Projects Agency, Janssen, and Gilead; and personal fees from IGM and AVVI Biotech; all outside the submitted work.

References

1. Fauci AS. An HIV vaccine is essential for ending the HIV/AIDS pandemic. *JAMA*. 2017; 318: 1535–1536
2. Stephenson K.E., D'Couto H.T., Barouch D.H. New concepts in HIV-1 vaccine development. *Curr Opin Immunol*. 2016; 41: 39–46
3. Bekker L-G, Moodie Z, Grunenberg N, et al. Subtype C ALVAC-HIV and bivalent subtype C gp120/MF59 HIV-1 vaccine in low-risk, HIV-uninfected, South African adults: a phase 1/2 trial. *Lancet HIV*. 2018; (published online June 10.) http://dx.doi.org/10.1016/S2352–3018(18)30071–7
4. Rerks-Ngarm S., Pitisuttithum P., Nitayaphan S., et al. Vaccination with ALVAC and AIDSVAX to prevent HIV-1 infection in Thailand. *N Engl J Med*. 2009; 361: 2209–2220
5. Haynes B.F., Gilbert P.B., McElrath M.J., et al. Immune-correlates analysis of an HIV-1 vaccine efficacy trial. *N Engl J Med*. 2012; 366: 1275–1286
6. Rolland M., Edlefsen P.T., Larsen B.B., et al. Increased HIV-1 vaccine efficacy against viruses with genetic signatures in Env V2. *Nature*. 2012; 490: 417–420

15.3

Broadly Neutralizing Antibodies for HIV-1 Prevention or Immunotherapy

Marina Caskey, M.D., Florian Klein, M.D., and Michel C. Nussenzweig, M.D., Ph.D.

DESPITE TREMENDOUS EFFORTS TO PREVENT transmission of human immunodeficiency virus type 1 (HIV-1), new infections and AIDS-related deaths continue to be a global problem. Antiretroviral therapy (ART) can effectively suppress HIV-1 replication and limit disease progression. However, ART fails to eradicate the virus, and suppression requires lifelong therapy, which may have side effects and poses a risk of the development of resistance. New approaches to preventing and treating HIV-1 infection are there fore necessary to contain the epidemic and to bolster nascent efforts to find a cure.

A new generation of highly potent broadly neutralizing antibodies (bNAbs) may represent a promising approach to combating HIV-1 infection.[1] Although antibodies that neutralize HIV-1 were discovered shortly after the disease was first described, most HIV-1–infected people produce nonneutralizing antibodies or antibodies that neutralize only a limited number of different HIV-1 strains. However, high serum titers of HIV-1 neutralizing activity develop in a small fraction of infected persons. In contrast to the typical antibody response, bNAbs can take years to develop, and it has not yet proved possible to elicit them by standard immunization strategies.

Isolation of bNAbs from infected persons with high levels of HIV-1–neutralizing serum activity (so-called elite neutralizers) was not easily achieved until the advent of single-cell–based anti-HIV-1 antibody cloning techniques.[2] The anti–HIV-1 antibodies obtained by this and subsequently developed related methods had a number of unusual characteristics that partially account for the difficulty of developing a vaccine that can elicit bNAbs. The most prominent of these features is a high level of somatic hypermutation, which is required to accommodate binding to the highly glycosylated viral envelope protein. Some of the new bNAbs can neutralize up to 90% of HIV-1 strains worldwide at low concentrations.[1] Moreover, bNAbs recognize many sites on the viral envelope spike (see diagram). Anti bodies currently being tested or under development for clinical use target the CD4-binding site, a glycan patch surrounding the V3 loop, and the apex of the HIV-1 spike.[3] It thus seems possible that they could be used in combination to prevent or control HIV-1 infection. As with other drugs, the efficacy of any single anti-HIV-1 antibody in preclinical and clinical trials is related to the potency and breadth of its activity against different HIV-1 isolates. Like monotherapy with small-molecule antiretroviral (ARV) drugs, the administration of a single anti-idiotypic bNAb selects for resistant variants. As recently reported,[3] in work that Bar et al. have extended, bNAbs are being studied as a potential way to suppress viremia during analytical treatment interruption. The degree of efficacy in maintaining viral suppression in these and other studies was most likely related to the potency of the bNAbs.[4,5]

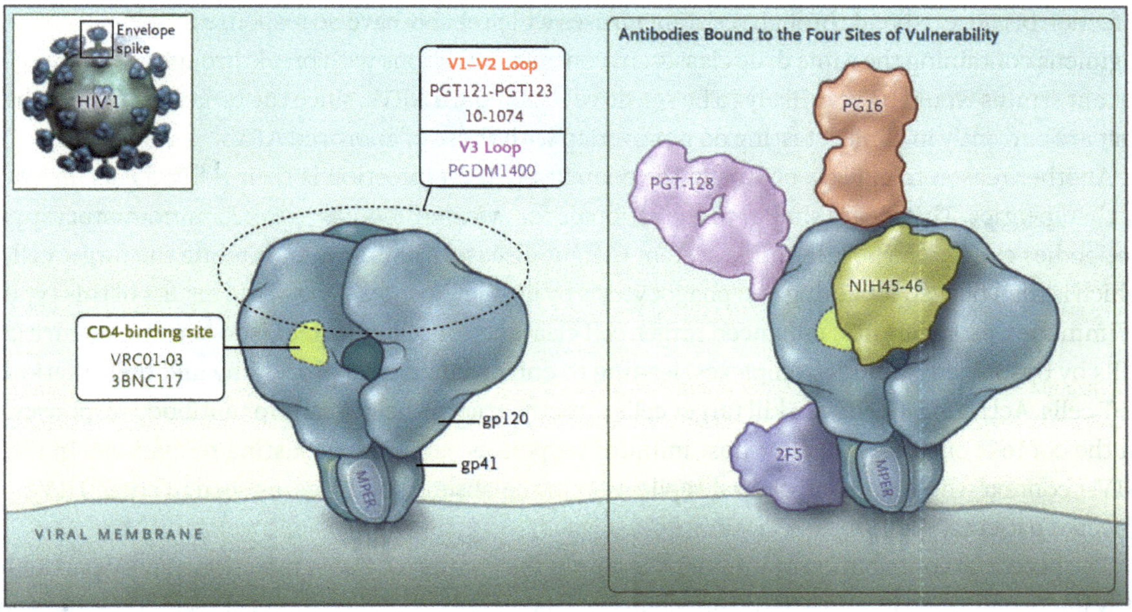

HIV-1 SPIKE Protein, Showing Sites Targeted by Broadly Neutralizing Monoclonal Antibodies.

The inset shows the virus with its surface spikes. The left panel shows target sites of monoclonal antibodies in clinical development. The right panel illustrates the binding of four different broadly neutralizing antibodies.

However, antibodies are currently expensive to produce and must be administered parenterally. In contrast, small-molecule ARV drugs can be synthesized at low cost, are administered orally, and are highly effective. So it is important to ask why we should bother investigating the use of antibodies for HIV-1 prevention or therapy.

Several unique features of antibodies make them interesting to explore as drugs for HIV-1 prevention and therapy. First, antibodies differ from small-molecule drugs in having naturally long half-lives of 2 to 3 weeks. It was this property that made it possible, before the advent of an active hepatitis vaccine, to administer pooled antihepatitis immunoglobulins as a passive vaccine to prevent infection in travelers for up to 3 months. The same is true for bNAbs and HIV-1 prevention. A single administration of anti-HIV-1 bNAbs can protect macaques for up to 23 sequential weekly challenges.[5] Moreover, the antibody half-life can be increased by a factor of 2 to 4 by point mutations in the constant (Fc) region of the molecule. For example, in clinical investigations, an anti–respiratory syncytial virus antibody that carries half-life extension mutations showed neutralizing activity for 240 days after administration in humans. When similar mutations were introduced into anti-HIV-1 bNAbs, they resulted in a prolonged half-life and extended the protective effects in macaques.[5]

The pharmacokinetic properties of anti-HIV1 bNAbs with half-life–extending mutations are currently being tested in humans. It is entirely possible that bNAbs could be used as passive vaccines administered subcutaneously on a quarterly or a biannual basis. In contrast, the best small-molecule drugs in late-stage clinical testing have to be administered intramuscularly every 2 months for prevention or therapy. More important, decaying levels of these long-acting drugs may allow selection of resistant viral strains, and persons in whom oral or injectable small-molecule drugs fail to prevent infection because of breakthrough resistant viruses will probably have no response to anti-retroviral regimens containing the same drug classes. In contrast, infections with breakthrough antibody-resistant strains would be very likely to be sensitive to standard ARVs, since the targets of the bNAbs that are currently in clinical testing do not overlap with those of approved ARVs.

Another reason to explore bNAbs in the context of HIV-1 infection is their potential as immunotherapeutics. This idea is similar to the rationale for using antibodies in cancer immunotherapy: antibodies engage the host immune system to fight disease. They do so by binding the target cell, which is then flagged for killing and phagocytosis by host leukocytes. One of the results of this type of immune opsonization is enhanced target-cell clearance. A second effect is to activate dendritic cells by opsonized immune complexes, leading to enhanced antigen processing and presentation to T cells. Activated T cells can kill target cells directly or act as helper cells for antibody responses. In the context of cancer therapy, host immune responses can produce lasting remissions. In the HIV-1 context, they can control viral replication in the absence of drugs, as seen in some HIV-1–infected patients.

The potential contribution of immunotherapy in the context of HIV-1 infection may be particularly important when it comes to the possibility of HIV-1 eradication. In phase 1 clinical trials, bNAbs enhanced clearance of HIV-1, infected cells, or both and boosted host humoral immunity to HIV-1.

These antibody-mediated immune-enhancing effects might lead to better control of viral replication and reduce the size of the long-lived latent reservoir that persists despite suppressive ART. It is important to note, however, that the immune-engaging features of antibodies are mediated through binding of antibody to available antigen. Suppressive ART may therefore dampen these potential effects by a nearly complete shutdown of viral replication. It will therefore be important to further evaluate the effects of bNAbs in combination with strategies aimed at reactivating latent pro-viruses in the presence or absence of standard ART.

Although bNAbs have attractive properties, particularly for HIV-1 eradication strategies, as compared with standard ART, resistance does develop during antibody monotherapy. Moreover, preexisting resistance to individual bNAbs, as described in our work[3,4] and by Bar and colleagues, may also pose a challenge to their use, especially during chronic HIV-1 infection. We speculate that a combination of bNAbs, like combinations of small-molecule ARV drugs, can avert selection of escape variants. Ongoing studies aim to explore their use for HIV-1 prevention and immunotherapy in infected persons.

Disclosure forms provided by the authors are available at NEJM.org.

From the Laboratory of Molecular Immunology (M.C., M.C.N.) and the Howard Hughes Medical Institute (M.C.N.), Rocke-feller University, New York; and the Laboratory of Experimental Immunology, Center for Molecular Medicine Cologne (CMMC), University of Cologne, Department I of Internal Medicine, Center of Integrated Oncology Cologne–Bonn, University Hospital Cologne, and the German Center for Infection Research, partner site Bonn–Cologne—all in Cologne, Germany (F.K.).

This article was published on November 9, 2016, at NEJM.org.

Klein F., Mouquet H., Dosenovic P., Scheid J.F., Scharf L., Nussenzweig M.C. Antibodies in HIV-1 vaccine development and therapy. Science 2013; 341: 1199-204.

Scheid J.F., Mouquet H., Feldhahn N., et al. A method for identification of HIV gp140 binding memory B cells in human blood. J Immunol Methods 2009; 343:65-7.

Caskey M., Klein F., Lorenzi J.C., et al. Viraemia suppressed in HIV-1-infected humans by broadly neutralizing antibody 3BNC117. Nature 2015; 522: 487-91.

Scheid J.F., Horwitz J.A., Bar-On Y., et al. HIV-1 antibody 3BNC117 suppresses viral rebound in humans during treatment interruption. Nature 2016; 535: 556-60.

Gautam R., Nishimura Y., Pegu A., et al. A single injection of anti-HIV-1 antibodies protects against repeated SHIV challenges. Nature 2016; 533: 105-9.

Section XVI

Therapies

16.1

HIV Treatment

The National Institutes of Health

What Is Antiretroviral Therapy?

Antiretroviral therapy (ART) is the use of HIV medicines to treat HIV infection. People on ART take a combination of HIV medicines (called an HIV treatment regimen) every day.

ART is recommended for everyone who has HIV. ART can't cure HIV, but HIV medicines help people with HIV live longer, healthier lives. ART also reduces the risk of HIV transmission.

How Do HIV Medicines Work?

HIV attacks and destroys the infection-fighting CD4 cells of the immune system. Loss of CD4 cells makes it hard for the body to fight off infections and certain HIV-related cancers.

HIV medicines prevent HIV from multiplying (making copies of itself), which reduces the amount of HIV in the body (also called the viral load). Having less HIV in the body gives the immune system a chance to recover. Even though there is still some HIV in the body, the immune system is strong enough to fight off infections and certain HIV-related cancers.

By reducing the amount of HIV in the body, HIV medicines also reduce the risk of HIV transmission. A main goal of ART is to reduce a person's viral load to an undetectable level. An undetectable viral load means that the level of HIV in the blood is too low to be detected by a viral load test. People with HIV who maintain an undetectable viral load have effectively no risk of transmitting HIV to their HIV-negative partner through sex.

When Is It Time to Start Taking HIV Medicines?

People with HIV should start ART as soon as possible. In people with the following conditions, it's especially important to start ART right away: pregnancy, AIDS, certain HIV-related illnesses and coinfections, and early HIV infection. (Early HIV infection is the period up to 6 months after infection with HIV.)

Source: https://aidsinfo.nih.gov/understanding-hiv-aids/.

What Is an HIV regimen?

An HIV regimen is a combination of HIV medicines used to treat HIV infection. HIV treatment begins with choosing an HIV regimen. People on ART take the HIV medicines in their HIV regimens every day.

There are more than 30 HIV medicines approved by the U.S. Food and Drug Administration (FDA) to treat HIV infection. Some HIV medicines are available in combination (in other words, two or more different HIV medicines combined in one pill).

The U.S. Department of Health and Human Services (HHS) provides guidelines on the use of HIV medicines. In general, the guidelines recommend starting ART with a regimen that includes three HIV medicines from at least two different drug classes.

What Are the HIV Drug Classes?

HIV medicines are grouped into seven drug classes according to how they fight HIV. The seven drug classes are:

- Non-nucleoside reverse transcriptase inhibitors (NNRTIs)
- Nucleoside reverse transcriptase inhibitors (NRTIs)
- Protease inhibitors (PIs)
- Fusion inhibitors
- CCR5 antagonists
- Integrase strand transfer inhibitors (INSTIs)
- Post-attachment inhibitors

In general, a person's first HIV regimen includes two NRTIs plus an INSTI, an NNRTI, or a PI boosted with cobicistat (brand name: Tybost) or ritonavir (brand name: Norvir). Cobicistat or ritonavir increase (boost) the effectiveness of the PI.

How Does Each Drug Class Work?

1. **Non-Nucleoside Reverse Transcriptase Inhibitor (NNRTI)**
These drugs bind to and block HIV reverse transcriptase (an HIV enzyme). HIV uses reverse transcriptase to convert its RNA into DNA (reverse transcription). Blocking reverse transcriptase and reverse transcription prevents HIV from replicating.

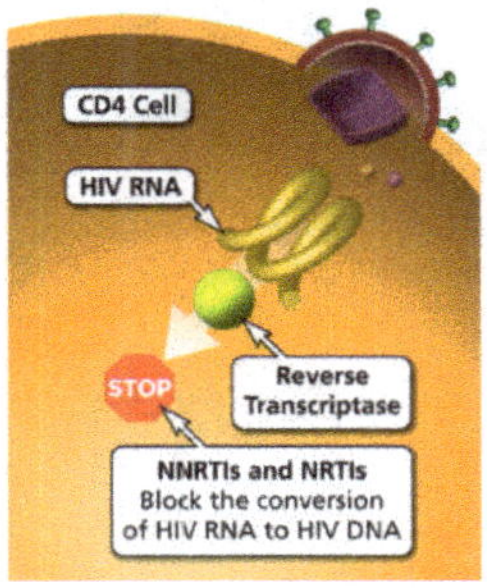

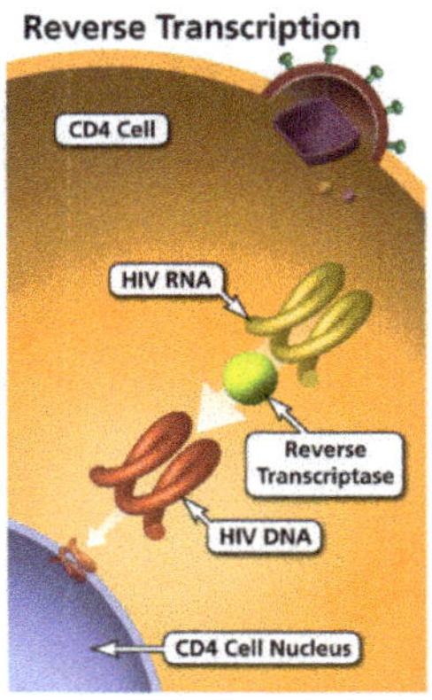

2. **Nucleoside Reverse Transcriptase Inhibitor (NRTI)**
These drugs block reverse transcriptase (an HIV enzyme). HIV uses reverse transcriptase to convert its RNA into DNA (reverse transcription). Blocking reverse transcriptase and reverse transcription prevents HIV from replicating.

3. **Protease Inhibitor (PI)**
Antiretroviral (ARV) HIV drug class. Protease inhibitors (PIs) block protease (an HIV enzyme). By blocking protease, PIs prevent new (immature) HIV from becoming a mature virus that can infect other CD4 cells.

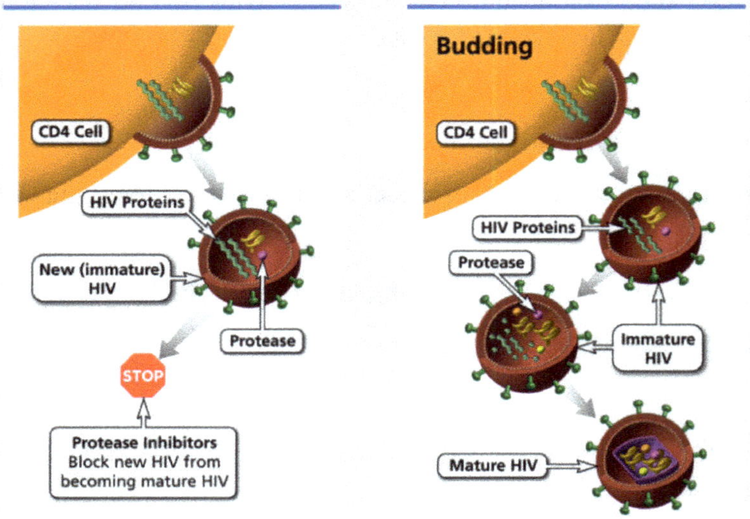

4. **Fusion Inhibitor**
Antiretroviral (ARV) HIV drug class. A fusion inhibitor blocks the HIV envelope from merging with the host CD4 cell membrane (fusion). This prevents HIV from entering the CD4 cell.

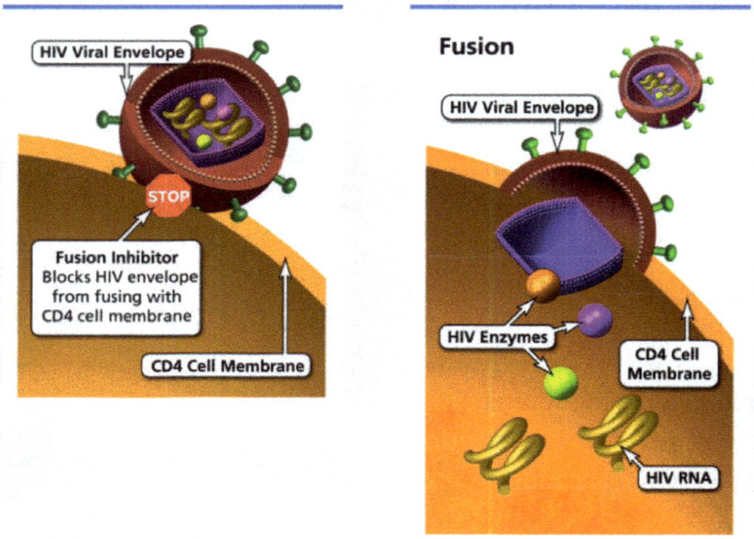

5. **CCR5 Antagonist**
Antiretroviral (ARV) HIV drug class. CCR5 antagonists block the CCR5 coreceptor on the surface of certain immune cells, such as CD4 T lymphocytes (CD4 cells). This prevents HIV from entering the cell.

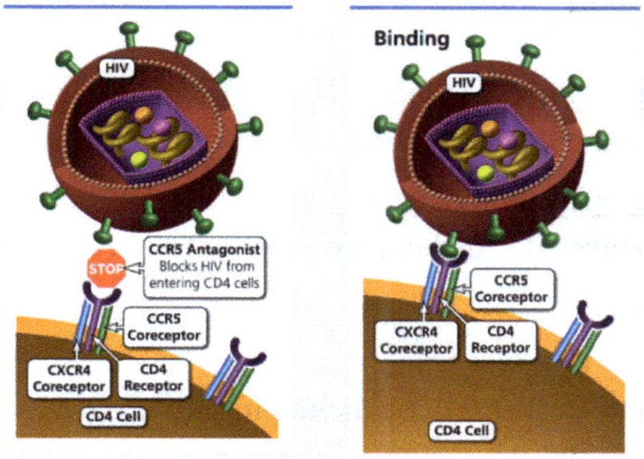

6. **Integrase Strand Transfer Inhibitor (INSTI)**
Antiretroviral (ARV) HIV drug class. Integrase strand transfer inhibitors (INSTIs) block integrase (an HIV enzyme). HIV uses integrase to insert (integrate) its viral DNA into the DNA of the host CD4 cell. Blocking integrase prevents HIV from replicating.

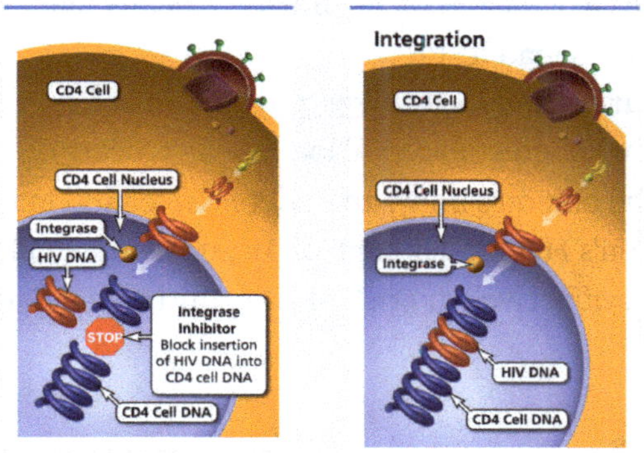

7. **Post-Attachment Inhibitor**
Post-attachment inhibitors are a class of drugs that block HIV from binding to the CCR5 and CXCR4 coreceptors after HIV binds to the CD4 receptor on the surface of a CD4 cell. This prevents HIV from entering the cell. Post-attachment inhibitors are part of a larger group of HIV drugs called entry inhibitors.

What Factors Are Considered When Choosing an HIV Regimen?

The choice of HIV medicines to include in an HIV regimen depends on a person's individual needs. When choosing an HIV regimen, people with HIV and their health care providers consider the following factors:

- Other diseases or conditions that the person with HIV may have, such as heart disease or pregnancy.

- Possible side effects of HIV medicines.
- Potential interactions between HIV medicines or between HIV medicines and other medicines the person with HIV is taking.
- Results of drug-resistance testing (and other tests). Drug-resistance testing identifies which, if any, HIV medicines won't be effective against a person's HIV.
- Convenience of the regimen. For example, a regimen that includes two or more HIV medicines combined in one pill is convenient to follow.
- Any issues that can make it difficult to follow an HIV regimen. For example, a busy schedule can make it hard to take HIV medicines consistently every day.
- Cost of HIV medicines.

The HHS guidelines on the use of HIV medicines in adults and adolescents recommend several regimens for people starting ART. The best regimen for a person depends on their individual needs.

How Long Does it Take For ART to Work?

Viral load is the amount of HIV in a person's blood. A main goal of ART is to reduce a person's viral load to an undetectable level. An undetectable viral load means that the level of HIV in the blood is too low to be detected by a viral load test.

Once effective ART is started, it usually takes 3 to 6 months for a person's viral load to reach an undetectable level. Having an undetectable viral load doesn't mean a person's HIV is cured. Although there is still some HIV in the person's body, an undetectable viral load shows that ART is working effectively to keep the person's HIV under control. In addition, people with HIV who maintain an undetectable viral load have effectively no risk of transmitting HIV to their HIV-negative partner through sex.

Can HIV Medicines Cause Side Effects?

HIV medicines can cause side effects. Most side effects from HIV medicines are manageable, but a few can be serious. Overall, the benefits of HIV medicines far outweigh the risk of side effects. In addition, newer HIV regimens cause fewer side effects than regimens used in the past. As HIV treatment options continue to improve, people are less likely to experience side effects from their HIV medicines.

Before starting HIV medicines, people with HIV discuss possible side effects from HIV medicines with their health care providers. They work together to select an HIV regimen based on the person's individual needs.

Do HIV Medicines Cause the Same Side Effects?

Different HIV medicines can cause different side effects. In addition, people taking the same HIV medicine can have different side effects.

Side effects from HIV medicines can last only a few days or weeks or continue for much longer. Some side effects may not appear until many months or even years after starting an HIV medicine.

What Are Some Short-Term Side Effects from HIV Medicines?

People starting an HIV medicine for the first time may have side effects that last a couple of weeks. These short-term side effects can include:

- Feeling tired
- Nausea (upset stomach)
- Vomiting
- Diarrhea
- Headache
- Fever
- Muscle pain
- Occasional dizziness
- Insomnia

Sometimes, side effects that may not seem serious, such as fever, rash, nausea, or fatigue, can be a sign of a life-threatening condition. Any swelling of the face, eyes, lips, throat, or tongue is considered a life-threatening side effect that requires immediate medical attention.

HIV infection itself, another medical condition, or other medicines a person is taking can also cause side effects. Drug interactions between HIV medicines or with other medicines a person is taking can also cause side effects.

What Are Some Long-Term Side Effects from HIV Medicines?

Some side effects from HIV medicines can appear months or even years after starting a medicine and can continue for a long time. Examples of long-term side effects include:

- Kidney problems, including kidney failure
- Liver damage (hepatotoxicity)
- Heart disease
- Diabetes or insulin resistance
- An increase in fat levels in the blood (hyperlipidemia)
- Changes in how the body uses and stores fat (lipodystrophy)
- Weakening of the bones (osteoporosis)
- Nerve damage (peripheral neuropathy)
- Mental health-related effects, including insomnia, depression, and thoughts of suicide

Why Is Adherence to an HIV Regimen Important?

Adherence to an HIV regimen gives HIV medicines the chance to do their job. Poor adherence to an HIV regimen allows HIV to destroy the immune system. Poor adherence also increases the risk of drug resistance and HIV treatment failure.

Why Is Medication Adherence Sometimes Difficult?

Adherence to an HIV regimen can be difficult for several reasons. For example, side effects from some HIV medicines, such as nausea or diarrhea, can make it hard to follow an HIV regimen. When an HIV regimen includes several HIV medicines, it's easy to forget how many pills to take and when to take them.

The following factors can also make medication adherence difficult:

- Side effects from interactions between HIV medicines and other medicines a person may take
- Trouble swallowing pills or other difficulty taking medicines
- A busy schedule, shift work, or travel away from home that makes it hard to take medicines on time
- Having an unstable living or housing situation
- Illness or depression
- Alcohol or drug use that interferes with the activities of daily life
- Fear of disclosing one's HIV-positive status to others
- Lack of health insurance to cover the cost of HIV medicines

What Is Drug Resistance?

When HIV multiplies, the virus sometimes mutates. Variations of HIV that develop while a person is taking HIV medicines can lead to new, drug-resistant strains of HIV. With drug resistance, HIV medicines that used to suppress the person's HIV are not effective against the new drug-resistant HIV. In other words, the person's HIV continues to multiply.

Once drug-resistant HIV develops, it remains in the body. Drug resistance limits the number of HIV medicines available to include in a current or future HIV regimen. Drug-resistant HIV can spread from person to person. People initially infected with drug-resistant HIV have drug resistance to one or more HIV medicines even before they start taking HIV medicines.

What Is the Connection Between Medication Adherence and Drug Resistance?

Taking HIV medicines every day prevents HIV from multiplying, which reduces the risk that HIV will mutate and produce drug-resistant HIV. Skipping HIV medicines allows HIV to multiply, which increases the risk of drug-resistant HIV developing.

Research shows that a person's first HIV regimen offers the best chance for long-term treatment success. So adherence is important from the start—when a person first begins taking HIV medicines.

What Is Cross Resistance?

Cross resistance is when resistance to one HIV medicine causes resistance to other medicines in the same HIV drug class. As a result of cross resistance, a person's HIV may be resistant even to HIV medicines that the person has never taken. Cross resistance limits the number of HIV medicines available to include in an HIV regimen.

What Is Drug-Resistance Testing?

Drug-resistance testing is done to identify which, if any, HIV medicines won't be effective against a person's strain of HIV. This testing is done using a sample of blood.

Drug-resistance testing is done when a person first begins receiving care for HIV infection. Resistance testing should be done whether the person decides to start taking HIV medicines immediately or to delay treatment. This can show whether the person was initially infected with a drug-resistant strain of HIV. Testing results are used to decide which HIV medicines to include in a person's first HIV regimen.

After treatment is started, drug-resistance testing is repeated if viral load testing indicates that a person's HIV regimen isn't controlling the virus. If drug-resistance testing shows that the HIV regimen isn't effective because of drug resistance, the test results can be used to select a new HIV regimen.

https://aidsinfo.nih.gov/understanding-hiv-aids/fact-sheets/21/51/hiv-treatment--the-basics
https://aidsinfo.nih.gov/understanding-hiv-aids/fact-sheets/21/53/what-to-start--choosing-an-hiv-regimen
https://aidsinfo.nih.gov/understanding-hiv-aids/fact-sheets/22/63/hiv-medicines-and-side-effects
https://aidsinfo.nih.gov/understanding-hiv-aids/fact-sheets/21/54/hiv-medication-adherence
https://aidsinfo.nih.gov/understanding-hiv-aids/fact-sheets/21/56/drug-resistance
https://aidsinfo.nih.gov/understanding-hiv-aids/glossary/513/non-nucleoside-reverse-transcriptase-inhibitor/
https://aidsinfo.nih.gov/understanding-hiv-aids/glossary/902/nucleoside-reverse-transcriptase-inhibitor/
https://aidsinfo.nih.gov/understanding-hiv-aids/glossary/603/protease-inhibitor/
https://aidsinfo.nih.gov/understanding-hiv-aids/glossary/258/fusion-inhibitor/
https://aidsinfo.nih.gov/understanding-hiv-aids/glossary/1549/ccr5-antagonist/
https://aidsinfo.nih.gov/understanding-hiv-aids/glossary/380/integrase-strand-transfer-inhibitor/
https://aidsinfo.nih.gov/understanding-hiv-aids/glossary/4696/post-attachment-inhibitor

16.2

Antiretroviral Drugs Used in the Treatment of HIV Infection

U.S. Food and Drug Administration

Drugs Used in the Treatment of HIV Infection

FDA-approved medicines used in the treatment of HIV can be found at Drugs@FDA or DailyMed. This list may not be comprehensive and it was last updated on April 12, 2018.

Multi-class Combination Products

Brand	Generic Name	Approval Date	Time to Approval
Atripla	efavirenz, emtricitabine and tenofovir disoproxil fumarate	12-July-06	2.5 months
Complera	emtricitabine, rilpivirine, and tenofovir disoproxil fumarate	10-August-11	6 months
Evotaz	atazanavir sulfate, cobicistat	29-January-15	9 months
Prezcobix	cobicistat, darunavir ethanolate	29-January-15	10 months
Stribild	elvitegravir, cobicistat, emtricitabine, tenofovir disoproxil fumarate	27-August-12	6 months

Nucleoside Reverse Transcriptase Inhibitors (NRTIs);

FDA-approved medicines used in the treatment of HIV can be found at Drugs@FDA or DailyMed.

Brand Name	Generic Name	Approval Date	Time to Approval
Combivir	lamivudine and zidovudine	27-Sep-97	3.9 months
Emtriva	emtricitabine, FTC	02-Jul-03	10 months
Epivir	lamivudine, 3TC	17-Nov-95	4.4 months
Epzicom	abacavir and lamivudine	02-Aug-04	10 months
Hivid	zalcitabine, dideoxycytidine, ddC (no longer marketed)	19-Jun-92	7.6 months
Retrovir	zidovudine, azidothymidine, AZT, ZDV	19-Mar-87	3.5 months
Trizivir	abacavir, zidovudine, and lamivudine	14-Nov-00	10.9 months
Truvada	tenofovir disoproxil fumarate and emtricitabine	02-Aug-04	5 months
Videx EC	enteric coated didanosine, ddI EC	31-Oct-00	9 months
Videx	didanosine, dideoxyinosine, ddI	9-Oct-91	6 months
Viread	tenofovir disoproxil fumarate, TDF	26-Oct-01	5.9 months
Zerit	stavudine, d4T	24-Jun-94	5.9 months
Ziagen	abacavir sulfate, ABC	17-Dec-98	5.8 months

Source: https://www.fda.gov/ForPatients/Illness/HIVAIDS/Treatment/ucm118915.htm.

Nonnucleoside Reverse Transcriptase Inhibitors (NNRTIs)

FDA-approved medicines used in the treatment of HIV can be found at Drugs@FDA or DailyMed.

Brand Name	Generic Name	Approval Date	Time to Approval
Edurant	rilpivirine	20-May-11	10 months
Intelence	etravirine	18-Jan-08	6 months
Rescriptor	delavirdine, DLV	4-Apr-97	8.7 months
Sustiva	efavirenz, EFV	17-Sep-98	3.2 months
Viramune (Immediate Release)	nevirapine, NVP	21-Jun-96	3.9 months
Viramune XR (Extended Release)	nevirapine, NVP	25-Mar-11	9.9 months

Protease Inhibitors (PIs)

FDA-approved medicines used in the treatment of HIV can be found at Drugs@FDA or DailyMed.

Brand Name	Generic Name	Approval Date	Time to Approval
Agenerase	amprenavir, APV (no longer marketed)	15-Apr-99	6 months
Aptivus	tipranavir, TPV	22-Jun-05	6 months
Crixivan	indinavir, IDV	13-Mar-96	1.4 months
Fortovase	saquinavir (no longer marketed)	7-Nov-97	5.9 months
Invirase	saquinavir mesylate, SQV	6-Dec-95	3.2 months
Kaletra	lopinavir and ritonavir, LPV/RTV	15-Sep-00	3.5 months
Lexiva	Fosamprenavir Calcium, FOS-APV	20-Oct-03	10 months
Norvir	ritonavir, RTV	1-Mar-96	2.3 months
Prezista	darunavir	23-Jun-06	6 months
Reyataz	atazanavir sulfate, ATV	20-Jun-03	6 months
Viracept	nelfinavir mesylate, NFV	14-Mar-97	2.6 months

Fusion Inhibitors

FDA-approved medicines used in the treatment of HIV can be found at Drugs@FDA or DailyMed.

Brand Name	Generic Name	Approval Date	Time to Approval
Fuzeon	enfuvirtide, T-20	13-Mar-03	6 months

Entry Inhibitors—CCR5 co-receptor antagonist

FDA-approved medicines used in the treatment of HIV can be found at Drugs@FDA or DailyMed.

Brand Name	Generic Name	Approval Date	Time to Approval
Selzentry	maraviroc	06-August-07	8 months

HIV integrase strand transfer inhibitors

FDA-approved medicines used in the treatment of HIV can be found at Drugs@FDA or DailyMed.

Brand Name	Generic Name	Approval Date	Time to Approval
Isentress	raltegravir	12-Oct-07	6 months
Tivicay	dolutegravir	13-August-13	6 months
Vitekta	elvitegravir	24-September-14	24 months

Approved and Tentatively Approved Antiretrovirals in Association with the President's Emergency Plan (PEPFAR)

16.3

HIV/AIDS Care Continuum

U.S. Center for Disease Control and Prevention

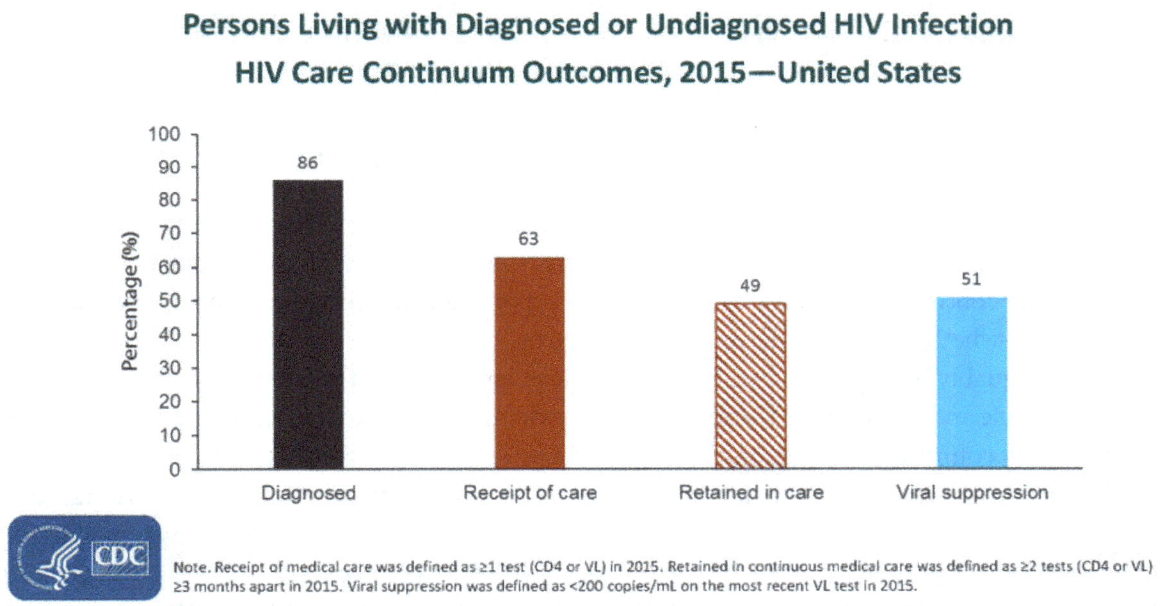

Source: https://www.cdc.gov/nchhstp/newsroom/2017/HIV-Continuum-of-Care.html.

16.4

HIV Drug Resistance—An Emerging Threat to Epidemic Control

Chris Beyrer, M.D., M.P.H., and Anton Pozniak, M.D.

There are now an estimated 19.5 million people worldwide living with HIV and receiving antiretroviral therapy (ART). That's approximately half of all people thought to be living with the virus in 2017—an extraordinary achievement in global health and human solidarity. The United Nations agencies, led by the Joint United Nations Program on HIV/AIDS (UNAIDS) and the World Health Organization (WHO), have committed to the goals of ending the AIDS pandemic as a public health threat by 2030 and ensuring that by 2020, 90% of people with HIV infection know they have it, 90% of those infected are receiving ART, and sustained viral suppression is achieved in 90% of those receiving treatment.[1] This last goal is critically important both to individual health and survival and to epidemic control of HIV, since data continue to mount showing that viral suppression greatly reduces the risk of continued transmission—whether sexual or perinatal—of the virus.

It would arguably be enormously difficult to achieve epidemic control simply by expanding ART. Too many people and communities—from adolescents in Africa, to sexual minorities and transgender people in many countries, to injection-drug users in Eastern Europe and Central Asia—are currently excluded from care. We believe that enhanced primary prevention of infection, by means of targeted use of preexposure prophylaxis (PrEP) for people at substantial risk and probably a preventive vaccine, will be required for ultimate control. Nevertheless, treatment can have—and is having—substantial effects on the rate of new infections, including in some of the world's most HIV-burdened countries, as shown by recent data from Swaziland.[2] The emergence of HIV drug resistance is a very real threat to these gains.

A recent report from the WHO, the Global Fund to Fight AIDS, Tuberculosis, and Malaria, and the Centers for Disease Control and Prevention (CDC) showed that the prevalence of HIV drug resistance has increased from 11% to 29% since the global rollout of ART in 2001.[1] The report was based on findings from 16 surveys in 14 countries that used the WHO's recommended approach to population-based sampling for HIV drug resistance among patients in public ART programs, supplemented by data from two population-based HIV impact assessments conducted through the President's Emergency Plan for AIDS Relief (PEPFAR) in Malawi and Zimbabwe.

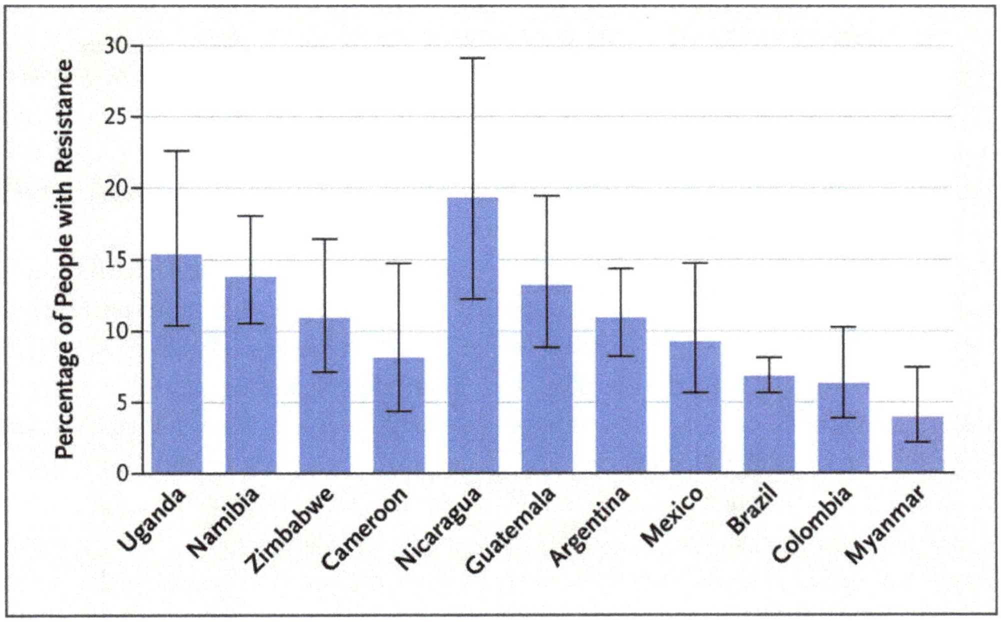

PRETREATMENT HIV Drug Resistance to Nonnucleoside Reverse Transcriptase Inhibitors in 11 Countries.

It is worrisome that in 6 of 11 countries surveyed—Argentina, Guatemala, Namibia, Nicaragua, Uganda, and Zimbabwe—the rate of pretreatment drug resistance surpassed 10% among people receiving ART for the first time (see graph). Here HIV drug resistance was defined as resistance to nonnucleoside reverse transcriptase inhibitors (NNRTIs), core drugs in most low- and middle-income countries' first-line regimens for HIV. Among people with past exposure to ART (those restarting treatment or women with past perinatal exposure) the rate of NNRTI resistance is even higher: 21.6% (95% confidence interval [CI], 13.8 to 32.2).[1] A recent report from South Africa revealed that among children 18 months old or younger identified through early infant diagnoses, NNRTI resistance was found in 63.7% (95% CI, 59.0 to 68.4).[1]

How significant is the increase in resistance to HIV treatment? And what can be done to mitigate it?

The WHO has proposed a five-point global action plan for monitoring, combating, and preventing drug resistance using a set of interventions and resources. The plan includes roles for communities, donors, and countries in prevention, monitoring and surveillance, research, expansion of laboratory capacity, and management and governance efforts. It outlines important, though not always easily implemented, ways to support and improve current programs. These include expanding the essential rollout of viral load monitoring capacity to ensure that patients are switched early to effective ART so that much drug resistance can be prevented, and an important focus on improving engagement in care and adherence to ART. Since HIV treatment, at least for now, continues to be daily oral therapy for life, adherence remains the Achilles' heel of therapy, as it has been for PrEP. But program failures, especially drug stock-outs and long wait times at clinics and drug dispensaries, must also be addressed, since they can undermine the efforts of even the most adherent patients.

One step beyond implementation of the WHO's proposals would be the rapid rollout to all HIV-infected people who have not yet received ART of newer regimens with higher genetic barriers to resistance. The integrase inhibitor dolutegravir, for instance, has an exceptionally high resistance barrier.[3] In patients receiving first-line treatment with dolutegravir-based ART, there has been only a single reported case of resistance selection.[4] Even in patients with virologic failure and acquired resistance to nonnucleoside-based regimens, treatment with dolutegravir and one fully active nucleoside achieved virologic undetectability rates of 82% at 48 weeks, and in those who had no response there were no emergent resistance mutations to integrase or nucleosides.

These regimens will be 20 to 50% cheaper and have fewer side effects than the WHO-recommended ones, although there have been reports of increased insomnia and other neuropsychiatric side effects (but not at the level or severity seen with other drugs and classes, including the NNRTI efavirenz). Data are accumulating on the use of such regimens during pregnancy and in patients with tuberculosis–HIV coinfection. Integrase-inhibitor–based regimens including dolutegravir are being rolled out in Botswana and Brazil, and other countries, including Kenya, Uganda, and Nigeria, are starting to adopt them. Although vigilance will be required, use of dolutegravir as first-line therapy could markedly reduce the incidence of HIV drug resistance. It will also be important to know whether the new regimens will work in patients with pretreatment drug resistance, and the data to answer that question will need to be collected as soon as practicable from these early-adopter countries.

A potential challenge to the widespread use of dolutegravir is the likely use of injectable cabotegravir, a long-acting integrase inhibitor, for both treatment and PrEP and in cases in which there is concern about cross-resistance to integrase inhibitors. Even in the confines of a randomized, controlled treatment trial, resistance to cabotegravir has occurred and could affect the activity of dolutegravir. In PrEP studies using these formulations, some participants had detectable cabotegravir levels up to a year after their last injection. This finding has raised concern that having stopped injectable PrEP, people who contract HIV after the drug has dropped below protective levels could have integrase-inhibitor–resistant virus.

What about people with HIV who have acquired drug resistance and have not had a response to an NNRTI-based regimen? Fortunately, both integrase inhibitors and boosted protease inhibitors have been shown to be effective for this population and can lead to sustained viral suppression and improved clinical outcomes. But deployment of these regimens urgently needs to be scaled up, and countries and programs will have to balance the sometimes conflicting imperatives to expand access for untreated patients and to improve quality for those already in care whose treatment is failing.

Vulnerable populations will continue to require special attention in the era of HIV drug resistance. We have to move most quickly on the WHO's recommendations for infants and children, the population with the highest resistance rates; adolescents and young adults, for whom adherence has been challenging; and stigmatized and criminalized populations, which face formidable social and structural barriers to prevention, treatment, and care.

Drug resistance is one of the markers of failure of HIV programs. The threat it poses is both that treatment will fail clinically in individual patients and that communities will be at risk from viremic patients whose disease continues to be infectious. Our newest and most effective prevention tool, PrEP with daily oral tenofovir–emtricitabine, is also at risk from HIV drug resistance. More robust drugs with higher resistance barriers may help solve some of these problems. But we will still face the many challenges of logistics, adherence, and the funding required to sustain the massive global treatment effort launched with the 2003 creation of PEPFAR and the Global Fund. Even in 2017, half of all HIV-infected people remain untreated.

The proposed multibillion-dollar cuts to U.S. federal funding for global health, for PEPFAR, the CDC, the U.S. Agency for International Development (USAID), the State Department, and the Global Fund, would devastate this effort and undercut many of the gains we've made against the pandemic.[5] The emergence of HIV drug resistance warrants a redoubling of our efforts, not a retreat from our commitments. But if President Donald Trump's proposed 2018 budget is any indication, U.S. leadership in global health and HIV response efforts is facing unprecedented threats.

From the Department of Epidemiology, Johns Hopkins Bloomberg School of Public Health, Baltimore (C.B.); and the Department of Genitourinary Medicine and HIV, Chelsea and Westminster Hospital, London (A.P.).

1. World Health Organization. HIV drug resistance report 2017 (www.who.int/hiv/pub/drugresistance/hivdr-report-2017/en/).
2. Nkambule R, Nuwagaba-Biribonwoha H, Mnisi Z, et al. Substantial progress in confronting the HIV epidemic in Swaziland: first evidence of national impact. Presented at the 9th International Conference on IAS Science, Paris, July 24, 2017. abstract.
3. Anstett K, Brenner B, Mesplede T, Wainberg MA. HIV drug resistance against strand transfer integrase inhibitors. Retrovirology 2017; 14: 36.
4. Fulcher JA, Du Y, Sun R, Landovitz RJ. Emergence of integrase resistance mutations during initial therapy with TDF/FTC/ DTG. Presented at the Conference on Retroviruses and Opportunistic Infections, Seattle, February 13–16, 2017. abstract.
5. Kates J, Wexler A, Michaud J, Stover J. What could U.S. budget cuts mean for global health? Kaiser Family Foundation Issue Brief. July 2017 (http://files.kff.org/attachment/Issue-Brief-What-Could-US-Budget-Cuts-Mean-for-Global-Health).

16.5

Can AIDS Be Cured?

Jerome Groopman

ONE MORNING IN THE WINTER OF 1981, my wife came home after her on-call shift at the U.C.L.A. Medical Center and told me about a baffling new case. Queenie was an eighteen-year-old prostitute, his hair dyed the color of brass. He had arrived at the emergency room with a high fever and a cough, and appeared to have a routine kind of pneumonia, readily treated with antibiotics. But the medical team retrieved a microbe from his lungs called *Pneumocystis carinii*. The microbe was known for causing a rare fungal pneumonia that had been seen in severely malnourished children and in adults undergoing organ transplants or chemotherapy.

Several specialists at the hospital were enlisted to make sense of the infection. Queenie had a critically low platelet count, which made him susceptible to hemorrhage, and I was called in to examine him. He was lying on his side and breathing with difficulty. His sheets were soaked with sweat. A herpes infection had so severely blistered his flesh that surgeons had cut away necrotic segments of his thighs. I couldn't explain his falling platelet numbers. His lungs began to fail, and he was placed on a ventilator. Soon afterward, Queenie died, of respiratory failure.

His was one of several cases of the same rare pneumonia seen by physicians on both coasts. Michael Gottlieb, a U.C.L.A. immunologist, studied the blood of some of these patients and made the key observation that they had lost almost all their helper T cells, which protect against infections and cancers. In June, 1981, the Centers for Disease Control published Gottlieb's cases in its *Morbidity and Mortality Weekly Report*, and, in July, Dr. Alvin Friedman-Kien, of New York University, reported that twenty-six gay men in New York and California had received diagnoses of Kaposi sarcoma, a cancer of the lymphatic channels and blood vessels. This, too, was strange: Kaposi sarcoma typically affected elderly men of Eastern European Jewish and Mediterranean ancestry.

I tended to our Kaposi-sarcoma patients. I was the most junior person on staff and had no expertise in the tumor, but none of the senior faculty wanted the job. My first patient, a middle-aged fireman nicknamed Bud, lived a closeted life in West Los Angeles. Not long before he checked in to the hospital, he had started to find growths on his legs that looked like ripe cherries. Then they appeared on his torso, on his face, and in his mouth. Despite strong doses of chemotherapy, the standard treatment for advanced Kaposi sarcoma, his tumors grew, disfiguring him and killing him in less than a year. By 1982, men with highly aggressive kinds of lymphoma had started to arrive at the hospital. They, too, failed to improve with chemotherapy. Patients were dying from an array of diseases that had overcome ravaged immune systems. All my patients had one disorder in common, which the C.D.C., that year, had named acquired-immunodeficiency syndrome, or *aids*. Scientists did not yet know what caused it.

The next year, two research teams—one led by Luc Montagnier and Françoise Barré-Sinoussi, of the Pasteur Institute, in Paris, the other by Robert Gallo, at the National Cancer Institute, in Maryland—published papers in *Science* that described a new retrovirus in the lymph nodes and blood cells of *aids* patients. A retrovirus has a pernicious way of reproducing: it permanently inserts a DNA copy of its genome into the nucleus of a host cell, hijacking the cell's machinery for its own purposes. When the retrovirus mutates, which it often does, its spawn becomes difficult for the body or a vaccine to target and chase out. Retroviral diseases were widely believed to be incurable. In May of 1986, after much dispute about credit for the discovery (the French finally won the Nobel, in 2008), an international committee of scientists agreed on the name H.I.V., or human immunodeficiency virus. By the end of that year, about twenty-five thousand of the nearly twenty-nine thousand Americans with reported *aids* diagnoses had died.

Since then, H.I.V. has been transformed into a treatable condition, one of the great victories of modern medicine. In 1987, the F.D.A. approved AZT, a cancer drug that had never gone to market, for use in H.I.V. patients. At first, it was extortionately priced and was prescribed in high doses, which proved toxic, provoking protest from the gay community. But AZT was able to insinuate itself into the virus's DNA as it formed, and later it was used in lower doses. Scientists have now developed more than thirty antiretroviral medicines that stop H.I.V. from reproducing in helper T cells.

The idea of combining medications into a "cocktail" came in the mid-nineteen-nineties, mirroring the way oncologists treated cancer. Cancer cells, like H.I.V. particles, can mutate quickly enough to escape a single targeted drug. The treatment regimen—*haart*, for highly active antiretroviral therapy—was put through clinical trials by prominent researchers such as David Ho, of the Aaron Diamond Institute, in New York. I gave the cocktail to one of my patients, David Sanford, and less than a month after beginning treatment his fever fell, his infections disappeared, his energy returned, and he started to gain weight. The H.I.V. in his bloodstream plummeted to an undetectable level, where it has remained. Later, in a Pulitzer Prize-winning article, Sanford wrote, "I am probably more likely to be hit by a truck than to die of *aids*." That now holds true for a great majority of people with H.I.V. in the United States. In the past five years, not one of the dozens of H.I.V. patients I've cared for has died of the disease.

There are still tremendous hurdles. Thirty-five million people in the world are living with the virus. In sub-Saharan Africa, where most new cases are reported, sixty-three percent of those eligible for the drug regimen do not receive it; those who do often fail to receive it in full. In the United States, a year's worth of *haart* costs many thousands of dollars per patient, and the long-term side effects can be debilitating.

Now researchers are talking more and more about a cure. We know as much about H.I.V. as we do about certain cancers: its genes have been sequenced, its method of infiltrating host cells deciphered, its proteins mapped in three dimensions. A critical discovery was made in 1997: the virus can lie dormant in long-lived cells, untouched by the current drugs. If we can safely and affordably eliminate the viral reservoir, we will finally have defeated H.I.V.

1997: discovered virus can lie dormant in cells
reservoir unaffected by drugs
-need to elim reservoir to cure HIV

Ward 86, the nation's first outpatient *aids* clinic, opened at San Francisco General Hospital on January 1, 1983. Recently, I went there to see Steven Deeks, an expert on the chronic immune activation and inflammation brought on by H.I.V. Deeks, a professor at the School of Medicine at U.C.S.F., also runs the *scope* Study: a cohort of two thousand H.I.V.-positive men and women in whom he measures the long-term effects of living with the virus. Each year, blood samples are sent to labs all over the world. Deeks's mission is to catalogue the damage that H.I.V. does to tissues and to test new drugs that might help.

The ward occupies the sixth floor of an Art Deco building on the north side of campus. I found Deeks in his office, wearing a flannel shirt and New Balance sneakers. He explained his concerns about the drug cocktail. "Antiretroviral drugs are designed to block H.I.V. replication, and they do that quite well," he said. But they don't enable many patients to recover fully. The immune system improves enough to prevent *aids*, but, because the virus persists, the immune system must mount a continuous low-level response. That creates chronic inflammation, which injures tissues.

The inflammation is exacerbated by side effects of the medicines. Early treatments caused anemia, nerve damage, and lipodystrophy—the wasting of the limbs and face, and the deposits of fat around the belly. Lipodystrophy is still a major problem. Deeks has observed many patients in the *scope* cohort with high levels of cholesterol and triglyceride, and these can lead to organ damage. One serious consequence is heart disease, which appears to be caused by inflammation of the artery walls. Deeks has also seen lung, liver, and skin cancers in his patients. In a disturbing echo of the early days of the epidemic, he has noticed that middle-aged patients develop diseases associated with aging: kidney and bone disease and possibly neurocognitive defects. A better definition for *aids,* according to Deeks, might be "acquired-inflammatory-disease syndrome."

He introduced me to one of his patients, whom I'll call Gordon. A tall, genial man with rimless glasses stood up to shake my hand, and I saw that he had the signature protruding belly. He has been H.I.V.-positive for almost forty years, and he said he felt lucky to be alive: "A ten-year partner of mine who had the same strain of H.I.V., who ate the same food, had the same doctors, took the same early H.I.V. meds, died in June, 1990, almost twenty-five years ago."

He told me, "I'm no longer that concerned about the virus itself. I'm more concerned about my internal organs and premature aging." In 1999, at fifty, he learned that fatty deposits had substantially constricted the blood flow in a major artery that supplies the heart's left ventricle. He began to experience crippling pain when he walked, because the blood supply to his bone tissue had diminished—a condition called avascular necrosis. In 2002, he had his first hip replacement, and the second in 2010. His muscles have shrunk, and sitting can be uncomfortable, so he sometimes wears special foam-padded underwear. Every other year, he has his face injected with poly-L-lactic acid, which replaces lost connective tissue.

Gordon's longevity, and the dozens of drugs he has taken to stay alive, exemplifies the experience of millions of infected *aids* patients. His state-of-the-art treatment costs almost a hundred thousand dollars a year. Although it's covered by his insurance and by the State of California, he calls it "a ransom: your money or your life." For Deeks, the question is "Can the world find the resources to build a system to deliver, on a daily basis, antiretroviral drugs to some thirty-five million people, many in very poor regions?" He is doubtful, which is why he is focussed on helping to find a cure. "Our philosophy is that in order to cure H.I.V., we need to know where and why it persists," he said.

In 1997, amid euphoria about *haart*, people first started thinking seriously about a cure. Sooner or later, all infected cells die on their own. Could the right drugs in the right combination rout the virus for good? That year, David Ho published a paper in *Nature* in which he mathematically predicted that an H.I.V. patient on the *haart* regimen should be able to conquer the detectable virus in twenty-eight to thirty-seven months. That issue also contained a very different report from Robert Siliciano, currently a Howard Hughes investigator at the Johns Hopkins School of Medicine. Using an uncommonly sensitive measurement technique that he'd invented, Siliciano located H.I.V. in a type of helper T cell that provides memory to our immune system and normally survives for decades. Memory T cells are uniquely important: they recognize the antigens in infections and orchestrate speedy responses. But the virus proved to be even cleverer. It lay dormant in strands of host DNA, untouched by the drug cocktail, later springing back to life and degrading the immune system.

At sixty-two, lanky and circumspect, Siliciano is highly regarded in the tight-knit community of H.I.V. researchers. He met his wife and collaborator, Janet, in the nineteen-seventies, when she was a graduate student at Johns Hopkins, studying the proteins that T cells release when they encounter microbes. Now fifty-nine years old, with curly red hair and a hint of a New Jersey accent, Janet joined Bob's lab after his paper appeared in *Nature*. She said that the idea was his, but Bob told me that Janet developed it over the next seven years, tracking the levels of dormant virus in patients consistently treated with *haart*. Her data confirmed his thesis: the virus could survive almost indefinitely. "We calculated that it would take seventy years of continuous *haart* for all the memory T cells to die," she said.

Siliciano told me about the first time he saw the latent virus emerge in the memory T cells of an H.I.V. patient on *haart*. The patient was thought to be cured. "He had been biopsied in every imaginable place, and nobody could find any virus," Siliciano said. Researchers took twenty tubes of the patient's blood, isolated the T cells, and divided them into multiple wells. The specimen was then intermixed with cells from uninfected people. If the healthy T cells became infected, the virus would reproduce and be released. Detection of the virus would be signalled by a color change to blue. Siliciano remembers sitting at his desk, talking with a visitor, when a graduate student burst in: "The wells are turning blue!" He said, "It was a very strange moment, because it was a confirmation of this hypothesis—so it was exciting—but it was also a disaster. Everybody came to the same conclusion: that these cells persisted despite the antiretroviral therapy."

The Siliciano laboratory occupies the eighth floor of the Miller Research Building, at the Johns Hopkins School of Medicine. The twenty-six-person research team—technicians, students, fellows, and faculty—works in an airy, open space and in a smaller Biosafety Level 3 facility on the north side of the building. There they handle the specimens of their clinic's H.I.V.-positive subjects and many more from labs like Deeks's worldwide. Inside a room with negative air pressure, researchers retrieve blood samples from an incubator and place them in a laminar flow hood, which draws up a stream of air. Nothing leaves the facility without being double-bagged and sterilized.

Much of the new *aids* research builds on the Silicianos' foundational discovery of H.I.V.'s hidden reservoirs. So does their own work. Using potent chemicals, they have been able to draw H.I.V. out of its hiding places in memory T cells, assess the reach of the virus within the body, and begin to map where else it might be lodged.

Several years ago, they began looking at "blips," the small, sudden jumps in viral load that sometimes occur in the blood of *haart* patients. Physicians had been concerned that blips might be particles of virus that had become resistant to *haart* and struck out on their own. The Silicianos believed otherwise: that the viral particles were released by latently infected cells that had become activated. They analyzed the blood of patients with blips every two to three days over three to four months, and their hypothesis proved correct: the virus had not become resistant to the drugs, but had been dormant in its reservoir within memory T cells. It could be intermittently released from the reservoir, even when the patient took antiretroviral drugs.

Although researchers were chastened by the realization that the drug regimen was not itself a cure, they recently found three unusual cases that were encouraging enough to make them keep trying. The first was that of Timothy Ray Brown.

Brown is known as the Berlin patient, after the city where he became the only person ever to have been cured of H.I.V. In 2006, more than a decade after he discovered he was H.I.V.-positive, he was given an unrelated diagnosis of acute myelogenous leukemia, a cancer of the bone marrow. After initial treatment, the leukemia returned. Brown needed a bone-marrow transplant. His hematologist, Gero Huetter, made the imaginative suggestion that they use a donor with a genetic mutation that shuts down the protein CCR5, a doorway for H.I.V. into helper T cells. On February 7, 2007, Brown received the transplant. One year later, he underwent the procedure again, and by 2009 biopsies of Brown's brain, lymph nodes, and bowel showed that the virus had not returned, and his T-cell count was back to normal.

Brown's cure was spectacular, but difficult to repeat. His doctor had twice destroyed all his native blood cells, with radiation and chemotherapy, and twice rebuilt his immune system with transplanted stem cells. It had been very dangerous and costly. Researchers wondered if they could create a scaled-down version. In 2013, physicians at Brigham and Women's Hospital, in Boston, reported on the outcome of a study in which two H.I.V.-positive men on *haart* had received bone-marrow transplants for lymphoma. Their marrow donors, unlike Brown's, did not have the CCR5 mutation, and their chemotherapy regimen was less intensive. *Haart* was stopped a few years after the transplants, and the virus remained undetectable for months, but then resurfaced.

This past July, results came in on the third case. In 2010, a girl known as the Mississippi baby was born to an H.I.V.-positive mother who had taken no antiretrovirals, and the baby had the virus in her blood. Thirty hours after delivery, the newborn started on antiretroviral therapy. Within weeks, the viral count fell below the limit of detection. The baby was eighteen months old when the treatment was interrupted, against medical advice. For two years, the girl's blood showed no trace of the virus, and researchers speculated that very early *haart* might prevent the virus from forming a dormant reservoir. Twenty-seven months after going off the drugs, however, the child tested positive for the virus. Though researchers were impressed that early intervention had temporarily banished H.I.V., she was not cured.

In August, Janet and Robert Siliciano wrote about the Brigham men and the Mississippi baby in *Science*, saying that the cases confirmed that researchers were on the right path in attacking latent infection. The Berlin patient was an even more compelling example. Karl Salzwedel, the chief of Pathogenesis and Basic Research in the Division of *aids* at the National Institute of Allergy and Infectious Diseases, told me that until Timothy Brown "it wasn't really clear how we would go about getting rid of the last bits of virus that remain in the reservoir." Brown's case provided "a proof of concept: it may be possible to eradicate latent H.I.V. from the body. It may be from a very risky and toxic method, but it's proof of concept nonetheless."

The new centerpiece of the American effort to cure H.I.V. is the Martin Delaney Collaboratories, funded by the N.I.H. Launched in 2011, the collaborative was formulated as a way to link clinical labs, research facilities, and pharmaceutical companies. Federal support was set at seventy million dollars for the first five years, on the premise of coöperation and open communication among all parties. Salzwedel told me that the N.I.H. funded three applications. "Each was taking a different complementary approach to trying to develop a strategy to eradicate H.I.V," he said: enhancing the patient's immune system, manipulating the CCR5 gene, and destroying the reservoirs themselves. They represented different responses to the Siliciano thesis and to the lessons of Timothy Brown.

Mike McCune, the head of the Division of Experimental Medicine at U.C.S.F., researches ways in which H.I.V. can be eradicated by the body's own immune system. He was prompted by an observation made in the early days of the epidemic: that babies born to mothers with H.I.V. become infected in utero only five to ten percent of the time, even though they are exposed to the virus throughout gestation. Recently, McCune and his colleagues observed that the developing fetal immune system does not react against maternal cells, which can easily cross the placenta and end up in fetal tissues. Instead, the fetus generates specialized T cells that suppress inflammatory responses against the mother, and that might also prevent inflammatory responses against H.I.V., thereby blocking the rapid spread of the virus in utero and sparing the child.

McCune has worked for many years with Steven Deeks and the *scope* Study. When I spoke with McCune in San Francisco, he said, "There is a yin and yang of the immune system. We are trying to recapitulate the orchestrated balance found in the fetus." McCune is now working on interventions that would prevent inflammation against H.I.V. in the adult, hoping to partly mimic the balance found in utero. He's also developing methods that would allow the immune system to better recognize, and destroy, the virus when it manifests itself. These studies are being carried out on nonhuman primates, and may lead to human trials within a year or two.

In Seattle, a group headed by Hans-Peter Kiem and Keith Jerome is taking a more futuristic approach. Using an enzyme called Zinc Finger Nuclease, they are genetically altering blood and marrow stem cells so as to disable CCR5, the doorway for infection in T cells. Researchers will modify the stem cells outside the body, so that when the cells are returned some portion of the T cells in the bloodstream will be resistant to H.I.V. infection. Over time, they hope, those cells will propagate, and the patient will slowly build an immune system that is resistant to the virus. Those patients might still have a small reservoir of H.I.V., but their bodies would be able to regulate the infection.

The largest Collaboratory, with more than twenty members, is led by David Margolis, at the University of North Carolina. Margolis, an infectious-disease expert, is targeting the reservoirs directly. The idea, which has come to be known as "shock and kill," is to reactivate the dormant virus, unmasking the cells that carry it, so that they can be destroyed. In 2012, he published the results of a clinical trial of the drug Vorinostat, which was originally developed for blood cancers of T cells, as a shock treatment. This October, "shock and kill" was widely discussed when the Collaboratory teams convened at the N.I.H., along with hundreds of other researchers, assorted academics, and interested laypeople. Margolis and his group explored in their talk new ways to shock the virus out of dormancy.

The killing stage is more challenging, because the shocked cells carry few H.I.V. antigens, the toxic flags released by pathogenic particles and recognized by the immune system prior to attack. One approach to the killing strategy comes from an unusual type of H.I.V.-positive patient who may carry the virus for decades yet seems not to be disturbed by it. Some of these so-called "élite controllers" possess cytotoxic, or killer, T cells that attack virus-producing cells. The objective is to make every H.I.V. patient into an élite controller through "therapeutic vaccination," enabling patients to generate killer T cells on their own.

Researchers are also trying to switch off a molecule called PD-1, which the body uses to restrain the immune system. Deactivating PD-1 has worked in clinical studies with melanoma and lung-cancer patients, and one patient seems to have been cured of hepatitis C by a single infusion of a PD-1 blocker from Bristol-Myers Squibb.

Groups outside the Collaboratories who are testing ways to cure *aids* share their results with the N.I.H. teams. In parallel with the Seattle group, Carl June, the director of translational research at the Abramson Cancer Center, at the University of Pennsylvania, and his colleagues have used genetic engineering to close off the CCR5 passageway. In the *New England Journal of Medicine* this past March, they reported on their recent clinical trial, which showed that the modified T cells could survive in people with H.I.V. for years. Similar work on knocking down CCR5 is being done by Calimmune, a California-based company devoted to curing *aids*. (One of its founders is David Baltimore, who received the Nobel Prize for the discovery of reverse transcriptase, a crucial enzyme in retroviral reproduction.) Groups in Denmark and Spain have made progress, too, and in 2012 researchers in France analyzed the Visconti study, which had put the early intervention received by the Mississippi baby to a formal test. A subset of fourteen H.I.V. patients had been treated within weeks of their infection, and then *haart* was interrupted. They remained free of the virus for several years.

The fight against *aids* is following a trajectory similar to that of the fight against many cancers. When I was growing up, in the nineteen-fifties, childhood leukemia was nearly always fatal. Eventually, drugs were developed that drove the cancer into remission for months or years, but it always came back. In the nineteen-seventies, researchers discovered that leukemic cells lay sleeping in the central nervous system, and developed targeted treatments that could eliminate them. Today, childhood leukemia is cured in nine out of ten cases.

This July, at the Twentieth International *aids* Conference, in Melbourne, Australia, Sharon Lewin, an infectious-disease expert at Monash University, said, "We probably are looking, at the moment, at trying to achieve long-term remission." Most experts agree that remission is feasible, and that, to some degree, we will be able to wean patients off lifelong therapies.

Even the most cautious *aids* researchers place remission along a continuum, with a cure at the end. Robert Siliciano told me, "The first goal is to reduce the reservoir. And this is not just for the individual but also has a public health consequence." For however long a person is off *haart*, doctors would be able to divert resources to patients who still needed treatment.

David Margolis believes that his "shock and kill" strategy will work, but that it could take ten to twenty years. The Silicianos agree that more research is needed. "Shock and kill," they said, will require more than a single drug like Vorinostat. And the optimal regimen can't be identified until it's clear precisely how much latent virus the body contains. The Silicianos have not yet developed a truly accurate measure. Only by following people who have been off all drugs for years would it be clear that a cure had been found. "The more we learn, the more questions there are to answer," Janet told me.

Still, the questions that have been answered astonish *aids* scientists. At U.C.L.A. during the brutal first years, I never would have imagined that future patients would live into their eighties. A fatal disease has been tamed into a chronic condition. The next step is to find a cure. Scientists are innately cautious, and *aids* researchers have learned humility over the years. Science operates around a core of uncertainty, within which lie setbacks, but also hope.

16.6

Barriers to HIV Cure

J. Stein[1], M. Storcksdieck genannt Bonsmann[80] and H. Streeck[80, 2]

Abstract

Since the beginning of the epidemic, more than 70 million people have been infected with human immunodeficiency virus (HIV) and about 38 million have died from acquired immune deficiency syndrome (AIDS)-related illnesses. While the discovery of highly active antiretroviral therapy (HAART) in the mid 90's has saved millions of lives, a complete eradication of HIV is still not possible as HIV can persist for decades in a small reservoir of latently infected cells. Once reactivated, these latently infected cells can actively produce viral particles. Recent studies suggest that several sanctuaries exist within infected individuals where HIV can remain undetected by the immune system. These cellular, anatomical and microanatomical viral reservoirs represent a major obstacle for the eradication of HIV. Here we review recent findings on potential sanctuaries of HIV and address potential avenues to overcome these immunological barriers.

Introduction

The discovery of highly active antiretroviral therapy (HAART) saved millions of lives in the wake of one of the biggest epidemics of the last century. The life expectancy of an human immunodeficiency virus (HIV)-infected individual, who can afford medication, increased from on average 6 years to that of an HIV-uninfected individual[1–3]. However, in spite of these groundbreaking advances in the treatment of HIV-infected individuals, HIV remains a chronic illness and neither a cure nor eradication of HIV is yet possible. Indeed, once HIV establishes infection, the virus persists indefinitely as an integrated part of the genome in a small population of latently infected cells. While the cellular population containing HIV DNA is small, it nevertheless remains relatively stable over time and interruption of antiretroviral treatment leads to in almost all cases a significant rebound of HIV viremia[4].

1 Institute for HIV Research, University Hospital Essen, University Duisburg-Essen, Essen, Germany

2 US Military HIV Research Program, Henry M. Jackson Foundation, Rockville, M.D., USA

J. Stein, M. Storcksdieck genannt Bonsmann and H. Streeck, "Barriers to HIV Cure," *HLA*, vol. 88, no. 4, pp. 155–163.

Interestingly, while antiretroviral treatment administered within hours after HIV exposure can completely avert HIV infection [post-exposure prophylaxis (PEP)][5], daunting data from animal models indicate that within days after infection the viral reservoir is already irrevocably established[6]. However, it is unknown at which point HIV turns from a 'curable' to a chronic 'uncurable' infection. In this review, we will describe potential barriers to HIV cure and determine factors that contribute to HIV's 'point of no return' in chronic persistence.

Seeding of the Reservoir

Most HIV infections occur during sexual intercourse[7] where HIV passes through the initial mucosal barrier either through micro lesions or by transcytosis of endothelial cells [7–9]. 'Hotspots' for HIV transmission have been shown to lie within the inner foreskin and the glans epithelium in men and at the cervix for women [10, 11]. Furthermore, traumatic abrasions may account for HIV transmission, in particular during anal intercourse[12]. Strikingly, 97% of all new infections occur from a single CCR5-tropic (R5-tropic) founder virus[13] while only in rare instances a CXCR4-tropic (X4-tropic) virus has been reported[14].

The first HIV-infected $CD4^+$ T cells establish a local founder population, which disseminates to other compartments within 1–3 days after initial infection. During this acute phase of HIV infection, viral loads rise exponentially to exceedingly high levels. As a consequence of massive viral replication, the majority of mucosal memory T helper cells, and up to 48% of all $CCR5^+$ memory $CD4^+$ T cells, are irreparably depleted [15–18].

It is likely that the latent reservoir is established during these early days of infection by seeding into long-lived $CD4^+$ T cells that enter a resting state (G0) or that inhibit HIV-1 gene expression by transcriptional interferences[19]. While there are reports of successful PEP in humans of up to 3 days after exposure, it has also been noted that the success rate of PEP rapidly declines within the first hours after HIV exposure[20]. The mechanism by which PEP prevents establishment of persistent HIV infection is not clear, but it is likely that HAART may prevent further dissemination of HIV into other cells.

Even though the window of opportunity to prevent HIV infection closes within a short period of time after infection, immediate HAART initiation may still have a beneficial effect as early exposure to therapy may limit the size of the latent viral reservoir and preserve critical immune functions[21]. Indeed, it has been demonstrated that the frequency of latently infected cells is dependent on the time of treatment initiation during the first days of infection[22] and that the reservoir is overall significantly lower in those individuals that were treated during acute HIV infection compared to chronic HIV infection[23]. Additionally, early HAART initiation may also be critical to boost antiviral HIV-specific $CD8^+$ T cell responses through the preservation of $CD4^+$ T helper signals[24]. Moreover, it has been reported that an estimated 5%–15% of the individuals treated during acute HIV infection are spontaneously able to control viral replication after treatment cessation [so called: post-treatment controller (PTC)] [25–28]. Interestingly, the ability to become a PTC has not been linked to host genetics[29] suggesting that early HAART may bolster the preservation of immune functions. Taken together, recent findings suggest that early HAART initiation can significantly limit the viral reservoir thereby potentially lowering the bar for future eradication attempts.

Cellular Compartmentalization

The time to eradicate HIV using current HAART regimens has been estimated to take between 60 and 80 years suggesting that HAART alone may not suffice to cure HIV[30,31]. To understand the nature of HIV persistence and to tailor future eradication strategies, it will be important to understand the anatomical, microanatomical and cellular location of HIV and to define the barriers preventing a cure from HIV infection. By analyzing the decay pattern of viremia after HAART initiation, some clues on cellular compartmentalization can be deducted:

After treatment initiation, the plasma viral load has an initial drop of several orders of magnitude, which suggests a depletion of short-lived, productively infected cells[32]. This is followed by a decrease in the rate of viral decay pointing to a long-lived cellular reservoir with low-level viremia. Since most antiretroviral medications act by preventing *de novo* infections, it is likely that the viral load decay after HAART initiation is mainly driven by the loss of viral producers[33,34]. $CD4^+$ T cells, the preferred target for HIV, possess varying degrees of half-lives, which can contribute to a stepwise decay characteristic. Naïve $CD4^+$ T cells, with an average lifespan of 1–8 years, represent a long-lived cellular reservoir whereas memory $CD4^+$ T cells, which possess on average a half-life of 1–12 months, may represent a more short-lived reservoir[35,36]. Interestingly, the majority of proviral HIV DNA can be found in $CD4^+$ memory T cells followed by naïve or effector $CD4^+$ T cell populations in individuals on HAART (Figure 16.6.1)[37]. Within the memory $CD4^+$ T cell compartment, central memory cells (Tcm, 51.7%), followed by transitional memory (Ttm, 34.3%) and effector memory $CD4^+$ T cells (Tem, 13.9%) have the largest viral burden[35]. Hence, it has been suggested that Tcm are a stable and long-lasting reservoir of HIV, due to their extremely low proliferation rate and relatively long half-life. In contrast, the major reservoir in treated individuals with a low viral burden and low $CD4^+$ T cell counts, has been detected in Ttm[35].

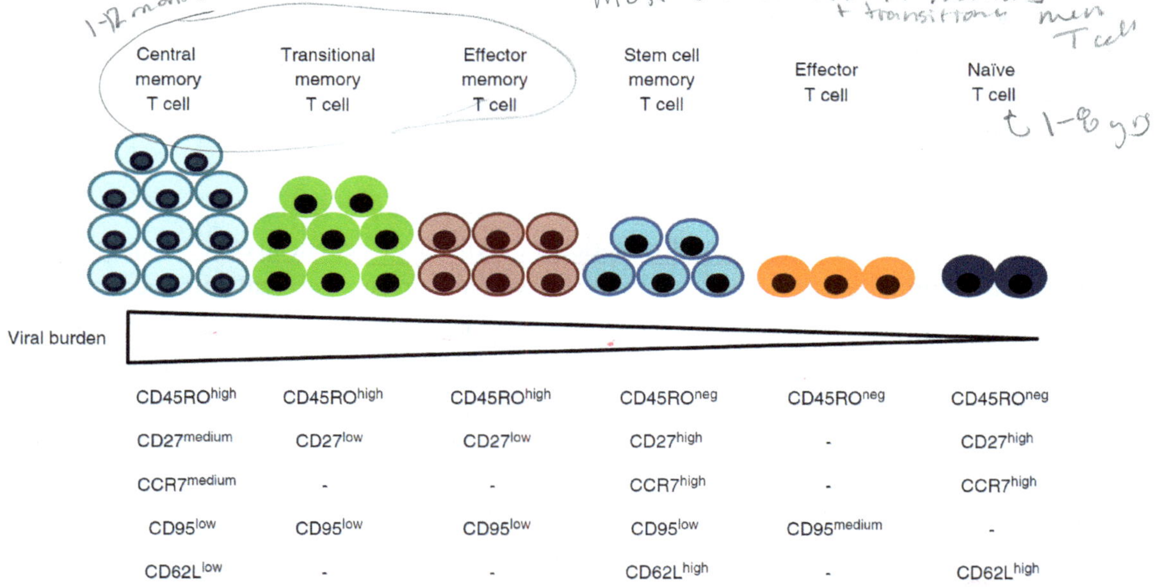

FIGURE 16.6.1 Latent viral reservoir in $CD4^+$ T cell subtypes—viral burden and surface phenotype. During highly active antiretroviral therapy (HAART), the viral reservoir differs between different $CD4^+$ T cell subtypes, as characterized by the indicated surface markers. The size of the viral reservoir ranges from central memory T cells being the largest to naïve T cells harboring the least amount of virus.

Recently, stem cell like memory T cells (Tscm) have also been suggested to be an important viral reservoir[38]. Tscm are a less differentiated memory T cell population, defined by the expression of CD45RA, CCR7, CD27 and CD62L, with the capacity to differentiate into central memory, effector memory or terminally differentiated T cells, and are capable of homeostatic self-renewal. The potential of proliferation and self-renewal makes Tscm comparably resistant to cell death and thus provides a very stable and long-lived cellular compartment[38].

HIV can potentially also infect macrophages. However, viral replicative capacity in macrophages is rather low in the absence of the HIV-2/SIV accessory protein Vpx[39]. It has been demonstrated that Vpx can block the host restriction factor SAMHD1, which in HIV-1 prevents the reverse transcription of viral genomes through depletion of intracellular dNTPs [40, 41]. In the presence of Vpx, macrophages can be a major viral reservoir. It has been shown in rhesus macaques that after $CD4^+$ T cell depletion, but prior to SIV infection, SIV replicated at exceedingly high levels and most viral RNA was detected in macrophages [42, 43]. Despite the lack of Vpx expression by HIV in humans, some studies have demonstrated HIV replication in human monocyte-derived macrophages after *in vitro* infection as well as in human tonsil biopsies or vaginal mucosa explants [44–50]. Moreover, some monocytes and macrophages can also enter immune privileged body compartments such as the central nervous system (CNS) and infect local macrophages such as microglia and perivascular macrophages[51]. However, the role of macrophages as a relevant viral reservoir is still under debate as most HIV DNA in myeloid cells of tissues showed traces of rearranged T-cell receptor sequences suggesting that the myeloid cells acquired viral DNA through phagocytosis of infected T cells[52]. Taken together, the main cellular compartments harboring HIV are $CD4^+$ T cells, especially central and transitional memory T cells.

Anatomical and Microanatomical Compartmentalization

Several regions of the human body are restricted in terms of permeability, cellular access and penetrability of immune cells to ensure their proper function and protect them from immune-mediated damage. However, as HIV can establish infection in these compartments, restricted access represents a major hurdle for eradication attempts (Figure 16.6.2).

Probably one of the most extensively studied compartments of HIV persistence is the central nervous system (CNS). The CNS is separated from the peripheral blood through the blood–brain-barrier, a layer of microvascular endothelial cells and a capillary basement membrane with embedded pericytes and astrocytes[53] that tightly regulate the influx of blood-borne molecules into the brain.

Surprisingly, HIV is already detectable in the CNS during the acute phase of infection [54, 55] and it has been suggested that HIV crosses the blood–brain-barrier by way of infected monocytes or macrophages[51]. Once passed the blood–brain-barrier, neurons, brain microvascular endothelial cells, oligodendrocytes, astrocytes, microglia and perivascular macrophages have been shown to be susceptible to HIV infection, but only microglia and perivascular macrophages are actively able to produce viral particles [56–58]. The life span of a microglia cell is comparably long and thus HIV may be able to persist in these cells for several years[59, 60].

A contributing factor to HIV's persistence in the CNS is that not all antiretrovirals (ARVs) have the equal capability to cross the blood–brain-barrier[61] as its permeability to ARVs is dependent on

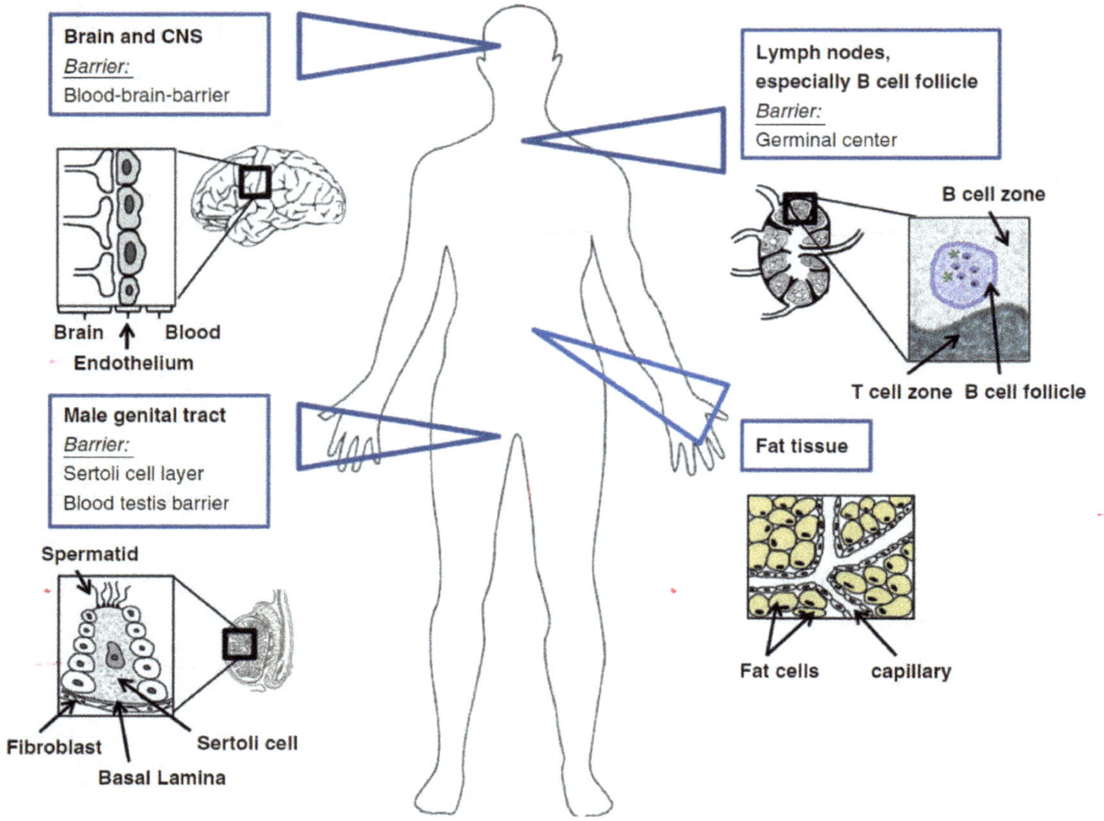

FIGURE 16.6.2 Anatomical compartmentalization of human immunodeficiency virus (HIV) persistence and barriers to cure. HIV is able to enter immune privileged sites of the human body such as the brain, the central nervous system (CNS), the male genital tract (MGT), lymph nodes or fat tissue, and persists in latently infected cells. Several of these sites of infection are protected by natural barriers including the blood–brain-barrier in the brain, the sertoli cell layer in the MGT or the B cell follicles within the lymph nodes.

molecular weight, protein binding and lipophilicity[62]. In addition, several efflux pumps also actively reduce the concentrations of ARVs within the CNS[62]. While only a fraction of ARVs have been tested for CNS penetration capacity[63], it is known that nucleoside reverse transcriptase inhibitors (NRTI) generally pass the blood–brain-barrier well, but protease inhibitors rather poorly.

Similar to the CNS, the male genital tract (MGT) separates the peripheral blood from the spermatocytes to protect their development. However, while viral HIV RNA and DNA have been found in the semen of the infected individuals[64], viral loads in plasma and semen do not appear to correlate suggesting different sources of viral replication in the MGT[65]. In addition, testes are also a pharmacological sanctuary that protects germ cell development against toxic or harmful agents thus causing HAART to be, at least in part, actively removed by drug efflux pumps, such as the ABC transporter P-glycoproteins, resulting in lowered antiretroviral concentrations in the testes compared to blood [66–69].

The MGT compartment is not an immunological sanctuary and HIV- or SIV-specific $CD8^+$ T cells have been detected in the testis interstitial tissue, in the stroma of the epididymis, seminal vesicles, prostate and urethra and within the epithelium of the epididymis, seminal vesicles and penile urethra [66,70,71]. However, it has been demonstrated that SIV-specific CD8+ T cells show dampened immune responses suggesting a local milieu of immunosuppression[72].

In addition, fat tissue has been suggested as a site of HIV persistence. Hazan et al. demonstrated that adipose tissue can express HIV's entry receptors CD4, CCR5 and CXCR4[73] and that HIV can be cultured from pre-adipocytes *in vitro*[74]. Moreover, it has been reported that fat-resident CD4+ T cells can contain latently integrated HIV[50]. A mode of HIV persistence in these cells may be an impairment of cytotoxic CD8+ T cells to reach HIV-infected CD4+ T cells, which may be due to secreted adipose tissue hormones like adiponectin. This hormone is known to act as anti-inflammatory by stimulating the secretion of IL-10 and reducing T-cell proliferation[75].

Probably one of the most critical microanatomical compartments of HIV is the B cell follicle within the lymph node. Already in 1997, it has been described that CD4+ T cells in germinal centers are productively infected during early infection and maintain high levels of HIV DNA even after HAART initiation[76]. These T follicular helper cells (Tfh) within the B cell follicles of lymphoid tissue are critical for the generation of humoral immune responses by driving the development of long-lived high-affinity matured antibodies. During chronic SIV infection of macaques and HIV infection of humans, Tfh cells are substantially expanded [77–79] and it has been demonstrated that Tfh cells contain comparably high levels of HIV DNA [80–82].

The presence of HIV-infected Tfh cells within B cell follicles has important implications with regard to the control and possible eradication attempts of the viral reservoir as the B cell follicle is relatively void of CD8+ T cells and thus unable to recognize and kill virally infected cells. It has been shown that only a small subset of CD8+ T cells is able to enter the B cell follicles[83]. However, these CD8+ T cells lack a classical 'killer' phenotype, most likely to avoid interference with the induction of the humoral immune responses in this antigen-rich environment[83]. Indeed, in HIV-infected individuals, SIV-infected rhesus macaques on HAART, or patients spontaneously able to control viral replication (elite controllers), HIV or SIV was exclusively found in the B cell follicle[84] suggesting that CD8+ T cells can recognize and kill virally infected cells in the T-cell zone and extrafollicular tissues, but are not able to clear infection from B cell follicles.

Taken together, HIV establishes latent reservoirs in several compartments of the human body that are separated and protected from immune recognition and antiretroviral treatment through physical or cellular barriers. Additionally, certain CD4+ T cell subsets may provide a sanctuary for HIV to avoid immune recognition and contribute to the establishment of latency.

Current Eradication Strategies to Overcome the Latent Reservoirs

It was a sobering moment when HIV researchers realized that HAART treatment alone does not suffice to eradicate HIV infection[85] and that the latent HIV reservoir was only marginally impacted by long-term HAART. During this time, a case report of a patient receiving HAART and hydroxyurea (HU) undergoing structured treatment interruption (STI) during acute HIV infection resulted in viremia levels becoming undetectable thus giving hope, that a cure may be possible[26]. Two hypotheses were deducted from this case: (1) STI may allow adequate exposure of the virus to the immune system during acute HIV infection which may result in better immune responses; (2) HU treatment may be beneficial as it inhibits viral DNA synthesis by acting synergistically with nucleoside reverse transcriptase inhibitors (NRTI) to increase antiviral activity [86,87]. Though 15 years later it was shown that the patient likely was able to control HIV replication due to a favorable genotype associated with spontaneous viral control (HLA-B57)[88], the single case report had a long-lasting scientific impact. The positive effect of STI strategies were most recently studied in the VISCONTI cohort. This cohort was assembled from about 2000 individuals treated during acute HIV infection. Of these, 14 individuals were identified that controlled viral replication after HAART interruption. Interestingly, none of the PTCs had any of the previously described protective HLA alleles or showed differences in their HIV-specific $CD8^+$ T cell responses[29]. One apparent prerequisite for the post-treatment control is the initiation of HAART during the early phase of HIV infection. However, only about 5 to 15% of the HIV positive individuals treated during acute HIV infection are able to control viremia after HAART interruption but the reason why some individuals have this ability is still unknown[29].

Although initially HAART treatment in combination with HU seemed to be successful in the case of the described patient, it disappointed in further prospective studies. Moreover, while HU supported HAART at low- and well-tolerated doses[89], a few studies have shown severe or even deadly side effects [90–92].

Similar results were obtained with other immunosuppressive agents such as Cyclosporin A (CsA), which inhibits activation of T cells and by this may prove effective in preventing viral replication, but CsA failed in clinical studies to improve HIV control [93–95].

However, a cure (or 'functional cure') can be potentially possible as shown by the case of the 'Berlin patient'. After diagnosis with B cell lymphoma, he underwent several rounds of chemotherapy as well as bone marrow transplantations[96]. The donor stem cells he received were homozygous for a 32 amino acid deletion in the CCR5 co-receptor (CCR5Δ32), which is protective against R5-tropic viruses[97]. Indeed, after transplantation followed by treatment interruption, no viral rebound was observed and HIV remained undetectable. Until today, several groups attempted to cure other patients using similar strategies, but all treated individuals either remained HIV positive or died of the underlying illness, that justified these treatment strategies. One of the most notable cases was an HIV-infected individual from Essen suffering from a T-cell lymphoma. Like the Berlin patient, he received chemotherapy and stem cell transplantation from a CCR5Δ32 homozygous donor. However, HAART treatment was interrupted prior to stem cell transplantation. In contrast to the Berlin patient, HIV rebounded shortly after stem cell transplantation. Analysis of the HIV variant showed an expansion of an X4-tropic virus[98].

To imitate the potential beneficial effect of CCR5Δ32 mutations, a CCR5 targeted zinc finger nuclease (ZFN) was developed and tested as a therapeutic approach. This DNA-binding protein enables double-strand breaks at specific locations, in this case the CCR5 gene. This gene editing leads to a permanent disruption of the CCR5 gene and subsequently to a nearly inexistent expression of CCR5 on the cell surface, thus protecting the cell from being infected. In a small clinical trial, HAART-treated individuals were adoptively transferred with autologous $CD4^+$ T cells, in which the CCR5 gene locus was modified by this enzyme. After HAART interruption, the treatment with CCR5 ZFN resulted in slower decay rates of the modified T-cells compared to unmodified T-cells. In a similar study with 12 participants, after ZFN treatment and HAART cessation, three individuals controlled viremia to undetectable levels. Notably, one patient showed complete viral suppression and stable $CD4^+$ counts for more than 1 year without HAART [99,100].

Furthermore, 'shock and kill' strategies have emerged as an eradication strategy, where 'viral inducers' drive latently infected cells to produce viral proteins that become detectable by the immune system under ongoing HAART[101]. Several substances have been tested as potential viral inducers including histone deacetylase inhibitors (HDACi), protein kinase C activators or activators of host transcription factors. However, none of these viral inducers have shown a significant effect on the viral reservoir in clinical trials [101–105, 112]. The reasons these shock and kill approaches failed may be multifactorial. Besides potential escape mutations in $CD8^+$ T-cell targeted epitopes [106, 107], it is possible that the microanatomical shielding of HIV as outlined above may be an important barrier to HIV cure.

In addition to the clinical trials there are many other approaches currently being tested *in vitro* by several laboratories. Mousseau et al. are attempting to establish a state of viral latency by inhibiting Tat using didehydro-cortistatin A (dCA)[108]. In contrast, a RNA-guided CRISPR/Cas9 and a specific recombinase (broad-range recombinase 1, Brec1) DNA editing system is being tested to remove the entire integrated HIV genome from latently infected human $CD4^+$ T cells [109, 110]. Whether these approaches will work *in vivo*, however, remain to be seen especially as recent reports have already demonstrated escape in those systems[111].

Outlook

During the last decades, we have gained significant understanding about HIV's latent viral reservoir and identified several barriers that currently prevent a cure. In particular, it became recently evident that not only cellular barriers and integration of HIV into the genome are a major hurdle, but also anatomical and microanatomical compartments that shield HIV-infected cells from recognition by the immune system. These sanctuaries of HIV represent serious immunological barriers and we are just beginning to understand how to drive HIV and HIV-infected cells out of these refuge sites. Over the last years, the HIV cure field was rejuvenated by a single case of an individual that was cured from HIV and several new promising approaches were developed. While we are still far away from eradicating HIV, there is hope that our generation will be able to end this epidemic.

Disclaimer

The views expressed are those of the authors and should not be construed to represent the positions of the U.S. Army or the Department of Defense.

Conflict of Interest

The authors have declared no conflicting interests.

References

1. Lifson AR, Hessol NA, Rutherford GW. Progression and clinical outcome of infection due to human immunodeficiency virus. *Clin Infect Dis* 1992: **14**: 966–72.

2. Samji H, Cescon A, Hogg RS et al. Closing the gap: increases in life expectancy among treated HIV-positive individuals in the United States and Canada. *PLoS One* 2013: **8**: –e81355.
3. May MT, Gompels M, Delpech V et al. Impact on life expectancy of HIV-1 positive individuals of $CD4^+$ cell count and viral load response to antiretroviral therapy. *AIDS* 2014: **28**: 1193–202.
4. JR. Davey RT, Bhat N, Yoder C et al. HIV-1 and T cell dynamics after interruption of highly active antiretroviral therapy (HAART) in patients with a history of sustained viral suppression. *Proc Natl Acad Sci USA* 1999: **96**: 15109–14.
5. Landovitz RJ, Currier JS. Clinical practice. Postexposure prophylaxis for HIV infection. *N Engl J Med* 2009: **361**: 1768–75.
6. Whitney JB, Hill AL, Sanisetty S et al. Rapid seeding of the viral reservoir prior to SIV viraemia in rhesus monkeys. *Nature* 2014: **512**: 74–7.
7. Hladik F, McElrath MJ. Setting the stage: host invasion by HIV. *Nat Rev Immunol* 2008: **8**: 447–57.
8. Gupta S, Gach JS, Becerra JC et al. The neonatal Fc receptor (FcRn) enhances human immunodeficiency virus type 1 (HIV-1) transcytosis across epithelial cells. *PLoS Pathog* 2013: **9**: e1003776.
9. Kohli A, Islam A, Moyes DL et al. Oral and vaginal epithelial cell lines bind and transfer cell-free infectious HIV-1 to permissive cells but are not productively infected. *PLoS One* 2014: **9**: e98077.
10. Carias AM, McCoombe S, McRaven M et al. Defining the interaction of HIV-1 with the mucosal barriers of the female reproductive tract. *J Virol* 2013: **87**: 11388–400.
11. Dinh MH, Anderson MR, McRaven M.D. et al. Visualization of HIV-1 interactions with penile and foreskin epithelia: clues for female-to-male HIV transmission. *PLoS Pathog* 2015: **11**: e1004729.
12. Baggaley RF, Dimitrov D, Owen BN et al. Heterosexual anal intercourse: a neglected risk factor for HIV? *Am J Reprod Immunol* 2013: **69** (Suppl 1): 95–105.
13. Keele BF, Giorgi EE, Salazar-Gonzalez JF et al. Identification and characterization of transmitted and early founder virus envelopes in primary HIV-1 infection. *Proc Natl Acad Sci USA* 2008: **105**: 7552–7.
14. Connor RI, Sheridan KE, Ceradini D, Choe S, Landau NR. Change in coreceptor use correlates with disease progression in HIV-1—infected individuals. *J Exp Med* 1997: **185**: 621–8.
15. Lim SG, Condez A, Lee CA, Johnson MA, Elia C, Poulter LW. Loss of mucosal CD4 lymphocytes is an early feature of HIV infection. *Clin Exp Immunol* 1993: **92**: 448–54.
16. Guadalupe M, Reay E, Sankaran S et al. Severe $CD4^+$ T-cell depletion in gut lymphoid tissue during primary human immunodeficiency virus type 1 infection and substantial delay in restoration following highly active antiretroviral therapy. *J Virol* 2003: **77**: 11708–17.
17. Brenchley JM, Schacker TW, Ruff LE et al. $CD4^+$ T cell depletion during all stages of HIV disease occurs predominantly in the gastrointestinal tract. *J Exp Med* 2004: **200**: 749–59.
18. Mattapallil JJ, Douek DC, Hill B, Nishimura Y, Martin M, Roederer M. Massive infection and loss of memory $CD4^+$ T cells in multiple tissues during acute SIV infection. *Nature* 2005: **434**: 1093–7.
19. Siliciano RF, Greene WC. HIV latency. *Cold Spring Harb Perspect Med* 2011: **1**: a007096.
20. Smith DK, Grohskopf LA, Black RJ et al. Antiretroviral postexposure prophylaxis after sexual, injection-drug use, or other nonoccupational exposure to HIV in the United States: recommendations from the U.S. Department of Health and Human Services. *MMWR Recomm Rep* 2005: **54**: 1–20.
21. Ananworanich J, Chomont N, Eller LA et al. HIV DNA set point is rapidly established in acute HIV infection and dramatically reduced by early ART. *EBioMedicine* 2016. DOI: http://dx.doi.org/10.1016/j.ebiom.2016.07.024 [Epub ahead of print].

22. Strain MC, Little SJ, Daar ES et al. Effect of treatment, during primary infection, on establishment and clearance of cellular reservoirs of HIV-1. *J Infect Dis* 2005: **191**: 1410–8.
23. Buzon MJ, Martin-Gayo E, Pereyra F et al. Long-term antiretroviral treatment initiated at primary HIV-1 infection affects the size, composition, and decay kinetics of the reservoir of HIV-1-infected CD4 T cells. *J Virol* 2014: **88**: 10056–65.
24. Oxenius A, Price DA, Easterbrook PJ et al. Early highly active antiretroviral therapy for acute HIV-1 infection preserves immune function of $CD8^+$ and $CD4^+$ T lymphocytes. *Proc Natl Acad Sci USA* 2000: **97**: 3382–7.
25. Goujard C, Girault I, Rouzioux C et al. HIV-1 control after transient antiretroviral treatment initiated in primary infection: role of patient characteristics and effect of therapy. *Antivir Ther* 2012: **17**: 1001–9.
26. Lisziewicz J, Rosenberg E, Lieberman J et al. Control of HIV despite the discontinuation of antiretroviral therapy. *N Engl J Med* 1999: **340**: 1683–4.
27. Rosenberg ES, Altfeld M, Poon SH et al. Immune control of HIV-1 after early treatment of acute infection. *Nature* 2000: **407**: 523–6.
28. Hocqueloux L, Prazuck T, Avettand-Fenoel V et al. Long-term immunovirologic control following antiretroviral therapy interruption in patients treated at the time of primary HIV-1 infection. *AIDS* 2010: **24**: 1598–601.
29. Sáez-Cirión A, Bacchus C, Hocqueloux L et al. Post-treatment HIV-1 controllers with a long-term virological remission after the interruption of early initiated antiretroviral therapy ANRS VISCONTI Study. *PLoS Pathog* 2013: **9**: e1003211.
30. Finzi D, Blankson J, Siliciano JD et al. Latent infection of $CD4^+$ T cells provides a mechanism for lifelong persistence of HIV-1, even in patients on effective combination therapy. *Nat Med* 1999: **5**: 512–7.
31. Chun TW, Stuyver L, Mizell SB et al. Presence of an inducible HIV-1 latent reservoir during highly active antiretroviral therapy. *Proc Natl Acad Sci USA* 1997: **94**: 13193–7.
32. Perelson AS, Neumann AU, Markowitz M, Leonard JM, Ho DD. HIV-1 dynamics in vivo: virion clearance rate, infected cell life-span, and viral generation time. *Science* 1996: **271**: 1582–6.
33. Perelson AS, Essunger P, Cao Y et al. Decay characteristics of HIV-1-infected compartments during combination therapy. *Nature* 1997: **387**: 188–91.
34. Palmer S, Maldarelli F, Wiegand A et al. Low-level viremia persists for at least 7 years in patients on suppressive antiretroviral therapy. *Proc Natl Acad Sci USA* 2008: **105**: 3879–84.
35. Chomont N, El-Far M, Ancuta P et al. HIV reservoir size and persistence are driven by T cell survival and homeostatic proliferation. *Nat Med* 2009: **15**: 893–900.
36. Farber DL, Yudanin NA, Restifo NP. Human memory T cells: generation, compartmentalization and homeostasis. *Nat Rev Immunol* 2014: **14**: 24–35.
37. Jaafoura S, de Goer de Herve MG, Hernandez-Vargas EA et al. Progressive contraction of the latent HIV reservoir around a core of less-differentiated $CD4^{(+)}$ memory T cells. *Nat Commun* 2014: **5**: 5407.
38. Buzon MJ, Sun H, Li C et al. HIV-1 persistence in $CD4^+$ T cells with stem cell-like properties. *Nat Med* 2014: **20**: 139–42.
39. Yu XF, Yu QC, Essex M, Lee TH. The vpx gene of simian immunodeficiency virus facilitates efficient viral replication in fresh lymphocytes and macrophage. *J Virol* 1991: **65**: 5088–91.

40. Lahouassa H, Daddacha W, Hofmann H et al. SAMHD1 restricts the replication of human immunodeficiency virus type 1 by depleting the intracellular pool of deoxynucleoside triphosphates. *Nat Immunol* 2012: **13**: 223–8.
41. Hrecka K, Hao C, Gierszewska M et al. Vpx relieves inhibition of HIV-1 infection of macrophages mediated by the SAMHD1 protein. *Nature* 2011: **474**: 658–61.
42. Micci L, Alvarez X, Iriele RI et al. CD4 depletion in SIV-infected macaques results in macrophage and microglia infection with rapid turnover of infected cells. *PLoS Pathog* 2014: **10**: e1004467.
43. Ortiz AM, Klatt NR, Li B et al. Depletion of CD4(+) T cells abrogates post-peak decline of viremia in SIV-infected rhesus macaques. *J Clin Invest* 2011: **121**: 4433–45.
44. Pelchen-Matthews A, Kramer B, Marsh M. Infectious HIV-1 assembles in late endosomes in primary macrophages. *J Cell Biol* 2003: **162**: 443–55.
45. Deneka M, Pelchen-Matthews A, Byland R, Ruiz-Mateos E, Marsh M. In macrophages, HIV-1 assembles into an intracellular plasma membrane domain containing the tetraspanins CD81, CD9, and CD53. *J Cell Biol* 2007: **177**: 329–41.
46. Jayakumar P, Berger I, Autschbach F et al. Tissue-resident macrophages are productively infected ex vivo by primary X4 isolates of human immunodeficiency virus type 1. *J Virol* 2005: **79**: 5220–6.
47. Shen R, Richter HE, Clements RH et al. Macrophages in vaginal but not intestinal mucosa are monocyte-like and permissive to human immunodeficiency virus type 1 infection. *J Virol* 2009: **83**: 3258–67.
48. Wang TH, Donaldson YK, Brettle RP, Bell JE, Simmonds P. Identification of shared populations of human immunodeficiency virus type 1 infecting microglia and tissue macrophages outside the central nervous system. *J Virol* 2001: **75**: 11686–99.
49. Yukl SA, Sinclair E, Somsouk M et al. A comparison of methods for measuring rectal HIV levels suggests that HIV DNA resides in cells other than $CD4^+$ T cells, including myeloid cells. *AIDS* 2014: **28**: 439–42.
50. Damouche A, Lazure T, Avettand-Fenoel V et al. Adipose tissue is a neglected viral reservoir and an inflammatory site during chronic HIV and SIV infection. *PLoS Pathog* 2015: **11**: e1005153.
51. Gonzalez-Scarano F, Martin-Garcia J. The neuropathogenesis of AIDS. *Nat Rev Immunol* 2005: **5**: 69–81.
52. Calantone N, Wu F, Klase Z et al. Tissue myeloid cells in SIV-infected primates acquire viral DNA through phagocytosis of infected T cells. *Immunity* 2014: **41**: 493–502.
53. Ballabh P, Braun A, Nedergaard M. The blood–brain barrier: an overview: structure, regulation, and clinical implications. *Neurobiol Dis* 2004: **16**: 1–13.
54. Davis LE, Hjelle BL, Miller VE et al. Early viral brain invasion in iatrogenic human immunodeficiency virus infection. *Neurology* 1992: **42**: 1736–9.
55. An SF, Groves M, Gray F, Scaravilli F. Early entry and widespread cellular involvement of HIV-1 DNA in brains of HIV-1 positive asymptomatic individuals. *J Neuropathol Exp Neurol* 1999: **58**: 1156–62.
56. Williams KC, Corey S, Westmoreland SV et al. Perivascular macrophages are the primary cell type productively infected by simian immunodeficiency virus in the brains of macaques: implications for the neuropathogenesis of AIDS. *J Exp Med* 2001: **193**: 905–15.
57. Cosenza MA, Zhao M, Si Q, Lee SC. Human brain parenchymal microglia express CD14 and CD45 and are productively infected by HIV-1 in HIV-1 encephalitis. *Brain Pathol* 2002: **12**: 442–55.
58. Fischer-Smith T, Croul S, Adeniyi A et al. Macrophage/microglial accumulation and proliferating cell nuclear antigen expression in the central nervous system in human immunodeficiency virus encephalopathy. *Am J Pathol* 2004: **164**: 2089–99.

59. Williams K, Alvarez X, Lackner AA. Central nervous system perivascular cells are immunoregulatory cells that connect the CNS with the peripheral immune system. *Glia* 2001: **36**: 156–64.
60. Ryzhova EV, Crino P, Shawver L, Westmoreland SV, Lackner AA, González-Scarano F. Simian immunodeficiency virus encephalitis: analysis of envelope sequences from individual brain multinucleated giant cells and tissue samples. *Virology* 2002: **297**: 57–67.
61. Letendre S, Marquie-Beck J, Capparelli E et al. Validation of the CNS Penetration-Effectiveness rank for quantifying antiretroviral penetration into the central nervous system. *Arch Neurol* 2008: **65**: 65–70.
62. Strazielle N, Ghersi-Egea J. Factors affecting delivery of antiviral drugs to the brain. *Rev Med Virol* 2005: **15**: 105–33.
63. Letendre SL, McCutchan JA, Childers ME et al. Enhancing antiretroviral therapy for human immunodeficiency virus cognitive disorders. *Ann Neurol* 2004: **56**: 416–23.
64. Mermin JH, Holodniy M, Katzenstein DA, Merigan TC. Detection of human immunodeficiency virus DNA and RNA in semen by the polymerase chain reaction. *J Infect Dis* 1991: **164**: 769–72.
65. Liuzzi G, Chirianni A, Clementi M et al. Analysis of HIV-1 load in blood, semen and saliva: evidence for different viral compartments in a cross-sectional and longitudinal study. *AIDS* 1996: **10**: F51–6.
66. Houzet L, Matusali G, Dejucq-Rainsford N. Origins of HIV-infected leukocytes and virions in semen. *J Infect Dis* 2014: **210** (Suppl 3): S622–30.
67. van Praag RM, Repping S, de Vries JW, Lange JM, Hoetelmans RM, Prins JM. Pharmacokinetic profiles of nevirapine and indinavir in various fractions of seminal plasma. *Antimicrob Agents Chemother* 2001: **45**: 2902–7.
68. Ghosn J, Chaix M, Peytavin G et al. Penetration of enfuvirtide, tenofovir, efavirenz, and protease inhibitors in the genital tract of HIV-1-infected men. *AIDS* 2004: **18**: 1958–61.
69. Taylor S, Jayasuriya AN, Berry A et al. Darunavir concentrations exceed the protein-corrected EC(5)(0) for wild-type HIV in the semen of HIV-1-infected men. *AIDS* 2010: **24**: 2583–7.
70. Quayle AJ, Coston WM, Trocha AK, Kalams SA, Mayer KH, Anderson DJ. Detection of HIV-1-specific CTLs in the semen of HIV-infected individuals. *J Immunol* 1998: **161**: 4406–10.
71. Winnall WR, Lloyd SB, de Rose R et al. Simian immunodeficiency virus infection and immune responses in the pig-tailed macaque testis. *J Leukoc Biol* 2015: **97**: 599–609.
72. Sheth PM, Danesh A, Shahabi K et al. HIV-specific $CD8^+$ lymphocytes in semen are not associated with reduced HIV shedding. *J Immunol* 2005: **175**: 4789–96.
73. Hazan U, Romero IA, Cancello R et al. Human adipose cells express CD4, CXCR4, and CCR5 corrected receptors: a new target cell type for the immunodeficiency virus-1? *FASEB J* 2002: **16**: 1254–6.
74. Munier S, Borjabad A, Lemaire M, Mariot V, Hazan U. In vitro infection of human primary adipose cells with HIV-1: a reassessment. *AIDS* 2003: **17**: 2537–9.
75. Koethe JR., Hulgan T, Niswender K. Adipose tissue and immune function: a review of evidence relevant to HIV infection. *J Infect Dis* 2013: **208**: 1194–201.
76. Stellbrink HJ, van Lunzen J, Hufert FT et al. Asymptomatic HIV infection is characterized by rapid turnover of HIV RNA in plasma and lymph nodes but not of latently infected lymph-node $CD4^+$ T cells. *AIDS* 1997: **11**: 1103–10.
77. Petrovas C, Yamamoto T, Gerner MY et al. CD4 T follicular helper cell dynamics during SIV infection. *J Clin Invest* 2012: **122**: 3281–94.

78. Lindqvist M, van Lunzen J, Soghoian DZ et al. Expansion of HIV-specific T follicular helper cells in chronic HIV infection. *J Clin Invest* 2012: **122**: 3271–80.
79. Hong JJ, Amancha PK, Rogers K, Ansari AA, Villinger F. Spatial alterations between CD4(+) T follicular helper, B, and CD8(+) T cells during simian immunodeficiency virus infection: T/B cell homeostasis, activation, and potential mechanism for viral escape. *J Immunol* 2012: **188**: 3247–56.
80. Perreau M, Savoye A, de Crignis E et al. Follicular helper T cells serve as the major CD4 T cell compartment for HIV-1 infection, replication, and production. *J Exp Med* 2013: **210**: 143–56.
81. Pallikkuth S, Sharkey M, Babic DZ et al. Peripheral T follicular helper cells are the major HIV reservoir within central memory CD4 T cells in peripheral blood from chronically HIV-infected individuals on combination antiretroviral therapy. *J Virol* 2016: **90**: 2718–28.
82. Pissani F, Streeck H. Emerging concepts on T follicular helper cell dynamics in HIV infection. *Trends Immunol* 2014: **35**: 278–86.
83. Quigley MF, Gonzalez VD, Granath A, Andersson J, Sandberg JK. CXCR5+ CCR7- CD8 T cells are early effector memory cells that infiltrate tonsil B cell follicles. *Eur J Immunol* 2007: **37**: 3352–62.
84. Fukazawa Y, Lum R, Okoye AA et al. B cell follicle sanctuary permits persistent productive simian immunodeficiency virus infection in elite controllers. *Nat Med* 2015: **21**: 132–9.
85. Deeks SG, Lewin SR, Havlir DV. The end of AIDS: HIV infection as a chronic disease. *Lancet* 2013: **382**: 1525–33.
86. Lisziewicz J, Foli A, Wainberg M, Lori F. Hydroxyurea in the Treatment of HIV Infection. *Drug Saf* 2003: **26**: 605–24.
87. Frank I, Bosch RJ, Fiscus S et al. Activity, safety, and immunological effects of hydroxyurea added to didanosine in antiretroviral-naive and experienced hiv type 1-infected subjects: a randomized, placebo-controlled trial, ACTG 307. *AIDS Res Hum Retroviruses* 2004: **20**: 916–26.
88. Jessen H, Allen TM, Streeck H. How a single patient influenced HIV research—15-year follow-up. *N Engl J Med* 2014: **370**: 682–3.
89. Lori F, Foli A, Groff A et al. Optimal suppression of HIV replication by low-dose hydroxyurea through the combination of antiviral and cytostatic ('virostatic') mechanisms. *AIDS* 2005: **19**: 1173–81.
90. Moore RD, Wong WM, Keruly JC, McArthur JC. Incidence of neuropathy in HIV-infected patients on monotherapy versus those on combination therapy with didanosine, stavudine and hydroxyurea. *AIDS* 2000: **14**: 273–8.
91. Moore RD, Keruly JC, Chaisson RE. Incidence of pancreatitis in HIV-infected patients receiving nucleoside reverse transcriptase inhibitor drugs. *AIDS* 2001: **15**: 617–20.
92. Havlir DV, Gilbert PB, Bennett K et al. Effects of treatment intensification with hydroxyurea in HIV-infected patients with virologic suppression. *AIDS* 2001: **15**: 1379–88.
93. Rizzardi GP, Harari A, Capiluppi B et al. Treatment of primary HIV-1 infection with cyclosporin A coupled with highly active antiretroviral therapy. *J Clin Invest* 2002: **109**: 681–8.
94. Lederman MM, Smeaton L, Smith KY et al. Cyclosporin A provides no sustained immunologic benefit to persons with chronic HIV-1 infection starting suppressive antiretroviral therapy: results of a randomized, controlled trial of the AIDS Clinical Trials Group A5138. *J Infect Dis* 2006: **194**: 1677–85.
95. Markowitz M, Vaida F, Hare CB et al. The virologic and immunologic effects of cyclosporine as an adjunct to antiretroviral therapy in patients treated during acute and early HIV-1 infection. *J Infect Dis* 2010: **201**: 1298–302.

96. Hutter G, Nowak D, Mossner M et al. Long-term control of HIV by CCR5 Delta32/Delta32 stem-cell transplantation. *N Engl J Med* 2009: **360**: 692–8.
97. Liu R, Paxton WA, Choe S et al. Homozygous defect in HIV-1 coreceptor accounts for resistance of some multiply-exposed individuals to HIV-1 infection. *Cell* 1996: **86**: 367–77.
98. Kordelas L, Verheyen J, Beelen DW et al. Shift of HIV tropism in stem-cell transplantation with CCR5 Delta32 mutation. *N Engl J Med* 2014: **371**: 880–2.
99. Tebas P, Stein D, Tang WW et al. Gene editing of CCR5 in autologous CD4 T cells of persons infected with HIV. *N Engl J Med* 2014: **370**: 901–10.
100. Wang CX, Cannon PM. The clinical applications of genome editing in HIV. *Blood* 2016: **127**: 2546–52.
101. Sebastian NT, Collins KL. Targeting HIV latency: resting memory T cells, hematopoietic progenitor cells and future directions. *Expert Rev Anti Infect Ther* 2014: **12**: 1187–201.
102. Remoli AL, Marsili G, Battistini A, Sgarbanti M. The development of immune-modulating compounds to disrupt HIV latency. *Cytokine Growth Factor Rev* 2012: **23**: 159–72.
103. Archin NM, Sung JM, Garrido C, Soriano-Sarabia N, Margolis DM. Eradicating HIV-1 infection: seeking to clear a persistent pathogen. *Nat Rev Microbiol* 2014: **12**: 750–64.
104. Prins JM, Jurriaans S, van Praag RM et al. Immuno-activation with anti-CD3 and recombinant human IL-2 in HIV-1-infected patients on potent antiretroviral therapy. *AIDS* 1999: **13**: 2405–10.
105. Lafeuillade A, Poggi C, Chadapaud S et al. Pilot study of a combination of highly active antiretroviral therapy and cytokines to induce HIV-1 remission. *J Acquir Immune Defic SynDr.* 2001: **26**: 44–55.
106. Shan L, Deng K, Shroff NS et al. Stimulation of HIV-1-specific cytolytic T lymphocytes facilitates elimination of latent viral reservoir after virus reactivation. *Immunity* 2012: **36**: 491–501.
107. Deng K, Pertea M, Rongvaux A et al. Broad CTL response is required to clear latent HIV-1 due to dominance of escape mutations. *Nature* 2015: **517**: 381–5.
108. Mousseau G, Kessing CF, Fromentin R, Trautmann L, Chomont N, Valente ST. The Tat inhibitor didehydro-cortistatin A prevents HIV-1 reactivation from latency. *MBio* 2015: **6**: e00465.
109. Kaminski R, Chen Y, Fischer T et al. Elimination of HIV-1 genomes from human T-lymphoid cells by CRISPR/Cas9 gene editing. *Sci Rep* 2016: **6**: 22555.
110. Karpinski J, Hauber I, Chemnitz J et al. Directed evolution of a recombinase that excises the provirus of most HIV-1 primary isolates with high specificity. *Nat Biotechnol* 2016: **34**: 401–9.
111. Wang Z, Pan Q, Gendron P et al. CRISPR/Cas9-derived mutations both inhibit HIV-1 replication and accelerate viral escape. *Cell Rep* 2016: **15**: 481–9.
112. Rasmussen TA, Tolstrup M, Sogaard OS. Reversal of Latency as Part of a Cure for HIV-1. *Trends in microbiology* 2016: **24**: 90–7.

16.7

Cure Summit Hears of New Remission Case

Liz Highleyman

THE PAST YEAR BROUGHT NO MAJOR breakthroughs in the search for an HIV cure, but a growing understanding of how the virus hides in the body is bringing people closer to strategies for long-term remission, researchers and advocates said at the 2017 HIV Cure Summit.

Since its founding in December 2015 with a $20 million grant from amfAR, the Institute for HIV Cure Research at UCSF has hosted an annual forum to mark World AIDS Day. Compared with past summits, this year's meeting focused less on nitty-gritty laboratory research and more on community participation in cure research.

"It is so important for the community to be involved in cure research so that they have the latest accurate information and reasonable expectations, especially if they want to volunteer to participate in HIV cure trials," Lynda Dee of the AIDS Treatment Activist Coalition, who spoke at the summit, told the Bay Area Reporter. "Personally, I believe it is also vital for the community to advocate for continued funding for all areas of HIV research, including cure research, as all things HIV are under a budget attack by the current administration."

Early Treatment Reduces Reservoir of the Virus

Summit participants heard about a case of HIV remission in a San Francisco man, Clark Hawley, who started antiretroviral treatment very soon after infection, shedding light on what might be needed to achieve a functional cure. Hawley has decided to be open about his experience and spoke at the summit in the hope of helping others. Another cure research participant, Luis Canales, also described his experience.

To date, only one person—former San Francisco resident Timothy Ray Brown, known as the Berlin Patient—appears to have been truly cured of HIV. Ten years after receiving bone marrow transplants to treat leukemia from a donor with a natural mutation that makes T-cells resistant to HIV infection, extensive testing has found no detectable functional virus in his blood or tissue samples.

Researchers have followed a number of cases over the years of people who appear to maintain control over HIV. Some have detectable virus but their immune system seems to be able to keep it in check naturally without antiretrovirals. Other individuals on treatment have reached the point where they had no detectable HIV according to the most sensitive tests, but the virus came roaring back when they tried stopping treatment.

As described in a special HIV edition of PLoS Medicine, Hawley, 54, enrolled in a PrEP demonstration project and started Truvada (tenofovir/emtricitabine). But it was later determined that he had very early HIV infection, during the "window period" when the so-called HIV reservoir is becoming established in CD4 T-cells and there is not yet enough of an immune response to produce antibodies against the virus.

When he had a detectable viral load test a week after starting PrEP, Hawley stepped up to a four-drug antiretroviral regimen, as Truvada alone is not enough to suppress the virus over the long term.

Study authors Dr. Timothy Henrich and Dr. Steve Deeks of UCSF and colleagues said that, to the best of their knowledge, this is the earliest documented case of HIV infection in an adult followed by immediate initiation of antiretroviral therapy (except for post-exposure prophylaxis, which involves starting preventive treatment after a known HIV exposure). San Francisco's RAPID program successfully gets people on treatment within days after diagnosis, but diagnosis typically does not happen immediately after infection.

Over the next three years, the researchers were unable to detect HIV in Hawley's blood plasma, brain fluid, samples of gut, lymph node, and bone marrow tissue, or in more than 500 million CD4 T-cells.

After 34 months on continuous antiretroviral therapy, Hawley decided to try a closely monitored treatment interruption. After stopping therapy his HIV remained undetectable for 225 days—around seven and a half months—but it then reappeared, rising steeply to nearly 80,000 copies. This is similar to the duration of off-treatment remission Henrich previously reported in a Boston bone marrow transplant recipient. Hawley went back on treatment, re-suppressed the virus, and is doing well.

This resurgence likely indicates that a rare residual virus became active and encountered no strong immune response to keep it in check, according to Deeks.

"By the time [Clark] stopped therapy, we think he had about 200 [HIV-infected T-cells]—that's a million-fold reduction in the amount of virus a typical person has," Deeks said. "It didn't cure him, but it got close, and it provided us a pathway to see what a near cure looks like. But at the end of the day, a low reservoir is insufficient, and we're going to need to stimulate the immune system at the same time."

Added Heinrich, "His case is important as it demonstrates that extremely early initiation of antiretroviral therapy can have a profound effect at limiting the overall burden of residual disease. Although early therapy did not completely abort or eradicate infection, it led to prolonged antiretroviral free remission."

To move forward, cure research will depend on people like Brown and Hawley, who will undergo extensive testing to look for residual virus, as well as individuals who are willing to interrupt treatment to see if experimental therapies can keep HIV under control without the help of daily antiretrovirals.

But this strategy is risky. Although study participants are monitored frequently, as soon as HIV starts replicating it can cause damage that is hard to undo. And anyone who stops treatment can lose their "undetectable equals untransmittable" status, with resurgent viral load putting their sex partners at risk of infection.

While there is ongoing debate within the community about whether treatment interruption studies and other types of cure research are ethical, a recent survey found that a substantial proportion of people living with HIV are willing to participate.

"One of the most encouraging things [in the HIV cure field] is that people living with HIV—including those who have had the infection for decades and have been through holy hell and back—are still willing to participate in these sometimes very intrusive studies and contribute to science for the health and well-being of not just themselves, but of people who haven't even been infected yet," science and policy consultant Judith Auerbach said at a summit media briefing.

Hawley offers a perfect example.

"When I was presented with the information that I was among the earliest detected HIV cases ever, and they felt they could learn a lot for the sake of humanity, I just agreed," he told the B.A.R. "When this started there was no one else's body that could give the researchers the information that mine could. When they tell you that you are the only person in the world where the disease was caught this early, and in a place where extensive testing is possible, it is far easier to step up and do what I can."

13.4.2 + 13.4.3

283-288

341-434

CPSIA information can be obtained
at www.ICGtesting.com
Printed in the USA
FSHW011856081221
86790FS